Diseases of the Liver and Biliary Tree

Annarosa Floreani
Editor

Diseases of the Liver and Biliary Tree

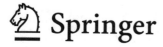 Springer

Editor
Annarosa Floreani
Scientific Consultant, Scientific Institute for Research
Hospitalization and Healthcare (IRCCS) Negrar
Verona
Italy

Senior Scholar University of Padova
Padova
Italy

ISBN 978-3-030-65910-3   ISBN 978-3-030-65908-0   (eBook)
https://doi.org/10.1007/978-3-030-65908-0

This Springer imprint is published by the registered company Springer Nature Switzerland AG
The registered company address is: Gewerbestrasse 11, 6330 Cham, Switzerland

Preface

Diseases of the biliary tree remain fascinating conditions. In the last decades there have been major advances in the understanding of the epidemiology, pathogenesis and treatment of these conditions. Given their particular importance (even for clinicians working with adults), paediatric conditions are now finally starting to translate into better diagnosis and management. Biliary atresia is a rare disease which occurs in newborn infants, its surgical treatment is most successful in babies younger than 3-months-old, so early diagnosis is important, and ongoing research will improve the outcomes. Congenital cystic lesions of the biliary tree and biliary hamartomas have been recently updated on the basis of new knowledge of the embryologic development of the biliary tree and the novel imaging findings which can better recognize the ductal plate malformations.

Part 2 provides an excellent overview of the genetic cholangiopathies with a summary of recent genetic discoveries in different conditions. One of the recent advances is the low phospholipid-associated cholelithiasis, a genetic disease associated with a mutation of the ABCB4 gene that codes for protein MDR3, a biliary carrier. This condition should be suspected in all patients with cholelithiasis before 40 years of age, but there also exist complicated forms involving extended intrahepatic lithiasis and its consequences. An excellent overview of immune cholangiopathies (primary biliary cholangitis, primary sclerosing cholangitis and overlap syndromes) is also presented. IgG4-related sclerosing cholangitis has emerged as one of the main differential diagnoses with primary sclerosing cholangitis. A chapter presents a comprehensive summary of current understanding of the pathophysiology, diagnosis, natural history and treatment of IgG4-related sclerosing cholangitis. One of the greatest challenges in the management of patients with primary sclerosing cholangitis lies on the significantly increased risk of malignancies, including cholangiocarcinoma, gallbladder neoplasia and colorectal neoplasia.

In terms of therapeutics, the area with greatest advances has been primary biliary cholangitis. Results of recent trials are discussed and we provide readers with up-date management. One chapter is dedicated to inflammatory cholangitis which is the most common form of secondary cholangitis, characterized by the proliferation of bacteria within the bile and with the secondary obstruction of biliary tracts. Another form, which in recent years has led to an increased interest in drug-induced liver injury, presents with a cholestatic pattern. In this view the current knowledge on this issue has been reviewed with a particular interest in monitoring specific

biomarkers and discussing the role of liver biopsy together with novel agents causing drug-induced cholestasis. The relationship between cholestatic liver disease and
pregnancy is discussed in another chapter considering the most relevant available
data in literature and recommendations reported by international societies. Finally,
much evidence has accumulated on liver transplantation and chronic cholangiopathies addressing the indications for liver transplantation, waitlist mortality, overall
results and disease recurrence.

Given its scope, the book offers a valuable guide for a broad range of practitio-
ners. Hepatology, gastroenterology, paediatrics and surgery are the disciplines
addressed by the book. I would like to sincerely thank all the contributors for taking
time from their extremely busy schedules.

Verona, Italy   Annarosa Floreani

Contents

Part I

Congenital Biliary Abnormalities

Biliary Atresia

1

Pietro Betalli, Maurizio Cheli, and Lorenzo D'Antiga

1.1 Introduction

Biliary atresia (BA) is the main cause of obstructive jaundice in the newborn, and it's defined as an obliterative disorder of the intra and extrahepatic biliary tree dependent on an inflammatory-destructive process of unknown etiology. Atresia of the biliary tract begins in the embryonic/perinatal period and has a variability in the atretic processes from case to case. It remains the most common cause of cirrhosis in children and the first indication for pediatric liver transplantation. No medical therapy is available for this condition. However, early diagnosis and early surgery can improve patient prognosis [1].

The earliest reference to what was probably an infant with BA was reported in 1817 by Dr. John Burns as an "incurable state of the biliary apparatus" [2]. Toward the end of the nineteenth century, John Thompson made the first accurate description of the clinical features and postmortem findings in an infant who appeared to have no common hepatic duct [3].

Treatment for BA is entirely surgical, being an attempt to restore bile flow from the native liver in the first instance, and is known as Kasai portoenterostomy (KPE); however, in approximately half of children who underwent KPE, bile flow is not restored, and liver transplantation is required shortly thereafter. The first surgical success was probably described by the Boston surgeon William E Ladd in 1935 in a series of patients with congenital biliary obstruction; Ladd anastomosed dilated proximal parts of the obstructed biliary tree with the intestines so restoring some kind of continuity [3]. It, however, became clear that in most infants recognized to

P. Betalli · M. Cheli
Department of Paediatric Surgery, Hospital Papa Giovanni XXIII, Bergamo, Italy

L. D'Antiga (✉)
Department of Child Health, Centre for Paediatric Hepatology, Gastroenterology and Transplantation, Hospital Papa Giovanni XXIII, Bergamo, Italy
e-mail: ldantiga@asst-pg23.it

© Springer Nature Switzerland AG 2021
A. Floreani (ed.), *Diseases of the Liver and Biliary Tree*,
https://doi.org/10.1007/978-3-030-65908-0_1

have BA, there was no proximal dilated remnant to find, irrespective of how high one dissected into the porta hepatis. They were, therefore, described as "uncorrectable" BA. In the late 1950s, Morio Kasai first began simply to transect high in the porta hepatis and join this up to a mobilized Roux loop even if there were no visible ducts present. In a proportion of cases, this enabled restoration of bile flow and clearance of jaundice [4, 5].

1.2   Epidemiology

The incidence of BA presents marked variation depending on geographic area, ranging from about 1 in 10,000 live births in Japanese population [6] to about 1 in 15,000–20,000 in mainland Europe [7], England and Wales [8], and North America [9]. The highest incidence is reported in French Polynesia (where it is reported in about 1:3000 live births) and Taiwan (1 in 5000) [10–12]. There is a female preponderance in those considered to have a "developmental" origin, whereas sex distribution is equal in the majority of patients with isolated BA [13, 14]. The incidence of BA with splenic malformation syndrome (BASM) is rarely reported in Asian series, but accounts for about 10% of European and North American cases [14–16].

1.3   Etiology and Pathogenesis

It is likely that a number of different mechanisms can lead to what we refer to as BA in the early postnatal life. At least four different subtypes of BA can be distinguished based on clinical or laboratory features.

1. Those with other congenital anomalies, and typically the BASM
2. Cystic BA, that is, extrahepatic cystic development within an obliterated biliary tree
3. Viral-associated BA—particularly CMV-IgM +ve-associated BA
4. Isolated BA, that is, none of the features described above

It is highly likely that BA with other congenital anomalies and cystic BA have in utero origins and can be regarded as "developmental" variants. BASM is associated with extrahepatic abnormalities, such as polysplenia or asplenia, cardiovascular anomalies, intestinal malrotation or nonrotation, preduodenal portal vein, and absence of the vena cava. About 1/3 also have situs inversus and are examples of so-called laterality defects, strongly suggesting their origin within the embryonic phase of human development. Given this, it also seems probable that a genetic or epigenetic etiology is involved [10, 11, 17, 18]. Genetic mouse models exist with defects of laterality and failure to form normal bile ducts, though the genes thought to be involved (*CFC-1, INV,* and others) have yet to be identified in humans. Some series identified maternal diabetes as a key clinical association, probably acting in an epigenetic manner. Other variants include an association with other major congenital malformations, such as esophageal or jejunal atresia, but without any sign of laterality defects (<5% overall) [19–22].

Cystic BA is seen in about 5–10% of most large series, irrespective of the geographic origin. The cyst may contain bile or mucus, implying onset after establishment of continuity between intra and extrahepatic bile ducts. Redkar et al. [23] showed that many cases of cystic BA can be detected by ultrasound during prenatal scanning, and that they have a good prognosis postsurgery.

Most infants with BA will simply appear as patients with isolated liver anomalies with a negative serological profile for common hepatotropic viruses. It is controversial whether a normal biliary tree can be damaged secondarily after birth, although large experimental research with animal models is based on this assumption. Harpavat et al. from Texas, USA retrospectively analyzed blood samples obtained from their BA patients series on day 1 or 2 of life and showed that all had elevated levels of conjugated bilirubin at this age, implying that all had biliary obstruction at the time of birth [24].

Nonetheless, there have been many theories regarding pathogenesis of isolated BA. The viral-induced, immune- or autoimmune-mediated inflammatory obstruction of the biliary tree has been the most commonly accepted theory, but largely based on experimental observations. Some groups have described infants with a different clinical and laboratory phenotype (later presentation, an inflammatory appearance in liver histology and a Th1-dominant T cell infiltrate) in their clinical series, linked with CMV (IgM+ve) infection [14–21].

From the pathology point of view, BA is as an occlusive panductular cholangiopathy affecting both intra and extrahepatic bile ducts that can be divided according to the extent of the fibrotic obliteration or absence of parts of the biliary tree. The most common classification divides BA into three types based on the most proximal level of occlusion of the extrahepatic biliary tree (Fig. 1.1).

In type 1, there is a patent biliary lumen from the liver to the common bile duct, which is then atretic; many cases are associated with cystic changes. In type 2, the patent biliary lumen extends to the common hepatic duct, which is atretic. In both types, there is a degree of preservation of structure in the intrahepatic bile ducts, but they are still irregular although not dilated (a key distinction from congenital choledochal malformation). Type 3 is the most common, characterized by no apparent connection and a "solid" proximal bile duct remnant at the level of the porta hepatis. In type 3 BA the intrahepatic bile ducts are usually grossly abnormal with a myriad of small ductules coalescing at the porta hepatis, which can be accessed at KPE (Fig. 1.1).

In BA, liver histology shows features suggestive of "large duct obstruction", with edematous expansion of the portal areas, bile ductular proliferation, and the appearance of bile plugs. The distinctive feature is ductular proliferation and portal fibrosis. There might be a marked inflammatory aspect with infiltration of activated mononuclear cells, such as CD4+ T cells and NK cells. As the disease progresses, monocytes/macrophages also appear prominent, along with progressive bridging fibrosis between portal areas. The extrahepatic remnant in type 3 BA is characterized by a multiplicity of microscopic bile ductules embedded within a fibro-inflammatory stroma—most evident at the level of the porta hepatis. Even in these, the

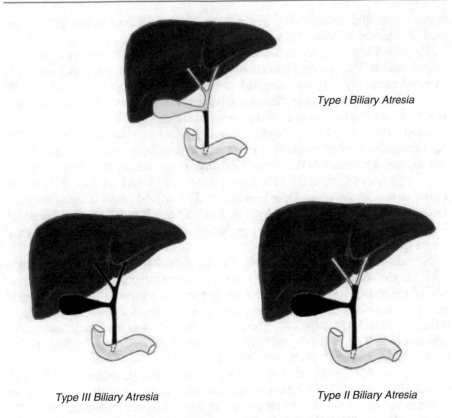

Fig. 1.1 Pathological classification of biliary atresia (in black the atretic biliary tract)

gallbladder and distal common bile duct may look completely normal, though the former contains clear "mucus."

A proinflammatory molecular profile was reported in a large-scale gene expression analysis of liver biopsies from infants with BA. This study suggested a genetic footprint in which genes involved in the Th1 helper cell response were activated at an early stage, with simultaneous but transient suppression of markers of humoral immunity [25, 26].

A novel mechanism of immune damage has been suggested by Muraji et al. [27] based on the observation that male BA infants have a three-fold increase in maternal-origin cells in their livers. These were later shown to be maternal-origin chimeric CD8+ T cells and CD45+ NK cells that appear capable of initiating immune cholangiolar damage. This has been termed *maternal microchimerism,* and it may explain why the destructive process seems time-limited and most potent shortly after birth.

Recently, an intriguing interpretation of outbreaks of BA in animals has been advanced, suggesting a possible environmental cause, which may have implications also for humans. Sheep farms around the Burrinjuck Dam, New South Wales, Australia, reported recurrent outbreaks of BA in lambs, where their pregnant mothers had been allowed to graze on the foreshores of the dam, which had become exposed by drought conditions [28]. It appeared that a particular weed known as the red crumbweed (*Dysphania glomulifera* subsp. *glomulifera*) in these conditions had proliferated and was the major source of maternal nutrition. In later years, whenever the exact combination of exposed foreshore, weed proliferation, and grazing pregnant livestock occurred, affected offsprings were born.

In conclusion, the etiology and pathogenesis of BA remains a field still unclear and unknown in most cases, though there are intriguing possibilities for the different clinical phenotypes or variants.

1.4   Clinical Features and Diagnosis

Pale stool is the key feature of BA (Fig. 1.2). This, together with dark urine in an otherwise healthy and well-nourished infant, is an alarm sign that must be investigated. Neonatal jaundice persisting for longer than 3 weeks in a breast-fed newborn or 2 weeks in a formula-fed newborn requires testing of total and conjugated bilirubin.

Such infants, despite the absence of gastrointestinal bile, initially thrive normally, masking the serious underlying disease. Jaundice persisting after 2 weeks in a term infant is not normal, therefore this should raise suspicion and lead to further examination of stool and urine. Urine at this age should be colorless and should not stain the nappy [29].

Screening programs have been developed in some countries, such as Taiwan and parts of Japan. These rely on stool color observation by the parents and return of a stool color card, which was given to all the mothers leaving the nursery. They have reported a remarkable improvement in the time it takes to diagnose BA, where there

Fig. 1.2 Acholic stool. The diaper contains cheesy, whitish stools completely lacking any bile pigment staining

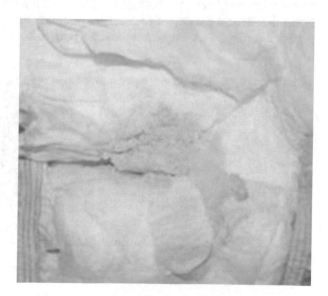

had been delays. Some European countries, such as Switzerland, or regions, such as North Netherlands, are also practicing screening though the results have not been published.

Apart from the jaundice, the physical signs at the first weeks of life may be minimal and consist only of soft hepatomegaly. Late signs include failure to thrive, ascites, and cutaneous signs of chronic liver disease with splenomegaly. In some infants, the presenting feature is fat-soluble vitamin K deficiency, leading to coagulopathy and bleeding. Sometimes, this is innocuous gastrointestinal hemorrhage but in some can be catastrophic intracranial hemorrhage.

The biochemical characteristics of BA include conjugated (direct) hyperbilirubinemia, raised hepatocellular enzymes, raised alkaline phosphatase, and γ-glutamyl transpeptidase, but there is a significant overlap with many other causes of neonatal-conjugated jaundice and no test is specific.

Ultrasonography (USS) is usually the next step. This typically shows absence of biliary tract dilatation with lack of display of the gallbladder. One feature that has been suggested as specific is the so-called "triangular cord sign" illustrating the cone-shaped periportal fibrous mass cranial to the bifurcation of the portal vein [30] (Fig. 1.3).

There is no single pathognomonic preoperative finding of BA, but reasonable suspicion necessitates progression to more invasive tests. In our practice, percutaneous liver biopsy is always performed after exclusion of medical causes of cholestatic jaundice (e.g., α-1 antitrypsin deficiency, Alagille syndrome) (Fig. 1.4).

USS and histology establish the diagnosis accurately in more of 85% of cases of BA [31]. Key histological features include bile duct proliferation, a small cell infiltrate, portal fibrosis, and absence of sinusoidal fibrosis [32].

Twenty-four hours duodenal aspiration and analysis of bile has been used for the diagnosis in some Asian centers, but its accuracy has never been published. Other noninvasive tests, such as radionuclide scans using a variety of technetium-labeled iminodiacetic acid derivatives, are now less commonly used because discrimination between medical and surgical causes is poor. Use of endoscopic retrograde

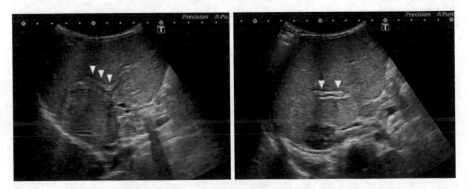

Fig. 1.3 Triangular cord sign: hyperechoic area, tube-shaped, anterior to the porta hepatis (arrowheads) representing the fibrotic residual of the biliary tree

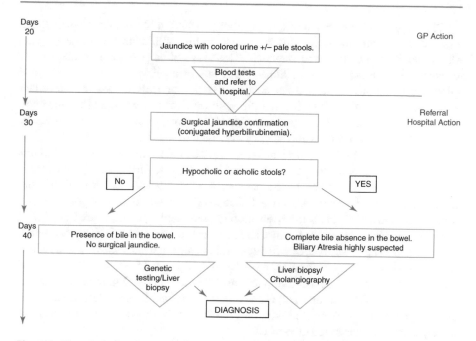

Fig. 1.4 Flowchart showing a timely and correct approach to the patient with suspected biliary atresia

cholangiopancreatography (ERCP) is possible in infants, but is currently confined to highly specialized centers [33]. In some centers, infants with equivocal biopsy results undergo ERCP, although it should be noted that this diagnosis depends crucially on failure to show a biliary tree, and hence, appropriate experience and judgment are essential. Furthermore, there is currently a dearth of appropriately sized endoscopes available, with manufacturers pulling out of production, and this doesn't bode well for being able to continue with this method in the future.

Operative visualization of biliary tree at laparotomy or laparoscopy with on-table cholangiography remains "the last resort" when all noninvasive methods do not allow a certain diagnosis.

1.5   Treatment

In most centers, the usual management of BA starts from a surgical attempt to restore bile flow through the KPE technique [4, 5]. If this fails liver transplantation is then considered. The aim of KPE is to restore, albeit imperfectly, the continuity of the residual intrahepatic biliary system with the gastrointestinal tract and alleviate any ongoing tendency to liver fibrosis.

The preoperative management includes correcting the coagulopathy and maybe an antibacterial bowel preparation. Perioperative antibiotics should be effective against aerobic and anaerobic flora.

The diagnosis is always confirmed initially through a limited right upper quadrant muscle-cutting incision, allowing access to the gallbladder. A cholangiogram should be done to confirm the diagnosis. This may not be possible in some, simply because the gallbladder has no lumen—but this in itself is indicative of BA and allows progression. Neonatal sclerosing cholangitis or various hypoplastic biliary appearances (typically seen with Alagille syndrome) can be detected in some cholangiograms, showing patency with proximal intrahepatic ducts. Little more can be done in these circumstances and surgery may be terminated.

Although visible bile-containing ducts may be evident in type 1 or 2 BA and a hepaticojejunostomy performed, it is probably better that further proximal tissue is resected completely, leading to the need of a portoenterostomy. Sometimes, on-table evidence of cirrhosis and variceal changes may seem to make a portoenterostomy futile. However, this is rarely absolutely predictable, and there are insufficient criteria to confidently decide when a late KPE is too late. Late KPE has been variably defined as age >90, 100, or 120 days, and the reported survival with native liver in these patients is 42% at 2 years, 23–45% at 4–5 years, 15–40% at 10 years, and <10% at 20 years. The decision to perform KPE after day 100 may be relevant, as KPE in infants with cirrhosis and ascites may precipitate hepatic decompensation, and the procedure is associated with an increased risk for bowel perforations and biliary complications at the time of LT.

Some authors have found that higher stages of fibrosis, a ductal plate configuration, and a moderate-to-marked bile duct injury at KPE were independently associated with a higher risk of transplantation. Nevertheless, there is uncertainty on whether liver histology can predict outcome after surgery, as the key determinant is restoration of bile flow, something that is only evident after surgery.

A reasonable working rule might be that in infants older than 100 days, primary LT may be considered more judicious (obviously where it is available), particularly, if there is clinical and USS evidence of nodularity on the liver surface and moderate to severe ascites [34–36].

If the BA diagnosis is confirmed, we believe that the most consistent and efficient dissection of the porta hepatis is facilitated by mobilization of the liver. This need not involve division of all the suspensory ligaments and can be limited to just the falciform and the left triangular, and still allows the entire organ to be everted onto the anterior abdominal cavity. The fibrotic remnant of the extrahepatic bile ducts is dissected free, dividing first the common bile duct to allow it to be tracked back to the porta hepatis. It is then transected at the level of the liver capsule. This transected portal plate is then anastomosed to a retrocolic 40 cm jejunal Roux loop to restore biliary continuity. A liver biopsy is performed at the conclusion of the operation in order to document hepatic histology. The goals of the operation are to restore the bile flow to the intestine, reduce jaundice, and halt ongoing liver damage.

Almost 15 years have now passed since Esteves et al. [37] reported the first laparoscopic KPE. Further reports have been published showing no significant advantage in performing this and in one German study worsening the outlook [38]. The laparoscopic approach has still not been taken up by the larger centers in Japan, Europe, and North America.

The use of steroids is controversial, but appealing, given the possible role of inflammation in the etiology of BA. Davenport et al. [39] in the first randomized placebo-controlled trial of oral prednisolone (2 then 1 mg/kg/day in first month) reported some improvements in early clearance of jaundice but a lack of real effect on final results and need for transplant. The same authors followed this using an open-label trial structure and a higher dose (starting at 5 mg/kg/day), which showed a statistically significant 15% increase in clearance of jaundice compared to control and placebo in those <70 days at KPE [40]. In 2014, Bezerra et al. [41] studied the effects of a 13-week course of steroids on clearance of jaundice with native liver at 6 months after Kasai. This was multicenter and had an older population than the UK trials, and although there was some difference between active and placebo groups, the authors found no statistical significance.

Ursodeoxycholic acid (UDCA) is widely thought to be beneficial, but only if surgery has already restored bile flow to reasonable levels. UDCA "enriches" bile and has a choleretic effect, increasing hepatic clearance of supposedly toxic endogenous bile acids and may confer a cytoprotective effect on hepatocytes.

1.6   Complications

Ascending cholangitis is the most frequent complication after KPE, especially in the first postoperative year, and is probably due to the restoration of direct communications between intrahepatic bile ducts and the small bowel [42]. Clinical presentation of cholangitis is with fever, jaundice, and abdominal pain. Acholic stool and deterioration in liver function tests should also be present. Early diagnosis is very important to prevent the loss of remaining patent bile ducts and to preserve the native liver function. In patients unresponsive to antimicrobial treatment a percutaneous liver biopsy may be cultured to identify the causative organism, but this is uncommonly required. Cholangitis should be treated aggressively with intravenous antibiotics against Gram-negative organisms.

A prophylactic regimen with oral antibiotics, such as amoxicillin, trimethoprim, and cefalexin, might be considered in all children who have undergone KPE in order to prevent cholangitis in the first months after the operation. In cases of children with recurrent cholangitis, following clearance of jaundice, liver scintigraphy may detect a Roux-loop obstruction. This is important, as it is surgically correctable.

Portal hypertension (PH) and esophageal varices are two serious complications after KPE, and they are due to the progressive liver fibrosis causing sustained elevation of portal venous pressure. Progressive hepatosplenomegaly, gastrointestinal bleeding, ascites, encephalopathy, and hepatopulmonary syndrome may all be signs of PH (Fig. 1.5). Among adult survivors with native liver, the incidence of PH varies from 50% to 90% [43].

Portal venous pressure is often already high before surgery. Some studies have shown that infants with this early high level of portal venous pressure have worse outcomes in terms of native liver survival and risk for varices and variceal bleeding.

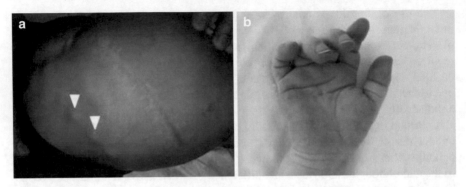

Fig. 1.5 Complications of failed Kasai portoenterostomy: (**a**) jaundice, abdominal distension, ascites, and rachitic rosary (arrowheads): (**b**) palmar erythema

Duche et al. also showed that the presence of ascites, serum bilirubin concentration >20 μmol/L, prothrombin ratio <80%, and portal vein diameter >5 mm are significant risk factors for bleeding [44]. Although bleeding is unusual before 9 months of age, from the first year of life each child should probably have periodic surveillance endoscopies and endoscopic variceal ligation if necessary. Sometimes, primary prophylaxis as prevention of variceal bleeding may be warranted. Occasionally, emergency treatment of bleeding varices using a Sengstaken tube is necessary.

There is a wide variation in estimation of the complications of portal hypertension. It is estimated that from 10 to 60% of patients present with at least one episode of gastrointestinal bleeding during 5 years of follow-up [45]. Developing fibrosis and cirrhotic nodules is the natural progression of the liver affected by BA. Perhaps, one of the most dangerous complications of cirrhosis is the development of hepatocellular carcinoma. Fortunately, it seems that only a small percentage of children with BA develop this kind of neoplasm and, in absence of the extrahepatic involvement, liver transplantation is the effective treatment [46].

1.6.1 Prognosis

Several factors may influence the outcome of patients with BA. Age at surgical intervention remains a critical issue, and it is widely accepted that late age at surgery contributes to a worse outcome in the long-term. The age at surgery also reflects on the effectiveness of the referring primary care system and efficacy of the diagnostic process [47]. The current accepted standard in Europe and North America is to perform KPE at the earliest possible age and carried out by an experienced biliary surgeon. The experience of the center performing the operation also appears as a major prognostic factor. Centralization of hepatobiliary services occurred in England and Wales at the end of the 1990s and results following this showed significant improvement on national outcome for this disease [48, 49].

1.6.2 Implications for Liver Transplantation

BA is the most common indication for liver transplantation (LT) in the pediatric population, accounting for about half of all liver transplants performed in children. Optimal timing is crucial to achieve a successful outcome and avoid deaths on the waiting list. The main factor affecting indication and timing of LT is the success of KPE (Table 1.1). Children not achieving clearance of jaundice in the first few months after surgery are usually transplanted by 2 years of age. If jaundice has resolved by 3 months after KPE, the 10-year transplant-free survival rate has been shown to range from 75% to 90%, whereas if jaundice persists after KPE, the 3-year transplant-free survival rate is only 20% [50]. In a recent North American study of the Children Liver Disease Research Network (ChiLDReN), infants with bilirubin >2 mg/dL ($\approx$34 µmol/L) at 3 months from KPE had diminished weight gain, greater probability of developing ascites, hypoalbuminemia, coagulopathy, and were more likely to die or require LT [51]. Thus, children who do not demonstrate good bile flow and clearance of jaundice by 3 months after KPE should be evaluated early for transplantation, ideally by 6–9 months of age [52].

Infectious complications may sometimes threaten the life of a child with BA who had a successful KPE. Repeated episodes of ascending cholangitis were associated with a three-fold increased risk for early failure after KPE. This complication should prompt listing to LT in case of recurrent episodes despite aggressive antibiotic therapy, multiresistant bacterial organisms, episodes of life-threatening sepsis, or severely impaired quality of life due to frequent hospitalizations [53].

PH accompanies the rapid progression of end-stage liver disease in children with a failed KPE, raising the issue of surveillance endoscopy of these patients while awaiting LT. However, in most patients, the risk of bleeding starts after the first year of life [54]. Considering that varices treatment is difficult in infants (due to the lack of a suitable banding device), that variceal bleed is rarely associated with death and that in most centers, LT is performed by 12–18 months of age, a conservative approach to PH based only on clinical observation in these patients seems reasonable. Despite a much slower course, PH develops almost invariably even after a successful KPE. A study from the USA, analyzing 163 children with BA who survived with their native liver to a mean age of 9.2 years, showed that PH could be identified in 67%. Variceal bleeding had occurred in 20% of subjects, although the

Table 1.1 Indications for liver transplantation in biliary atresia

• Failed KPE
• Late diagnosis: primary LT
• Failure to thrive despite aggressive nutritional support
• Recurrent or life-threatening bacterial cholangitis
• Recurrent hospitalizations impairing quality of life
• Refractory variceal bleeding
• Hepatopulmonary syndrome
• Portopulmonary hypertension
• Significant ascites and episodes of spontaneous bacterial peritonitis
• Hepatorenal syndrome
• Hepatic malignancy

majority (62%) had only one episode [55]. In Canada and Europe, up to 96% of adult patients with BA had features of PH, with 65% having evidence of varices, 91% had splenomegaly, and 14% ascites. A French study showed that 99% of BA survivors with their native liver into adulthood had evidence of cirrhosis and 70% had significant PH [43, 56]. Extrahepatic complications of PH, such as spontaneous bacterial peritonitis, hepatopulmonary syndrome, portopulmonary hypertension, represent a clear indication to promptly place the patient on the transplant list [57].

Deciding the best timing to list for LT a patient who had a failed Kasai may be challenging, and probably depends more on the transplant program setting rather than on an individual patient's features. A tool validated in children with chronic liver disease is the pediatric end-stage liver disease score (PELD). PELD score is calculated based on the age, growth failure, albumin, international normalized ratio, and total bilirubin level and is an excellent predictor for the outcome of pediatric patients listed for LT. However, it has been reported that the PELD score in BA patients does not accurately reflect the true mortality risk associated with complications of PH, variceal bleeding, refractory ascites, and hepatopulmonary syndrome. The US experience showed that BA patients have a median wait time on the list of 90 days and a median calculated PELD score of 15 at the time of transplant (UNOS data); 15% of children with chronic liver disease have either died on the waiting list or been removed because they were too ill to transplant. These figures are probably related to the fact that in the US network, only approximately 10% of eligible donor livers are split, missing an opportunity to expand access to transplant for BA patients, and leading to a high mortality on the list in children younger than 2 years of age [58–60]. This is not the case in countries, such as Italy, where the split technique is widely adopted, thus many left lateral segments grafts are offered to the centers, and the mortality on the list of recipients below 2 years of age is close to 0% [61]. Following transplantation, survival of children with BA is very satisfactory, being greater than 90% at 5 years (Fig. 1.6).

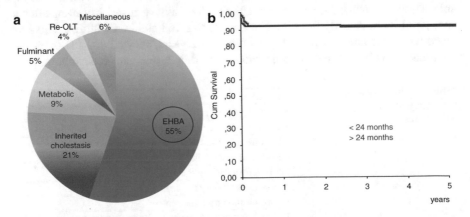

Fig. 1.6 Liver transplantation (OLT) in biliary atresia (EHBA). (**a**) Main indications to OLT; (**b**) posttransplant survival of children with EHBA according to the age at transplantation in the Bergamo center

References

1. Betalli P, Davenport M. Atresia and other congenital disorders of the extrahepatic biliary tree. Textbook of pediatric hepatology and liver transplantation. New York: Springer; 2019. p. 129–44.
2. Burns J. Principles of midwifery, including the diseases of women and children. London: Longman; 1817.
3. Thomson J. On congenital obliteration of the bile ducts. Edinb Med J. 1891;37:523–31.
4. Ladd WE. Congenital obstruction of the bile ducts. Ann Surg. 1935;102:742–51.
5. Kasai M, Kimura S, Asakura Y, Suzuki H, Taira Y, Ohashi E. Surgical treatment of biliary atresia. J Pediatr Surg. 1968;3:665–75.
6. Kasai M, Watanabe I, Ohi R. Follow-up studies of long-term survivors after hepatic portoenterostomy for "noncorrectable" biliary atresia. J Pediatr Surg. 1975;10:173–82.
7. Wada H, Muraji T, Yokoi A, Okamoto T, Sato S, Takamizawa S, et al. Insignificant seasonal and geographical variation in incidence of biliary atresia in Japan: a regional survey of over 20 years. J Pediatr Surg. 2007;42:2090–2.
8. Chardot C, Carton M, Spire-Bendelac N, Le Pommelet C, Golmard JL, Auvert B. Epidemiology of biliary atresia in France: a national study 1986–96. J Hepatol. 1999;31:1006–13.
9. Livesey E, Cortina Borja M, Sharif K, Alizai N, McClean P, et al. Epidemiology of biliary atresia in England and Wales (1999–2006). Arch Dis Child Fetal Neonatal Ed. 2009;94:451–5.
10. Schreilber RA, Barker CC, Roberts EA, Martin SR, Canadian Pediatric Hepatology Research Group. Biliary atresia in Canada: the effect of centre caseload experience on outcome. J Pediatr Gastroenterol Nutr. 2010;51:61–5.
11. Girard M, Jannot AS, Besnard M, Leutenegger AL, Jacquemin E, Lyonnet S, et al. Polynesian ecology determines seasonality of biliary atresia. Hepatology. 2011;54(5):1893–4.
12. Chen SM, Chang MH, Du JC, Lin CC, Chen AC, Lee HC, et al. Screening for biliary atresia by infant stool color card in Taiwan. Pediatrics. 2006;117(4):1147–54.
13. Chen SM, Chang MH Hsiao CH, Chang MH, Chen HL, et al. Universal screening for biliary atresia using an infant stool color card in Taiwan. Hepatology. 2008;47:1233–40.
14. Davenport M, Savage M, Mowat AP, Howard ER. The biliary atresia splenic malformation syndrome. Surgery. 1993;113:662–8.
15. Davenport M, Tizzard SA, Underhill J, Mieli-Vergani G, Portmann B, Hadzić N. The biliary atresia splenic malformation syndrome: a 28-year single-center retrospective study. J Pediatr. 2006;149:393–400.
16. Fischler B, Ehrnst A, Forsgren C, Orvell C, Nemeth A. The viral association of neonatal cholestasis in Sweden: a possible link between cytomegalovirus infection and extrahepatic biliary atresia. J Pediatr Gastroenterol Nutr. 1998;27:57–64.
17. Rauschenfels S, Krassmann M, Al-Masri AN, Verhagen W, Leonhardt J, Kuebler JF, et al. Incidence of hepatotropic viruses in biliary atresia. Eur J Pediatr. 2009;168:469–76.
18. Zani A, Quaglia A, Hadzić N, Zuckerman M, Davenport M. Cytomegalovirus-associated biliary atresia: an etiological and prognostic subgroup. J Pediatr Surg. 2015;50:1739–45.
19. Davenport M. Biliary atresia: clinical aspects. Semin Pediatr Surg. 2012;21:175–84.
20. Lakshminarayanan B, Davenport M. Biliary atresia: a comprehensive review. J Autoimmun. 2016;76:1–9.
21. Asai A, Miethke A, Bezzerra JA. Pathogenesis of biliary atresia: defining biology to understand clinical phenotypes. Nat Rev Gastroenterol Hepatol. 2015;12:342–52.
22. Verkade HJ, Bezerra AJ, Davenport M, Schreiber RA, Mieli-Vergani G, Hulscher JB, et al. Biliary atresia and other cholestatic childhood diseases: advances and future challenges. J Hepatol. 2016;65:631–42.
23. Redkar R, Davenport M, Howard ER. Antenatal diagnosis of congenital anomalies of biliary tract. J Pediatr Surg. 1998;33:700–4.
24. Harpavat S, Finegold MJ, Karpen SJ. Patients with biliary atresia have elevated direct/conjugated bilirubin levels shortly after birth. Pediatrics. 2011;128:1428–33.

25. Hill R, Quaglia A, Hussain M, Hadzic N, Mieli-Vergani G, Vergani D, et al. Th-17 cells infiltrate the liver in human biliary atresia and are related to surgical outcome. J Pediatr Surg. 2015;50:1297–303.
26. Bezzerra JA, Tiao G, Ryckman FC, Alonso M, Sabla GE, Shneider B, et al. Genetic induction of proinflammatory immunity in children with biliary atresia. Lancet. 2002;360:1563–659.
27. Muraji T, Hosaka N, Irie N, Yoshida M, Imai Y, Tanaka K, et al. Maternal microchimerism in underlying pathogenesis of biliary atresia: quantification and phenotypes of maternal cells in the liver. Pediatrics. 2008;121:517–21.
28. Harper P, Plant JW, Unger DB. Congenital biliary atresia and jaundice in lambs and calves. Aust Vet J. 1990;67:18–22.
29. Hussein M, Howard ER, Mieli-Vergani G, Mowat AP. Jaundice at 14 days: exclude biliary atresia. Arch Dis Child. 1991;66:1177–9.
30. Imanieh MH, Dehghani SM, Bagheri MH, Emad V, Haghighat M, Zahmatkeshan M, et al. Triangular cord sign in detection of biliary atresia: is it valuable sign? Dig Dis Sci. 2010;55:172–5.
31. Davenport M, Betalli P, D'Antiga L, Cheeseman P, Mieli-Vergani G, Howard ER. The spectrum of surgical jaundice in infancy. J Pediatr Surg. 2003;38:1471–9.
32. Russo P, Magee JC, Boitnott KE, Bove T, Raghunathan T, Finegold M, et al. Design and validation of the biliary atresia research consortium histologic assessment system for cholestasis in infancy. Clin Gastroenterol Hepatol. 2011;9:357–62.
33. Shanmugam NP, Harrison PM, Devlin P, Peddu P, Knisely AS, Davenport M, et al. Selective use of endoscopic retrograde cholangiopancreatography in the diagnosis of biliary atresia in infants younger than 100 days. J Pediatr Gastroenterol Nutr. 2009;46:1689–94.
34. Davenport M, Puricelli V, Farrant P, Hadzic M, Mieli-Vergani G, Portmann B, et al. The outcome of the older (>100 days) infant with biliary atresia. J Pediatr Surg. 2004;39:575–81.
35. Neto JS, Feier FH, Bierrenbach AL, Toscano CM, Fonseca EA, Pugliese R, et al. Impact of Kasai portoenterostomy on liver transplantation outcomes: a retrospective cohort study of 347 children with biliary atresia. Liver Transpl. 2015;21:922–7.
36. Russo P, Magee JC, Anders RA, Bove KE, Chung C, Cummings OW, et al. Childhood Liver Disease Research Network (ChiLDReN). Key histopathologic features of liver biopsies that distinguish biliary atresia from other causes of infantile cholestasis and their correlation with outcome: a multicenter study. Am J Surg Pathol. 2016;40:1601–15.
37. Esteves E, Clemente Neto E, Ottaiano Neto M, Devanir J Jr, Esteves Pereira R. Laparoscopic Kasai portoenterostomy for biliary atresia. Pediatr Surg Int. 2002;18:737–40.
38. Ure BM, Kuebler JF, Schukfeh N, Engelmann C, Dingemann J, Petersen C. Survival with the native liver after laparoscopic versus conventional Kasai portoenterostomy in infants with biliary atresia: a prospective trial. Ann Surg. 2011;253:826–30.
39. Davenport M, Stringer MD, Tizzard SA, McClean P, Mieli-Vergani G, Hadzic N. Randomized, double-blind, placebo-controlled trial of corticosteroids after Kasai portoenterostomy for biliary atresia. Hepatology. 2007;46:1821–7.
40. Davenport M, Tizzard SA, Parsons C, Hadzic N. Single surgeon, single centre: experience with steroids in biliary atresia. J Hepatol. 2013;59:1054–8.
41. Bezzerra JA, Spino C, Magee JC, Schneider BL, Rosenthal P, Wang KS, et al. Use of corticosteroids after hepatoportoentrostomy for bile drainage in infants with biliary atresia: the START-randomized clinical trial. JAMA. 2014;311:1750–9.
42. Hartley JL, Davenport M, Kelly DA. Biliary atresia. Lancet. 2009;374:1704–13.
43. Lykavieris P, Chardot C, Sokhn M, Gauthier F, Valayer J, Bernard O. Outcome in adulthood of biliary atresia: a study of 63 patients who survived for over 20 years with their native liver. Hepatology. 2005;41(2):366–71.
44. Duche M, Ducot B, Tournay E, Fabre M, Cohen J, Jacquemin E, Bernard O. Prognostic value of endoscopy in children with biliary atresia at risk for early development of varices and bleeding. Gastroenterology. 2010;139:1952–60.
45. Miga D, Sokol RJ, Mackenzie T. Survival after first esophageal variceal hemorrhage in patients with biliary atresia. J Pediatr. 2001;139:291–6.

46. Hadzic N, Quaglia A, Portmann B, Paramalingam S, Heaton ND, Rela M, Mieli-Vergani G, Davenport M. Hepatocellular carcinoma in biliary atresia: King's College Hospital experience. J Pediatr. 2011;159:617–22.
47. Kvist N, Davenport M. Thirty-four years experience with biliary atresia in Denmark: a single center study. Eur J Pediatr Surg. 2011;21:224–8.
48. Davenport M, De Ville de Goyet J, Stringer MD, Mieli-Vergani G, Kelly DA, McClean P, et al. Seamless management of biliary atresia in England and Wales (1999-2002). Lancet. 2004;363:1354–7.
49. Davenport M, Ong E, Sharif K, Alizai N, McClean P, Hadzic N, et al. Biliary atresia in England and Wales: results of centralization and new benchmark. J Pediatr Surg. 2011;46:1689–94.
50. Shneider BL, Brown MB, Haber B, Whitington PF, Schwarz K, Squires R, et al. Biliary Atresia Research Consortium. A multicenter study of the outcome of biliary atresia in the United States, 1997 to 2000. J Pediatr. 2006;148:467–74.
51. Shneider BL, Magee JC, Karpen SJ, Rand EB, Narkewicz MR, Bass LM, et al. Childhood Liver Disease Research Network (ChiLDReN). Total serum bilirubin within 3 months of hepatoportoenterostomy predicts short-term outcomes in biliary atresia. J Pediatr. 2016;170:211–7.
52. Nightingale S, Stormon MO, O'Loughlin EV, Shun A, Thomas G, et al. Early post-hepatoportoenterostomy predictors of native liver survival in biliary atresia. J Pediatr Gastroenterol Nutr. 2017;64:203–9.
53. Qiao G, Li L, Cheng W, Zhang Z, Ge J, Wang C. Conditional probability of survival in patients with biliary atresia after Kasai portoenterostomy: a Chinese population-based study. J Pediatr Surg. 2015;50:1310–5.
54. Duché M, Ducot B, Ackermann O, Baujard C, Chevret L, Frank-Soltysiak M, et al. Experience with endoscopic management of high-risk gastroesophageal varices, with and without bleeding, in children with biliary atresia. Gastroenterology. 2013;145:801–7.
55. Sundaram SS, Mack CL, Feldman AG, Sokol RJ. Biliary atresia: indications and timing of liver transplantation and optimization of pretransplant care. Liver Transplant. 2017;23(1):96–109.
56. Kumagi T, Drenth JP, Guttman O, Ng V, Lilly L, Therapondos G, et al. Biliary atresia and survival into adulthood without transplantation: a collaborative multicentre clinic review. Liver Int. 2012;32:510–8.
57. Di Giorgio A, D'Antiga L. Portal hypertension in children. Textbook of pediatric gastroenterology, hepatology and nutrition. New York: Springer International Publishing; 2016. p. 791–817.
58. Arnon R, Leshno M, Annunziato R, Florman S, Iyer K. What is the optimal timing of liver transplantation for children with biliary atresia? A Markov model simulation analysis. J Pediatr Gastroenterol Nutr. 2014;59:398–402.
59. Utterson EC, Sheperd RW, Sokol RJ, Bucuvalas J, Magee JC, McDiarmid SV, et al. Biliary atresia: clinical, profiles, risk factors, and outcomes of 755 patients listed for liver transplantation. J Pediatr. 2005;147:180–5.
60. Barshes NR, Lee TC, Udell IW, O'Mahoney CA, Karpen SJ, Carter BA, et al. The pediatric end-stage liver disease (PELD) model as a predictor of survival benefit and posttransplant survival in pediatric liver transplant recipients. Liver Transpl. 2006;12:475–80.
61. Gridelli B, Spada M, Petz W, Bertani A, Lucianetti A, Colledan M, et al. Split-liver transplantation eliminates the need for living-donor liver transplantation in children with end-stage cholestatic liver disease. Transplantation. 2003;75:1197–203.

Congenital Cystic Lesions of the Biliary Tree

2

Alberto Lasagni, Giovanni Morana, Mario Strazzabosco,
Luca Fabris, and Massimiliano Cadamuro

2.1 Introduction

Fibropolycystic liver diseases (FPLDs) designate a complex group of disorders affecting the biliary tree, characterized by dysgenesis of the bile ducts, resulting in the formation of segmental dilations or real cysts, eventually associated to cysts in other organs, including kidney, pancreas, and ovaries. Common traits of these disorders are the rare incidence, the congenital origin, and the unique pathogenesis driven, at least in most of them, by an abnormal development of the ductal plate (the embryonic structure originating the intrahepatic bile ducts) called ductal plate malformation (DPM). In this heterogeneous group, it is important to keep the polycystic liver diseases (PLDs)—autosomal-dominant polycystic liver disease (ADPLD) or autosomal-dominant polycystic kidney disease (ADPKD)—distinct from the rarer

A. Lasagni
General Medicine Division, Azienda Ospedale-Università di Padova, Padova, Italy
e-mail: alberto.lasagni@aopd.veneto.it

G. Morana
Radiology Unit, Treviso Regional Hospital, Azienda ULSS2 Marca Trevigiana, Treviso, Italy
e-mail: giovanni.morana@aulss2.veneto.it

M. Strazzabosco
Digestive Disease Section, Yale University, New Haven, CT, USA
e-mail: mario.strazzabosco@yale.edu

L. Fabris (✉)
General Medicine Division, Azienda Ospedale-Università di Padova, Padova, Italy

Digestive Disease Section, Yale University, New Haven, CT, USA

Department of Molecular Medicine-DMM, University of Padova, Padova, Italy
e-mail: luca.fabris@unipd.it, luca.fabris@yale.edu

M. Cadamuro
Department of Molecular Medicine-DMM, University of Padova, Padova, Italy
e-mail: massimiliano.cadamuro@unipd.it

© Springer Nature Switzerland AG 2021
A. Floreani (ed.), *Diseases of the Liver and Biliary Tree*,
https://doi.org/10.1007/978-3-030-65908-0_2

Table 2.1 Fibrocystic liver disease classification according to the level of biliary tree involvement

Disease	Biliary tree level affected	Size
von Meyenburg complex	Small intralobular bile ducts	<20 μm
PLDs[a]	Interlobular and septal bile ducts	20–50 μm
Congenital hepatic fibrosis (CHF)	Interlobular and septal bile ducts	20–50 μm
Autosomal-recessive polycystic kidney disease (ARPKD)	CHF associated to nonobstructive fusiform dilations of the renal-collecting ducts	20–50 μm
Caroli's disease (CD)	Larger intrahepatic bile ducts	>50 μm
Caroli's syndrome (CS)	Both interlobular and larger intrahepatic bile ducts (CHF+CD)	>20 μm
Choledochal cysts (CC)	Extrahepatic bile ducts	2–8 mm

[a]Cystic formations disconnected from biliary tree

fibrocystic liver disease (FLDs), as different clinical, genetic, and pathophysiological aspects depict these entities. PLDs are inherited disorders characterized by the development of multiple (>20) fluid-filled biliary cysts widespread throughout liver parenchyma and disconnected from biliary tree [1]. FLDs encompass von Meyenburg complex (VMC), autosomal-recessive polycystic kidney disease (ARPKD), congenital hepatic fibrosis (CHF), Caroli disease (CD) and syndrome (CS), and choledochal cysts (CCs). The distinctive feature of FLDs is the presence of cyst-like dilatations of the biliary tree embedded by a macrophage-dominant immune infiltrate and dense fibrosis [2]. Schematically, each condition can be led back to a distinct anatomical level of biliary involvement, as outlined in Table 2.1.

However, the demarcation line between these conditions is actually not sharp, as the intrahepatic biliary tree can be simultaneously affected at multiple levels, depending on the degree of DPM. For instance, CS is characterized by the presence of both large duct ectasia and CHF, typically affecting the smaller bile ducts. Moreover, biliary dysgenesis can be part of a multisystemic disease involving other ductal epithelia, such as kidney and pancreas. Combination of renal and hepatic disease may vary, and different liver diseases can overlap in the same patient, suggesting common underlying mechanisms.

Ciliopathies. FPLDs belong to a much wider group of developmental diseases affecting the ductal epithelia, collectively called in the last decade as ciliopathies, to highlight the notion that cilium dysfunction plays a key role in their pathogenesis [3, 4]. Cellular cilia are categorized as motile or nonmotile. Motile cilia are expressed by the respiratory, fallopian tube, sperm, and ependymal epithelial cells, whereby they are involved in the regulation of fluid transport across the epithelial surfaces. Their dysfunction causes a variety of conditions, including bronchiectasis, *situs inversus viscerum,* and infertility [5, 6]. Nonmotile cilia are sensory organelles expressed by most polarized eukaryotic cells, including cholangiocytes and renal tubular epithelial cells. They lay on basal bodies (centrioles) and extend outward from the cell surface to serve as signal transducers between extracellular fluids (e.g., urine, bile) and the intracellular environment [7]. Upon entry in the cell cycle, nonmotile cilia are disassembled, leaving the basal bodies free to arrange the mitotic spindle that will drive separation of chromosomes. Cilia harbor a group of proteins (polycystins, fibrocystin, polaris) mediating cell-cell and cell-matrix interactions that are crucial for tissue development, regeneration/repair, and homeostasis. Thus, alterations of these proteins during embryogenesis can explain clinical and histological findings in human ciliopathies with early onset [8]. As most polarized eukaryotic cells, cholangiocytes and renal tubular epithelial cells express primary cilia. Thus, these cells are the most frequently targeted by genetic defects in humans. Ciliopathies caused by defects in primary nonmotile cilia are characterized by a wide degree of ductal dysgenesis that may result in the development of cystic lesions. For instance, in ciliopathies targeting the kidneys, clinical manifestations hugely range from mild urinary concentration defects in normal appearing kidneys to kidney with a clear, abnormal morphology and severe functional impairment. The most common renal ciliopathies are autosomal-dominant and recessive polycystic kidneys disease (ADPKD and ARPKD), but nephronophthisis, cystic dysplastic kidneys, medullary sponge kidney, and various overlap syndromes are also worth mentioning [3].

Embryology. Since DPM represents a key feature of the hepatic phenotype in ciliopathies [9, 10], we will now briefly overview the main steps of the biliary morphogenesis. The biliary system starts to develop at the 8th week of gestation from the endodermal hepatic diverticulum of the ventral foregut endoderm. The intrahepatic bile duct epithelium originates from the cranial part, while the extrahepatic portion of the biliary tree derives from the caudal part of the ventral foregut endoderm. In the liver parenchyma, the primordial biliary structure is the "ductal plate," a single layer of immature epithelial-like cells derived from the differentiation of hepatoblasts (cells with bipotential capabilities), localized in the area abutting the nascent portal area. Ductal plates evolve to bilayered structures expressing a dual epithelial identity, resembling cholangiocytes on the side facing the portal tract, and hepatocytes on the parenchymal side. In these structures, the further duplication couples with a progressive dilation encircling a lumen to generate tubular structures, whereby hepatoblasts are progressively replaced by cholangiocytes, and thus may migrate into the portal mesenchyme. Once the lumen is created, around the 30th week, intrahepatic bile ducts mature along cross-sectional and craniocaudal axis directed from the hilum to the periphery. Progressive elongation of the bile ducts is critically regulated by an intricate mechanism that orientates mitosis along the right axis and maintains the tubular architecture within the ductal plane, the so-called "planar cell polarity." This process is finely orchestrated by mutual interactions between ductal plate and mesenchymal cells under the control of a huge number of growth and transcription factors, stimulating cell migration and cholangiocyte differentiation. When defective, this mechanism leads to abnormal dilated or disconnected bile ducts, resulting into biliary cystic or "cyst-like" lesions. Depending on the time when this embryological development is hampered, DPM can lead to different liver phenotypes. At an early stage of ductal plate remodeling, the largest intra or extrahepatic bile ducts are affected, resulting in CD, CS, or choledochal cyst. In the intermediate period, medium-sized intrahepatic bile ducts are involved, and this perturbation leads to ADPKD and ADPLD. Only in the later stages, small interlobular bile ducts are affected, giving rise to VMC or CHF [9, 11].

Genetics and molecular pathogenesis. Ciliopathies encompass a wide range of diseases caused by different genetic defects, though clinically characterized by similar features.

ADPKD is caused by mutations in PKD1 (80–85%) or PKD2 (10–15%) [12, 13]. Liver is affected in 85% of patients [1, 14]. PKD1–2 encode the ciliary proteins polycystin-1 (PC1) and PC2 that form a functional complex regulating intracellular calcium homeostasis [15] composed by PC1, a mechanoreceptor involved in calcium signaling and PC2, a nonselective calcium channel. However, ADPLD is the result of mutations in several genes, including PRKCSH that is the most frequent, present in around 15% cases, SEC63, SEC61B, GANAB, ALG8, LRP5 [16–20]. Nonetheless, these gene mutations are found only in half of ADPLD patients. All of these genes encode for proteins located in endoplasmic reticulum (ER), involved in protein biogenesis, except for LRP5 that is a plasma membrane coreceptor participating in Wnt signaling. As shown in experimental models, cystogenesis is supervised by PC1. Thus, affections of PKD1 or in the aforementioned ER-related genes result in impaired ciliary structure and, therefore, cholangiocyte proliferation and cystogenesis [21]. Moreover, PC1 is also involved in controlling Wnt signaling, linking to LRP5 mutations.

PLDs are an autosomal-dominant disease that is recessive on a cellular level. A somatic mutation on the wild-type allele or a mutation on a second PLD-associated gene is necessary to initiate cyst development [22]. Thus, cystogenesis originates both from DPM and second-hit mutations in the wild-type allele of PLD-related genes in intrahepatic cholangiocytes with loss of heterozygosity [22]. Patients with PKD1, particularly truncating mutations, present a more severe phenotype with earlier progression to end-stage renal failure than PKD2-mutated patients [23]. In ADPLD, a worse clinical course is associated to mutations in PRKCSH or SEC 63 [24].

According to different models, cystogenesis arise either from cystic cholangiocyte proliferation or through the recruitment and biliary differentiation of nearby hepatoblasts [25–27]. Anyway, the natural history of PLDs is characterized by growth of cyst during adult age, and these processes require cell proliferation [2]. Through different mechanism, PC1- and/or PC2-defective cholangiocytes alter calcium concentrations increasing cAMP production, and thereby activating PKA-dependent cell proliferation and hypersecretion. Meanwhile, increased cAMP stimulates vascular endothelial growth factor (VEGF) via an mTOR-ERK1/2-HIF1α-mediated pathway [28, 29]. VEGF has autocrine and paracrine proliferative effects on cystic cholangiocytes and vascular endothelial cells, resulting in cyst expansion and pericystic vascularization [30–32].

PKHD1 is the most frequently involved gene in FLD, such as CHF/CD and ARPKD. It is a complex gene of 500 kb located on the chromosome 6p21.1p12 encoding for fibrocystin/polyductin (FPC). FPC is a receptor-like protein localized in the basal body of cilia and centromeres, predominantly in collecting ducts and thick ascending loop epithelium in the kidney, and in ductal epithelium of liver and pancreas. Its function is yet far to be deciphered, but it is likely involved in multiple cell activities, such as proliferation, secretion, terminal differentiation, and hetero-typic interactions with the extracellular matrix. Recently, it has been suggested that FPC may control the "planar cell polarity," acting together with β-catenin indepen-dently of Wnt activation [2, 9]. Recent studies have unveiled that in cholangiocytes, FPC exerts an inhibitory tone on a pro-inflammatory phenotype, which is likely reminiscent of a developmental behavior of epithelial cells necessary to accomplish cell-cell communications during embryogenesis. When FPC is defective, β-catenin is overactivated, leading to an uncontrolled secretion of cyto/chemokines (CXCL1, CXCL10, CXCL12) able to attract macrophages and mesenchymal cells in the peribiliary area, ultimately resulting in a progressive collagen deposition around the dysgenetic ducts. In FPC-defective cholangiocytes, chemokine secretion is further enhanced by a local, self-perpetuating feed-forward loop sustained by IL-1β through the activation of the JAK-signal transducer and activator of transcription 3 (STAT3) pathway, which operates through an activated inflammasome [2, 33, 34]. Genetic structure of *PKHD1* has been analyzed, leading to the identification of over 300 mutations, with a detection rate ranging from 42 to 87% [35]. However, the overall picture is even more complex, as clinical features and progression rate of renal or hepatic disease are independent and may vary within a given *PKHD1* mutation, sug-gesting the intervention of other unknown phenotype modifying genes. Of note, current mutation analysis is not predictive of outcome. Missense, deletion/insertion, and splicing mutations have been described in ARPKD patients. The most frequent pathogenic variants of *PKHD1* gene are nonsense truncating mutations (around 60%), while missense mutations account for 40% [36]. Moreover, mutation detec-tion rates are higher for patients with severe, early-onset disease because they usu-ally show truncating mutations that are easier to detect [37]. Given the high frequency of missense mutations, in particular single nucleotide mutations, ·an ARPKD mutation database has been created to support genetic studies and interpre-tation of genetic testing in view to predict the severity of the disease [38]. Other genes can be involved in the pathogenesis of CHF and CD, and they are reported in Table 2.2. Among them, mutations in IFT88/polaris—encoding a component of the intracellular transport system, involved in cell cycle and ciliogenesis—cause a liver phenotype similar to FPC deficiency, as shown in rodent models [39].

Table 2.2 Genetics of FLD-related syndromes. Adapted from [37]

Mutated gene	Associated syndrome	Liver disease
PKHD1	ARPDK	CHF, CD
PDK1–2	ADPDK	CHF, biliary cysts
NPHP1–15	NPHP	CHF
JBTS1–20	Joubert	CHF, CD
BBS1–15	Bardet-Biedl	CHF
MKS1–10	Meckel-Gruber	CHF
OFD1	Oral-facial-digital 1	CHF
ATD1–5	Jeune	CHF, CD

2.2   Polycystic Liver Disease

PLD is characterized by more than 20 fluid-filled liver cysts [40], even if recently a consensus experts suggested to consider PLD in the context of >10 cysts [1]. Cysts could be located to one or more segments or spread throughout liver. Presence of large and numerous cysts lead to hepatomegaly as shown in Fig. 2.1. The natural history is characterized by growth of cyst during adult age. PLD occurs in the context of two distinct hereditary disorders, more frequently associated with polycystic kidney disease in ADPKD rather than as primary ADPLD. Its prevalence is 1:500–1000 and 1:100,000, respectively in ADPKD and ADPLD [41].

Polycystic kidneys are the primary lesion in ADPKD, and PLD is associated up to 83% cases [14]; whereas in ADPLD, even if renal disease is absent, asymptomatic renal cysts could be found in 28–35% of patients [42].

There is a large variation in the severity of liver disease, from few cysts to incapacitating severe hepatomegaly. This clinical heterogeneity may be partially explained by the different effects of each mutation on PC1 expression/function, as well as on the other proteins that contribute to the process of cystogenesis [18, 43]. Family studies suggest a disease penetrance around 80%, so 20% of mutation carriers will have only mild or absent disease [41].

Etiology, age, and gender have been associated with severity of disease. Women affected by ADPKD have larger hepatomegaly in terms of height-adjusted total liver volume (hTLV) (see below) than those with ADPLD, even after age correction [1]. Young women (<48 years) appeared to present a more rapid progression and much

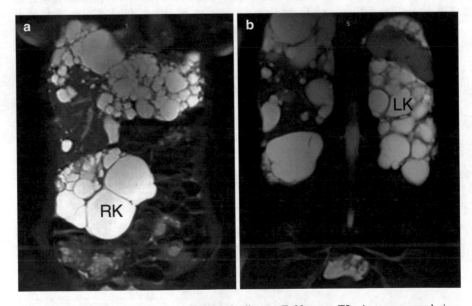

Fig. 2.1 (a, b) Autosomal-dominant polycystic disease. F, 32 years. T2w images, coronal view, two different slices. A diffuse cystic involvement of the liver and the kidneys (RK; LK) can be appreciated

larger increase in liver volume compared to older woman or man. These gender-dependent differences could be linked to the hormonal status of the woman. Indeed, massive hepatomegaly in ADPKD is more frequent with a prior pregnancy and, in postmenopausal women, liver growth appeared to slow down [44]. The effect of estrogen use in oral contraceptives has also been questioned, but results from studies are contradictory, possibly due to progressive decrease in the dosage during last decades. Anyway, even requiring further elucidation, in clinical practice avoiding oral contraceptives containing estrogen is the main lifestyle adjustment suggested. Longitudinal studies comparing natural course of ADPKD and ADPLD are needed to develop a prediction model based on age, gender, etiology, and hormonal status. Such model, able to select patients at risk for severe hepatomegaly, is still warranted to offer better counseling and management advice [44].

In most patients, PLD courses asymptomatic and routine surveillance are not recommended. Indeed, clinical presentation is related to the number, volume of cysts, and especially to the development of hepatomegaly that triggers symptoms and prompt-imaging testing. Symptoms are related to the compression that the enlarged liver exert on close organs, including stomach, lungs, and intestines. Accordingly to liver shape and volume, symptoms may range from pain to the back or flank in mild PLDs to dyspnea, debilitating abdomen-flank-back pain, early satiety, gastro-esophageal reflux, decreased food intake resulting in weight loss and sarcopenia in severe PLDs [45]. Regardless of liver upheaval, liver function remains preserved. However, recent findings suggest that compression of hepatic veins or inferior vena cava causes hepatic venous outflow obstruction (HVOO). This was found in 92% of patients who underwent liver resection or transplantation. Furthermore, histology on these samples revealed liver fibrosis in 56.8% of patients. Clinical impact of HVOO remains unclear, but it may be related to ascites and liver failure in the postoperative [46]. Elevated alkaline phosphatase (ALP) or gamma-glutamyl transferase (GGT) is not uncommon in the moderate or severe disease, but they do not have any clinical significance. Finally, quality of life is also severely impacted by physical appearance, especially in young female patients who, in severe PLDs, bear a protruding abdomen similar to full-term pregnancy.

Associated disease and syndromes. ADPKD is a multisystemic disorder. Renal function is severally affected in ADPKD with onset of hypertension and progressive renal failure in most patients. Moreover, intracranial and arterial aneurysms, cardiac valvular alterations, especially mitral valve prolapse [42, 47] may coexist, thus early assessment of cardiovascular risk factor and screening with cerebral MRI angiography are advised [48]. Cysts in other organs, such as pancreas or seminal vesicles in testis, have been demonstrated but remain silent [41]. Arachnoid cysts, present in 8% of patients, may occasionally lead to subdural hematoma [48]. Finally, a multi-specialist patient-centered approach in specialized centers is warranted in these patients [49].

Diagnosis. Diagnostic criteria for ADPLD and ADPKD are summarized in Table 2.3. Imaging is pivotal in the diagnostic, staging, and prognostic process. Abdominal ultrasound (US) is the first level test in case of abdominal pain, physical examination suggesting hepatomegaly or abnormal liver test. Cysts appear as

Table 2.3 ADPLD and
ADPKD diagnostic criteria

ADPLD	Liver cysts
Positive family history	
<40 years	≥1
≥40 years	≥4
Negative family history	
30–70 years	>10
ADPKD	**Kidney cysts**
Positive family history	
15–39 years	3[a]
40–59 years	2[b]
≥60 years	4[b]
Negative family history	
≤60 years	5[c]
>60 years	8[c]

[a]Unilaterally or bilaterally
[b]Bilaterally
[c]Per kidney

homogeneous anechoic fluid-filled well-circumscribed round space. US also per-
mits to differ between ADPLD and ADPKD based on finding of either liver and/or
kidney multiple cysts. Moreover, US is the first mean for screening in at-risk individuals or asymptomatic first-degree relatives. On computed tomography (CT) or
magnetic resonance imaging (MRI), cysts have nonenhancing, well-circumscribed
round walls with hypodense content, while on T2w MRI scans, they appear as
homogeneously spherical lesions. Furthermore, by using semiautomatic software,
CT and MRI add the possibility to estimate liver volume that is a prognostic marker
and the main endpoint for novel therapeutic strategies, as it impacts both on symptom burden and quality of life [1]. MRI showed better performance in detecting
small cyst in young individuals [50].

Genetic testing and counseling are not required for diagnosis of ADPKD, unless
in selected cases, including atypical renal imaging and sporadic PKD without family history. PKD1/2 mutation is detectable in most cases with current techniques.

Once identified, hepatomegaly needs to be further categorized in order to assess
severity, prognosis, and eventual therapeutic recommendation. Several classifications have been implemented and are outlined in Table 2.4. The Gigot classification
is based on number, size of the cyst, and extent of liver parenchyma involved and
can help for a crude differentiation of phenotypes. Since it does not include symptoms, it is inappropriate for evaluating progression of the disease or considering to
start treatment [51]. The Schnelldorfer's classification aims to select patients that
could benefit from resection (Type C) or transplantation (Type D) [52]. Two specific
questionnaires, POLCA and PLD-Q, have been validated to assess the burden of
symptoms along time and after treatment and may serve as new clinical endpoints
[53, 54]. As aforementioned, liver volume is a mainstay feature in the course of
PLD. Among different classifications based on hTLV, the one described by Kim
better correlates with reported symptoms and need for therapy [45]. Although, it is

Table 2.4 PLDs classifications

Gigot classification	
Type I	<10 large hepatic cysts with diameter >10 cm
Type II	Diffuse multiple cysts with remaining large areas of noncystic parenchyma
Type III	Diffuse small, medium-size multiple cysts with remaining few areas of noncystic parenchyma
Schnelldorfer's classification	
Type A	Absent to mild symptoms
Type B	Moderate to severe symptoms and ≥2 spared liver segments
Type C	Moderate to severe symptoms and ≥1 spared liver segment
Type D	Moderate to severe symptoms and portal vein occlusion
Kim classification	**Ht-TLV (mL/m)**
Mild	<1600
Moderate	1600–3200
Severe	>3200

important to highlight that different shapes could strongly impact on symptoms, even in similar hTLV.

Complications. Complications in PLD appeared to be more frequent in ADPKD than ADPLD and can be divided in intracystic, hemorrhage, infection or rupture, or liver volume related [42]. Cyst hemorrhage usually occurs in large solitary cyst (>11 cm) and manifests with acute pain in the upper abdomen or flank. Diagnosis is made by imaging, and typical findings, intracystic inhomogeneity due to fibrin wires and clots internal septa and higher attenuation value, are regularly seen by US. Color-doppler US, CT, or MRI help to differentiate benign from malignant disease in case of suspect of cystadenoma or cystoadenocarcinoma ruling out vascularization in septa or capsule. Treatment is usually conservative with antipain. In severe symptomatic patients, surgical cyst deroofing or enucleation can be considered [55]. Cyst infection is characterized by right upper quadrant pain and fever; without treatment, it can complicate with life-threatening sepsis. The gold standard for diagnosis is cyst aspirate containing inflammatory cells and bacteria. Most infections arise from bacterial translocation across intestinal barrier, where *E. coli* or *Klebsiella* spp. are the most common agents. Treatment needs a combination of antimicrobial agents and is guided by culture and aspirate results. In case of antibiotic failure, cyst drainage could be considered. FDG-PET may help in diagnosis or follow-up in selected cases [56]. Cyst rupture is very rare and is usually associated to triggers, including hemorrhage, trauma, and rapid growth. Clinical presentation is usually characterized by severe abdominal pain and can progress to hemodynamic instability. Imaging shows perihepatic free fluid and often a residual cyst in the liver. Prompt recognition is essential for treatment that consists in percutaneous ascites drainage and eventually surgical intervention [57]. Liver volume-related complications can result in several different symptoms according to the site of compression; among them, the most feared ones push liver vascularization or bile duct.

Portal vein occlusion, Budd-Chiari syndrome, inferior vena cava compression, leading to peripheral edema and ascites, portal hypertension with splenic varices, and obstructive jaundice have been noticed and need individualized treatment [58].

Treatment. Asymptomatic PLDs does not need any treatment. Unfortunately, natural history remains mainly unknown, and it is not possible to predict if a patient will become symptomatic and in which time frame. Nevertheless, PLD does not bear the risk of serious complications like liver failure, malignant insufficiency, or cyst rupture. Symptomatic PLDs patients with hepatomegaly need treatment aiming to reduce liver volume in order to improve quality of life and relief symptoms. According to cyst size, location, and disease extent in liver parenchyma, different strategies could be considered, even if generally an unmet need for treatments still remains and liver transplantation is the only curative option. Currently, somatostatin analogues (SA) are the only medical treatment able to reduce liver volume. SA inhibits the production of cAMP in cystic cholangiocytes, leading to decreased fluid secretion and proliferation. Monthly injections of long-acting SA, lanreotide or octreotide, for a period between 6 months and 3 years, showed liver volume reduction and improvement of quality of life with few side effects [1]. New therapeutic strategies aiming to interrupt pathologic liver cystogenesis and VEGF signaling are under development and are mentioned in Table 2.5 [2, 59]. Surgical management

Table 2.5 Experimental therapeutic targets in FPLD. Adapted from [2, 59]

Target	Mechanism	Agent	References
Somatostatin receptors[a]	Block of cAMP signaling through binding to somatostatin receptors	Pasireotide[a,b]	[137]
		Octreotide[a,b]	[137, 138]
		Lanreotide[b,c]	[1, 40]
Inhibition of VEGFR2[c]	Inhibition of VEGF pathway proliferative activation	SU5416	[31, 32]
BRAF[c]	Inhibition of VEGF pathway proliferative activation	Sorafenib	[28]
Inhibition of AC5[c]	Inhibition of production of cAMP	SQ22,536	[29]
p-mTOR[c]	Inhibition of mTOR pathway	Rapamycin	[139]
Intracellular Ca^{++} levels and toxic bile acids[a]	Block of cAMP signaling by increasing intracellular Ca^{++}	UDCA TRPV4 agonist	[140] [141]
Matrix metalloproteases (MMPs)[d]	Inhibition of MMP function decreasing hepatic cystogenesis	Marimastat	[142]
PPARγ[d]	Inhibition of ERK1/2 and mTOR–S6 kinase signaling pathways	Pioglitazone	[143]
		Telmisartan	[143, 144]
Macrophages[d]	Direct inhibition of monocyte–macrophage transdifferentiation	Clodronate	[34]
CXCR3[d]	Inhibition of monocyte recruitment acting on the CXCL10 receptor	AMG-487	[33]

[a]Both PLDs and FLDs
[b]Clinical trials in phase I–II are currently ongoing in PLD (octreotide in NCT00426153, pasireotide in NCT01670110)
[c]Only PLDs
[d]Only FLDs

includes aspiration sclerotherapy, fenestration, and liver resection or transplantation. In case of symptoms caused by one dominant cyst (>5 cm), aspiration sclerotherapy is the option of choice. It is a minimally invasive approach consisting in punction under radiological guidance, cyst fluid aspiration, and temporarily injection of sclerosing agent in order to destroy the inner epithelial cells lining cysts. It is safe and effective technique, no mortality has been reported, and the most frequent side effects are postprocedural pain and intracystic bleeding [60]. Cyst fenestration approach is chosen when symptoms arise from multiple larger cysts located in the anterior segments of the liver. Aspiration and surgical deroofing are carried out through laparoscopic approach with instant symptoms relief. Unfortunately, recurrence occurs in 20% of patients, and complications, including postoperative ascites, pleural effusion, and bleeding, are not uncommon. Mortality rates range around 2% [61]. Furthermore, hepatic resection is an option for symptomatic patients with multiple cysts in few liver segments with other segments less affected, but it is burdened by high morbidity and mortality [62]. In some cases, dual therapy with segmental resection and fenestration can be carried out. Finally, liver transplantation is the only curative option but reserved to a selected minority of patients. Outcome is excellent and similar to those for other indications [63]. Clinical criteria include massive hepatomegaly, severe malnutrition, low serum albumin, sarcopenia, severe recurrent complications as cyst infection or portal hypertension. MELD score is not representative of disease severity in these patients, thus exception guidelines warrant extra points to these patients after a certain time in the waiting list [64]. Combined liver-kidney transplant in patients with ADPKD and severe renal failure should be considered [65].

2.3 Congenital Hepatic Fibrosis, Caroli's Disease, and Caroli's Syndrome

Congenital hepatic fibrosis (CHF), Caroli's disease (CD), and Caroli's syndrome (CS), namely when CHF presents dilations also in the larger intrahepatic bile ducts, often coexist. CD is presented in Chap. 5. Thus, we will discuss their clinical aspects together, highlighting the differences.

CHF is a rare autosomal-recessive disease. DPM affects interlobular bile ducts leading to progressive peribiliary fibrosis, portal hypertension, and its life-threatening complications. Although epidemiological data on the prevalence of CHF and CD/CS are lacking, conditions associated with CHF seem to affect around 1:10–20,000 subjects, whereas CD/CS is even rarer, affecting around 1:1000,000 subjects. The natural history of this disease is variable, as the severity of clinical manifestations depends not only on portal hypertension, but also on the renal function impairment, given the close association CHF with ARPKD. Clinical onset is highly variable, ranging from childhood to the sixth decade, though diagnosis is mainly performed in adolescence or young adulthood. However, since clinical manifestations are nonspecific, diagnosis can be challenging and deferred until the appearance of complications. Most patients are asymptomatic, while some can complain of mild right upper abdominal quadrant pain, eventually accompanied by hepatosplenomegaly or nephromegaly if associated to polycystic renal disease [66]. At the biochemical level, liver function is usually preserved as it does in most cholangiopathies. Mild elevation of liver enzymes can be observed, but marked cholestasis occurring in cholangitic forms are rare. Moreover, renal function must be evaluated regardless of the presence of renal disease. CHF can be classified in different clinical types based on the predominance of portal hypertension, more frequent, and/or cholestasis, usually associated to CS and a late-onset phenotype.

In CD, DPM involvement extends beyond the small interlobular bile ducts to affect the larger intrahepatic bile ducts or even the segmental portions of a single lobe, usually the left one, or more rarely, the whole biliary tree as a bilobar disease (Fig. 2.2). This results in a bile-duct ectasia that can be recognized by imaging studies to support early detection. CD is sporadic and less common than CS, which is inherited as autosomal-recessive disease, and as CHF, is frequently associated with kidney polycystic disease. In CD, clinical course is usually oligosymptomatic or asymptomatic for all lifelong. As CHF, onset occurs in childhood or teen, but it can be diagnosed many years later as well, in the fifth decade. Symptoms are mostly related to complications, such as acute bacterial cholangitis or intrahepatic biliary stones, keeping the attention on the fact that recurrent cholangitic episode can evolve to secondary biliary cirrhosis [37, 67]. In younger ages, before 40, symptoms

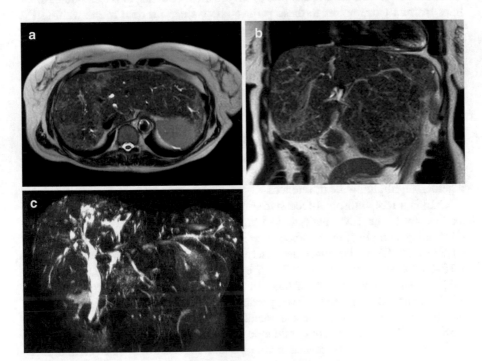

Fig. 2.2 (a–c) Caroli's disease. F, 70 years. Axial, coronal T2-weighted MRI (**a**, **b**), and MRCP (**c**) showing cirrhotic liver with multifocal dilatations of segmental intrahepatic bile ducts

are more likely related to portal hypertension due to concomitant CHF in the context of CS.

Associated diseases and syndromes. FLD often occurs with a spectrum of both inherited and noninherited disorders, mainly associated to renal disease, collectively grouped as hepatorenal fibrocystic diseases (HRFCD). HRFCD shows some peculiar features but with a variable overlap in causative genes and clinical features. Extrahepatic manifestations include cystic dysplastic kidney degeneration, pancreatic cysts, polydactyly, mid and hindbrain abnormalities, retinal degeneration, and iris or retinal colobomas. Among them, ARPKD is the most frequently associated disease as well as the most common ciliopathy in childhood with a prevalence of 1:20,000 live births [68–70]. Genetic defect is mainly related to mutations in *PDKHD1* gene. ARPKD is characterized by nonobstructive fusiform dilations of the renal-collecting ducts with progressive renal insufficiency. In about 40% of patients, liver and renal disease coexists, but it is still unclear if severity of both diseases correlates [71]. Prognosis is poor with about 30% of affected infants dying during the neonatal period for pulmonary complications. Nevertheless, in the last decade, thanks to the constant improvements in neonatal respiratory support and in renal replacement therapy, the 10-year survival has risen up to 80% of patients with a time shift of CHF/CS-related complication occurrence in adolescence and adulthood [72].

Diagnosis. Color-doppler ultrasound (US) is the first step of the radiological diagnostic workup of both primary liver and kidney disease and their related complications. Typical US findings in FLDs are outlined in Table 2.6. Second-line imaging studies as contrast-enhanced CT scan and MRI coupled with MR cholangiopancreatography (MRCP) allow a better visualization of the vasculature and biliary tree, as shown in Fig. 2.2, as well as provide a better staging of fibrosis. At imaging, a pathognomonic sign of CD is the "central dot sign," consisting of a small enhancing focus containing a dilated intrahepatic duct with a cystic configuration observed at contrast-enhanced CT and MR. At the histological level, it is related to dense fibrovascular bundles embedding the portal vein and hepatic artery branches, localized around abnormally dilated intrahepatic bile ducts [73]. Moreover, the initial approach must also include a brain CT scan or MRI to rule out cerebral malformations that could be associated to HRFCD (e.g., Joubert or COACH syndromes) [74, 75]. Recent observations derived from some case reports suggest that radiology can be helpful also in the antenatal diagnosis of CD by means of 3D ultrasound and MRI that show the congenital saccular dilations of fetal liver [76]. During follow-up, ultrasound with acoustic radiation force impulse elastography

Table 2.6 Typical US findings in FPLDs

Increased or heterogeneous liver echogenicity with hyperechoic portal triad and periportal thickening
Hypertrophy of left lateral and caudate segment (and atrophic right lobe in cases with advanced fibrosis)
Splenomegaly (if portal hypertension)
Dilated intrahepatic bile ducts (eventually hosting stones in CD)

may provide a noninvasive tool to stage fibrosis and portal hypertension in children [77].

Although radiological findings have diagnostic value in most patients, liver biopsy can be of help in uncertain cases. Histology may have a role, especially in adults with portal hypertension and chronic liver disease of unknown origin since childhood [78]. Typical histological findings are thick portal/peribiliary fibrosis embedding dysgenetic bile ducts eventually evolving to cystic dilations when CD coexists. In CHF, peribiliary fibrosis progresses to porto-portal rather than porto-central bridging as seen in cirrhosis of more common etiologies. Another histological lesion strongly suggesting DPM is the persistence of $CD56^+$ ductal plate remnants, together with an increase in hepatic artery branches and hypoplasia or abnormal branching of the portal vein, leading to a picture originally described as "pollard willow" pattern. Of note, these distinctive features are well phenocopied by experimental models, as shown in the *PKHD1*-defective mouse.

Complications. The main determinants of clinical progression of CHF and CD/CS are portal hypertension with the related manifestations, recurrent acute cholangitis, and intrahepatic cholangiocarcinoma (iCCA). Of note, all of them can lead to liver transplant since childhood. Moreover, it is crucial to monitor renal function and the progression of renal disease, which affect liver prognosis and response to treatments.

Portal hypertension is the most frequent complication, and it usually occurs as variceal bleeding, often the first manifestation of CHF at any age, or as splenomegaly with thrombocytopenia. Ascites is uncommon in these patients, whereas portal vein thrombosis can be reported. The management of portal hypertension does not differ from that of other etiologies according to the standard guidelines [79].

Acute cholangitis is more typical of CD, but it is a life-threatening complication, also in CHF, for the high risk of sepsis. It is generally caused by bacterial infections sustained by Gram$^-$ Enterobacteria (*E. coli, K. Pneumoniae, Enterobacter* spp.) [80] and must be suspected in case of fever that could be the only sign of disease in these patients.

iCCA is the most feared complication not only for CD/CS, but also for CHF, whose pathogenesis is related to progressive fibrosis developing in close vicinity of dysgenetic biliary structures as observed in other inflammatory cholangiopathies, particularly in primary sclerosing cholangitis (PSC) [81]. In CD/CS, it is often incidentally diagnosed at the time of liver surgery. Incidence ranges from 2.5 to 16% with a median age at diagnosis of 58.8 years [82]. Despite remarkable improvements in the radiological approach, no surveillance guidelines for CCA have been generated so far in these patients.

Treatment. Clinical management in FLDs is challenging, and well-established guidelines are lacking. Thus, a multidisciplinary approach involving hepatologist, nephrologist, radiologist, endoscopist, and surgeon is even more eagerly needed. Liver and renal diseases, when coexisting, progress at different rates and may variably affect the outcome of ongoing treatments. No effective strategies to reverse, stop or dampen disease progression are available in CHF/CS/CD, which can be thus considered as "orphan" diseases. New therapeutic strategies, summarized in

Table 2.5, still are under development at initial step. Therefore, current therapy aims at treating complications, in particular, those related to portal hypertension.

Endoscopic treatment, particularly bind ligation, is the current standard of care in esophagus varices, whereas unselective β-blockers are hitherto not recommended due to the lack of specific studies in the CHF/CS pediatric population [83]. In recurrent variceal bleeding, a portal decompressive shunt can be considered in highly specialized hepatological surgical centers, though unusually performed in children. Small series showed it was effective when performed in patients with preserved hepatic synthesis [84]. On the contrary, shunts in ARPKD/CHF should be considered with caution in patients with end-stage kidney disease for the reported higher risk of terminal encephalopathy and the increased surgical complexity when prospecting future kidney transplantation [71, 84]. In the long-term, transjugular intrahepatic portosystemic shunt (TIPS) can be a reasonable alternative to surgical shunt, given its feasibility in children. Results from small series are encouraging, as they show regression of portal hypertension (ascites, esophageal varices) and reduction in spleen size, with an increase in the platelet count. Of note, TIPS might delay the time of transplantation, notwithstanding the close monitoring of complications [85].

Intrahepatic lithiasis is a common complication of CS/CD, often associated with bacterial infections responsible for recurrent cholangitis, liver abscess, and sepsis. In case of high suspicion, antibiotic treatment should be started without hesitation because of the risk of quick deterioration, which is further increased in patients with ARPKD or under immunosuppressive therapy following renal transplantation. In transplanted patients, a 6–12-week antibiotic prophylaxis is recommended immediately after transplant, and anytime in case of enhanced immunosuppression [86]. Ursodeoxycholic acid showed only limited efficacy in reducing the risk of cholangitis or in treating hepatolithiasis [87].

As aforementioned, these patients present a 100-fold increased risk of iCCA than the general population with prevalence in CD/CS as high as 7% [88, 89]. Unfortunately, no surveillance programs have been developed yet, thus, the early detection of iCCA is difficult [90]. In general, in iCCA, surgical resection still represents the unique curative possibility, though only less than one-third of patients are eligible at diagnosis and 5-year survival is poor, ranging from 22 to 44% [89]. Furthermore, liver transplantation is associated with rapid tumor recurrence and low survival (10–25%), and it is not considered in the treatment algorithm of iCCA [91]. Whether genetic alterations amenable of personalized targeted interventions might identify distinctive subgroups of iCCA arising in CHF/CD/CS is yet an unexplored topic.

Liver resection of hepatic segments affected by sac-like intrahepatic bile duct dilation showed excellent long-term results in selected patients with symptomatic monolobar disease without underlying chronic liver disease [92]. The largest surgical series—111 patients, 90% of them with left lobe involvement—reported no perisurgical mortality and good control of complications by 25 months of median follow-up. To maximize the beneficial effects of resection, a thorough preliminary evaluation of the real extension of liver disease is mandatory, since incomplete resection is associated with poor outcome [93]. Surgical treatment should be planned as early as possible due to the dual risk of CCA and infections (as mutually interacting factors) that increase over time [94]. In the last few years, endoscopic, radiological, and laparoscopic approaches have been improved to perform abscess drainage and stone clearance in easier and less invasive ways.

Liver transplantation (LT) remains the only curative option in CHF/CS, with strict indications limited to patients with bilobar involvement, complicated by recurrent cholangitis or portal hypertension [94–96]. In the largest published series, collected from the European Transplant Liver Registry and the United Network of Organ Sharing data, similar survival rates were reported, being 89%, 86%, 76% and 88.5%, 81%, and 78% at 1, 5, and 10 years, respectively. Poor outcome was related to older age and to superinfections at the time of transplant [97]. These studies reported a 10% of perioperative mortality, mainly caused by severe infections further facilitated by the immunosuppressive therapy. Therefore, it is recommended to avoid preoperative invasive biliary procedures that can enhance the risk of infections, and to undergo prolonged antibiotic prophylaxis before and after LT.

Another transplant issue is the indication to the double liver-kidney transplantation, including its timing. In fact, it must be underlined that patients with HRFCD usually present a more severe involvement in one organ, and both diseases progress at independent rate without any genotype-phenotype association [66]. Indeed, only a small subset of these patients seems to require double transplantation, either sequentially or in combination. In a large series of 716 HRFCD patients receiving a liver (LT) and/or kidney transplant (KT) between 1990 and 2010, most received KT (86%), while only small numbers LT (10%) or both (6%), in accordance with the concept that the functional impairment more frequently affects the kidney. Moreover, only few patients needed a second transplant of the other organ (7% of LT and 5% of KT recipients). However, mortality rate was higher after LT (23%) than KT (10%) or double transplant (12%) [98]. In the posttransplant setting, it is of utmost importance to preserve the function of the nontransplanted organ still left in place. Therefore, after LT, calcineurin inhibitors must be kept at the lowest effective dose to protect the kidney [99]. On the other side, after KT, chronic immunosuppression may favor the development of cholangitis, thus supporting indication to combined KT+LT in patients with end-stage renal failure with history of cholangitis or with marked abnormalities of the biliary tree. Furthermore, simultaneous transplant provides the kidney with an immunological advantage that improves outcome and graft survival in both adults and children [100, 101]. There are a number of key questions needing consideration by future studies. Since we are dealing with a rare and clinically heterogeneous disease, we must bear in mind that data on LT-generated so far have been obtained in patients transplanted for complications related to portal hypertension or recurrent cholangitis rather than for end-stage liver disease due to the low MELD/PELD typically scored by these patients. Thus, criteria supporting indications to LT/LT+KT lack standardized protocols, making these studies difficult to be analyzed. Moreover, there is no consensus yet if asymptomatic patients with diffuse bilobar disease can be considered a good indication for prophylactic LT. Similarly, a candidacy with prophylactic intent must be also considered in view of the risk of CCA development, as hotly debated for PSC [102], since LT indication becomes much weaker when iCCA develops [94].

2.4 Choledochal or Bile Duct Cysts

Choledochal cysts (CC) are congenital alterations resulting from DPM involving the largest intra or extrahepatic bile ducts. The most quoted classification is the Todani's system, outlined in Table 2.7 that describes site, extent, and shape of biliary tree [103, 104]. Different revisions of this classification have been proposed, suggesting to separate cystic and fusiform variants (type I CCs) and to remove CD (type V) [105].

It is a rare disease with prevalence 1:13–20,000 live birth, higher in Asia, especially in Japan (1:1000 live birth, 33–50% of cases) [106, 107]. There is a slight female predominance $F{:}M{=}3{:}1$ [108] and the prevalence is increasing in the last decades due to improving and spreading of noninvasive imaging [104]. Diagnosis usually occurs during childhood, in a quarter of cases within 1st year and only in 20% in adulthood. Clinical features, such as presentation and malignancy risk, could present differences between Eastern (Asiatic) and Western populations. Particularly, Eastern population is more often symptomatic at diagnosis and seems to present higher malignancy rate [109]. Moreover, management is still driven by Asiatic literature, where prevalence is higher. Thus, multiinstitutional studies in the Western countries with decades of follow-up are needed to better understand the natural history of CC disease, and in particular, the risk of biliary tract cancer [109].

The main pathogenetic hypothesis is based on a defective biliopancreatic junction—present in 96–100% of children affected—where pancreatic and bile ducts join upstream to the Oddi sphincter. Thus, pancreatic enzymes can reflux into biliary tree, leading to increases in intraductal pressure, inflammation, and ultimately to secondary ductal dilation [110]. A different theory focuses on functional or anatomic obstruction of the distal part of extrahepatic biliary tree due to inadequate autonomic innervation that results in dysmotility, worsening duct lumen dilation as

Table 2.7 Todani's classification of CCs

	Site of dilation
Type I[a]	Common bile duct (subtypes: cystic, segmental and fusiform)
Type II[b]	Supraduodenal area
Type III (choledochocele)	Within duodenal wall
Type IVa	Multiple dilations of intrahepatic and extrahepatic bile ducts
Type IVb	Multiple and segmental dilations of extrahepatic bile ducts
Type V[b] (Caroli's disease)	Largest intrahepatic biliary tree

[a]The most frequent (70–90%)
[b]Rare (<2%)

in achalasia or Hirschprung's diseases [111]. As previously discussed, DPM in CD is limited to the largest intrahepatic bile ducts.

CCs course asymptomatic for years, thus diagnosis arrives incidentally after imaging performed for a different purpose. Nevertheless, around 80% of patients show suspicious symptoms, usually belonging to the classic triad of jaundice, right upper quadrant abdominal pain, and palpable abdominal mass, before 10 years old. Adults usually present abdominal pain, pancreatitis, or history of cholecystectomy for biliary stones [112].

Diagnosis. Gold standard is MRI coupled with MRCP. This imaging ensures assessment of cyst anatomy, extension, and definition of the intrahepatic involvement. Moreover, it is very accurate in detecting anomalies at biliopancreatic junction without risk of complications of invasive imaging. ERCP and transhepatic cholangiography remain as second-level test in case of failure of noninvasive imaging or for those alterations that could need a concomitant endoscopic treatment (i.e., hepatolithiasis, ductal stricture, carcinoma) [113, 114]. Recently, endoscopic ultrasonography (EUS) showed a promising potential in differentiating choledochal from pancreatic cysts, especially in patients with type II choledochal cysts. When radiological imaging is equivocal, EUS is able to better define anatomical borders of adjacent structures with also the possibility of EUS-guided fluid aspiration [115].

Complications. Symptoms are often due to complications. Besides infections, CCs could complicate with obstructive frame, ab extrinsico compression, rupture or malignant evolution.

Acute cholangitis and pancreatitis are triggered by bile stasis and secondary-stone formation, followed by chronic inflammation, ductal strictures, and cyst dilation [106]. Additionally, chronic inflammation and bile lithiasis in the distal portion of common bile duct and pancreatic duct lead to obstructive protein-plug formation [116]. Recurrent cholangitis and chronic biliary obstruction evolve to secondary biliary cirrhosis in 40–50% of patients, especially when intrahepatic involvement is present [117]. Mechanical compression exerted by CCs on portal vein can bring to portal hypertension even without cirrhosis; moreover, gastric outlet can be affected and compression of type III lesions might favor wall intussusception [118]. Another acute dreadful complication is cyst rupture with acute abdomen due to biliary peritonitis. It occurs spontaneously, mostly in young infants, thus, it may be the first manifestation of the disease in 1–12% of patients. Ductal fragility, secondary to chronic inflammation, enables rupture that is precipitated by conditions that increase ductal pressure (i.e., pregnancy, ascites). Most often, rupture happens at level of confluence between common bile and cystic duct [119]. A case series identified GGT levels—higher than 615 U/L—as independently predictive of forthcoming perforation [120]. Diagnosis is intraoperative with the detection of bile-stained ascites. Ultrasound often shows a misleading normal biliary tree for cyst decompression secondary to rupture.

Chronic inflammation leads to higher risk of hepatobiliopancreatic tumoral transformation. CCA is the most frequent, with a 20–30-fold higher risk than normal population [121]. Nevertheless, hepatocarcinoma and pancreatic malignancy have been also reported. According to a metaanalysis accounting articles from both

Western and Eastern center, world incidence of CCA in these patients is around 11% [122]. Instead, in a large Japanese multicentric series incidence of CCA was 17.5% compared to 0.01–0.39% reported in autoptic series in normal population [108]. The risk is age-related, but it starts since childhood, reaching 14.3% after 20 years old [123]. Thus, diagnosis is often two decades earlier with a median age of 32 years old. Tumorigenesis may spread beyond the cystic area, so CCA may arise in either normal tissue, highlighting the role of extracellular milieu [103, 122, and 124]. Although all CCs may develop CCA, Type I and IVA cyst showed a stronger association. Cyst drainage procedure is also a risk factor for malignancy; indeed, a report pinpointed that around 18.6% patients developed CCA after such intervention with a latency of 10 years [125]. Thus, elective cyst excision in asymptomatic patients is to take into account in previously treated with cyst enterostomy [113]. The short postoperative follow-up in the available literature makes difficult to extrapolate life-time risk of malignancy. Also for this reason, it has been inconclusive the attempt to identify a group of risk factors. Hence, surveillance continues to be nonselective and annual controls of CA19–9, abdominal ultrasound, and eventual invasive investigations should be planned in all treated children and adolescents [105].

Treatment. Definitive treatment in CCs is cyst surgical excision. This procedure showed better outcome and less morbidity than classical drainage procedures, choledochus-cysto-duodenostomy, or choledochus-cysto-jejunostomy. Besides, a complete resection avoids also the risk of malignant degeneration, a central point in a considerable pediatric population with a long-life expectancy.

Symptoms are a strong indication for surgery at any age. In asymptomatic patients, it is recommended to perform a surgery with reconstruction from the age of 6 months, though there is some evidence suggesting anticipating as early as the first month of life [126]. Laparoscopic cyst excision with reconstruction has been performed in children as young as 3 months and as small as 6 kg [127]. Intervention is elective and patient should be medically optimized priorly. Specific approach depends on cyst type, but common target is to remove the entire cyst and to restore the enteric biliary drainage either into duodenum or via Roux-en-Y hepaticojejunostomy (RYHJ) [128]. RYHJ seems to be affected by bile reflux in a fewer number of cases than hepaticoduodenostomy. Surgery can be either open or laparoscopic, depending on patient features and center experience. Laparoscopy presents longer intraoperative time, but shorter hospital admission and outcome are comparable [129]. Evidences are increasing on robot-assisted resection with RYHJ. This appeared to be a safe and feasible option with short-term results that are comparable to laparoscopic surgery. Advantages include better intracorporeal suturing and provision of a good 3D visual field [130].

In type I and IVb cysts, management is resection of extrahepatic biliary tree with cholecystectomy and hepaticoenterostomy [131]. Type II cysts require diverticulectomy or simple cyst excision. In type III cysts, the choice is endoscopic sphincterotomy without excision of the cyst. Whether or not possible, lateral duodenotomy with sphincteroplasty and marsupialization of the cavity may be performed. Various papers report good symptom control through endoscopic management, even if long-term follow-up is still lacking [132]. Type IVa cysts need a more complex treatment due to intrahepatic and extrahepatic involvement. Preoperative extension of disease has to be precisely assessed differentiating real intrahepatic cysts from secondary upstream ductal dilation. In adults, percutaneous biliary drainage is suggested to decompress intrahepatic biliary ductal tree before surgery. Intrahepatic disease needs hepatectomy to prevent carcinogenesis. If staging imaging is not conclusive, a strict follow-up of intrahepatic ducts is recommended. Indeed, in some cases, intrahepatic dilation resolved 3–6 months after adequate drainage [104, 125, and 131].

Early postsurgical complications include anastomotic leak, bleeding, wound infection, acute pancreatitis, and pancreatic or biliary fistula [133]. Subsequently, benign anastomotic strictures can occur in 10–25% of patients, with restarting of biliary stasis, chronic inflammation, and related complications [101, 102, 134, 135]. Finally, screening for biliary carcinoma, especially CCA, is a cornerstone of long-term follow-up because even after CC excision, the risk remains more elevated than general population with a rate up to 14%, and it is the most frequent case of late mortality in pediatric series [112, 125, 136].

2.5   Conclusions

The rising interest recently drawn to FPLDs has pointed out the considerable translational significance of genetic cholangiopathies, further supported by the large availability of animal and cellular models that phenocopy the disease [2]. By deciphering the multiple dysfunctions derived from single ciliary protein defects in cholangiocytes, new insights into the pathophysiology may pave the way to innovative therapies, a concept that is even more important in these rare diseases, given their "orphan" condition. Furthermore, basic pathologic mechanisms uncovered in genetic cholangiopathies might be applicable to understanding of acquired cholangiopathies and, more broadly, of chronic liver diseases. Although future directions addressed by the most recent translational observations are promising, there are a number of clinical issues deserving consideration by the next studies. LT represents a valuable therapeutic option, especially in view of the search for "alternative indications to LT" in the near future, but the limited data collected so far indicate that these patients have low priority due to indications generally related to recurrent complications rather than to end-stage cirrhosis, thus with lower MELD/PELD scores than the other candidates do have. These patients might benefit from living-donor LT with consequently shorter waiting times and a lower risk of life-threatening complications [94, 95, 104]. New studies on surgical series are claimed to standardize LT protocols and to better investigate feasibility and ethical issues about living-donor procedures. Finally, the increased risk of developing CCA is currently one of the major gaps in knowledge, especially in children, where cancer is the most frequent cause of late mortality [109]. Unfortunately, no standard protocols of surveillance have been produced, and therefore, research studies are strongly recommended to clarify the real CCA incidence, long-term follow-up, and additional risk factors with related predictive biomarkers.

References

1. van Aerts RMM, van de Laarschot LFM, Banales JM, Drenth JPH. Clinical management of polycystic liver disease. J Hepatol. 2018;68(4):827–37.
2. Fabris L, Fiorotto R, Spirli C, Cadamuro M, Mariotti V, Perugorria MJ, et al. Pathobiology of inherited biliary diseases: a roadmap to understand acquired liver diseases. Nat Rev Gastroenterol Hepatol. 2019;16(8):497–511.
3. Gunay-Aygun M. Liver and kidney disease in ciliopathies. Am J Med Genet C Semin Med Genet. 2009;151C(4):296–306.
4. Gascue C, Katsanis N, Badano JL. Cystic diseases of the kidney: ciliary dysfunction and cystogenic mechanisms. Pediatr Nephrol. 2011;26(8):1181–95.
5. Avidor-Reiss T, Maer AM, Koundakjian E, Polyanovsky A, Keil T, Subramaniam S, et al. Decoding cilia function: defining specialized genes required for compartmentalized cilia biogenesis. Cell. 2004;117(4):527–39.
6. Fliegauf M, Benzing T, Omran H. When cilia go bad: cilia defects and ciliopathies. Nat Rev Mol Cell Biol. 2007;8(11):880–93.
7. Mahjoub MR. The importance of a single primary cilium. Organogenesis. 2013;9(2):61–9.
8. Rock N, McLin V. Liver involvement in children with ciliopathies. Clin Res Hepatol Gastroenterol. 2014;38(4):407–14.
9. Strazzabosco M, Fabris L. Development of the bile ducts: essentials for the clinical hepatologist. J Hepatol. 2012;56(5):1159–70.
10. Roskams T, Desmet V. Embryology of extra and intrahepatic bile ducts, the ductal plate. Anat Rec (Hoboken). 2008;291(6):628–35.
11. Santiago I, Loureiro R, Curvo-Semedo L, Marques C, Tardáguila F, Matos C, et al. Congenital cystic lesions of the biliary tree. AJR Am J Roentgenol. 2012;198(4):825–35.
12. The European Polycystic Kidney Disease Consortium. The polycystic kidney disease 1 gene encodes a 14 kb transcript and lies within a duplicated region on chromosome 16. Cell. 1994;78(4):725.
13. Mochizuki T, Wu G, Hayashi T, Xenophontos SL, Veldhuisen B, Saris JJ, et al. PKD2, a gene for polycystic kidney disease that encodes an integral membrane protein. Science. 1996;272(5266):1339–42.
14. Strazzabosco M, Somlo S. Polycystic liver diseases: congenital disorders of cholangiocyte signaling. Gastroenterology. 2011;140(7):1855–1859.e1.
15. Masyuk AI, Masyuk TV, Splinter PL, Huang BQ, Stroope AJ, LaRusso NF. Cholangiocyte cilia detect changes in luminal fluid flow and transmit them into intracellular Ca2+ and cAMP signaling. Gastroenterology. 2006;131(3):911–20.
16. Drenth JPH, te Morsche RHM, Smink R, Bonifacino JS, Jansen JBMJ. Germline mutations in PRKCSH are associated with autosomal-dominant polycystic liver disease. Nat Genet. 2003;33(3):345–7.
17. Davila S, Furu L, Gharavi AG, Tian X, Onoe T, Qian Q, et al. Mutations in SEC63 cause autosomal-dominant polycystic liver disease. Nat Genet. 2004;36(6):575–7.
18. Besse W, Dong K, Choi J, Punia S, Fedeles SV, Choi M, et al. Isolated polycystic liver disease genes define effectors of polycystin-1 function. J Clin Invest. 2017;127(5):1772–85.
19. Porath B, Gainullin VG, Cornec-Le Gall E, Dillinger EK, Heyer CM, Hopp K, et al. Mutations in *GANAB*, encoding the glucosidase IIα subunit, cause autosomal-dominant polycystic kidney and liver disease. Am J Hum Genet. 2016;98(6):1193–207.
20. Cnossen WR, te Morsche RHM, Hoischen A, Gilissen C, Chrispijn M, Venselaar H, et al. Whole-exome sequencing reveals LRP5 mutations and canonical Wnt signaling associated with hepatic cystogenesis. Proc Natl Acad Sci U S A. 2014;111(14):5343–8.
21. Fedeles SV, Tian X, Gallagher A-R, Mitobe M, Nishio S, Lee SH, et al. A genetic interaction network of five genes for human polycystic kidney and liver diseases defines polycystin-1 as the central determinant of cyst formation. Nat Genet. 2011;43(7):639–47.

22. Janssen MJ, Waanders E, Te Morsche RHM, Xing R, Dijkman HBPM, Woudenberg J, et al. Secondary, somatic mutations might promote cyst formation in patients with autosomal-dominant polycystic liver disease. Gastroenterology. 2011;141(6):2056–2063.e2.

23. Chebib FT, Jung Y, Heyer CM, Irazabal MV, Hogan MC, Harris PC, et al. Effect of genotype on the severity and volume progression of polycystic liver disease in autosomal-dominant polycystic kidney disease. Nephrol Dial Transplant. 2016;31(6):952–60.

24. Van Keimpema L, De Koning DB, Van Hoek B, Van Den Berg AP, Van Oijen MGH, De Man RA, et al. Patients with isolated polycystic liver disease referred to liver centres: clinical characterization of 137 cases. Liver Int. 2011;31(1):92–8.

25. Banales JM, Masyuk TV, Gradilone SA, Masyuk AI, Medina JF, LaRusso NF. The cAMP effectors Epac and protein kinase a (PKA) are involved in the hepatic cystogenesis of an animal model of autosomal-recessive polycystic kidney disease (ARPKD). Hepatology. 2009;49(1):160–74.

26. Masyuk AI, Masyuk TV, Pisarello MJL, Ding JF, Loarca L, Huang BQ, et al. Cholangiocyte autophagy contributes to hepatic cystogenesis in polycystic liver disease and represents a potential therapeutic target. Hepatology. 2018;67(3):1088–108.

27. Beaudry J-B, Cordi S, Demarez C, Lepreux S, Pierreux CE, Lemaigre FP. Proliferation-independent initiation of biliary cysts in polycystic liver diseases. PLoS One. 2015;10(6):e0132295.

28. Spirli C, Morell CM, Locatelli L, Okolicsanyi S, Ferrero C, Kim AK, et al. Cyclic AMP/PKA-dependent paradoxical activation of Raf/MEK/ERK signaling in polycystin-2 defective mice treated with sorafenib. Hepatology. 2012;56(6):2363–74.

29. Spirli C, Mariotti V, Villani A, Fabris L, Fiorotto R, Strazzabosco M. Adenylyl cyclase 5 links changes in calcium homeostasis to cAMP-dependent cyst growth in polycystic liver disease. J Hepatol. 2017;66(3):571–80.

30. Fabris L, Cadamuro M, Fiorotto R, Roskams T, Spirlì C, Melero S, et al. Effects of angiogenic factor overexpression by human and rodent cholangiocytes in polycystic liver diseases. Hepatology. 2006;43(5):1001–12.

31. Amura CR, Brodsky KS, Groff R, Gattone VH, Voelkel NF, Doctor RB. VEGF receptor inhibition blocks liver cyst growth in pkd2(WS25/-) mice. Am J Physiol Cell Physiol. 2007;293(1):C419–28.

32. Spirli C, Okolicsanyi S, Fiorotto R, Fabris L, Cadamuro M, Lecchi S, et al. ERK1/2-dependent vascular endothelial growth factor signaling sustains cyst growth in polycystin-2 defective mice. Gastroenterology. 2010;138(1):360–371.e7.

33. Kaffe E, Fiorotto R, Pellegrino F, Mariotti V, Amenduni M, Cadamuro M, et al. β-Catenin and interleukin-1β–dependent chemokine (C-X-C motif) ligand 10 production drives progression of disease in a mouse model of congenital hepatic fibrosis. Hepatology. 2018;67(5):1903–19.

34. Locatelli L, Cadamuro M, Spirlì C, Fiorotto R, Lecchi S, Morell CM, et al. Macrophage recruitment by fibrocystin-defective biliary epithelial cells promotes portal fibrosis in congenital hepatic fibrosis. Hepatology. 2016;63(3):965–82.

35. Paka P, Huang B, Duan B, Li J-S, Zhou P, Paka L, et al. A small molecule fibrokinase inhibitor in a model of fibropolycystic hepatorenal disease. World J Nephrol. 2018;7(5):96–107.

36. Rossetti S, Harris PC. Genotype-phenotype correlations in autosomal-dominant and autosomal-recessive polycystic kidney disease. J Am Soc Nephrol. 2007;18(5):1374–80.

37. Hartung EA, Guay-Woodford LM. Autosomal-recessive polycystic kidney disease: a hepatorenal fibrocystic disorder with pleiotropic effects. Pediatrics. 2014;134(3):e833–45.

38. humgen.rwth-aachen.de—Database [Internet]. [cited 2020 Mar 31]. http://www.humgen.rwth-aachen.de/index.php?page=database.

39. Cano DA, Murcia NS, Pazour GJ, Hebrok M. Orpk mouse model of polycystic kidney disease reveals essential role of primary cilia in pancreatic tissue organization. Development. 2004;131(14):3457–67.

40. Gevers TJG, Drenth JPH. Diagnosis and management of polycystic liver disease. Nat Rev Gastroenterol Hepatol. 2013;10(2):101–8.

41. Cnossen WR, Drenth JP. Polycystic liver disease: an overview of pathogenesis, clinical manifestations and management. Orphanet J Rare Dis. 2014;9(1):69.
42. Hoevenaren IA, Wester R, Schrier RW, McFann K, Doctor RB, Drenth JPH, et al. Polycystic liver: clinical characteristics of patients with isolated polycystic liver disease compared with patients with polycystic liver and autosomal-dominant polycystic kidney disease. Liver Int. 2008;28(2):264–70.
43. Perugorria MJ, Banales JM. Genetics: novel causative genes for polycystic liver disease. Nat Rev Gastroenterol Hepatol. 2017;14(7):391–2.
44. van Aerts RMM, Kievit W, de Jong ME, Ahn C, Bañales JM, Reiterová J, et al. Severity in polycystic liver disease is associated with aetiology and female gender: results of the International PLD Registry. Liver Int. 2019;39(3):575–82.
45. Kim H, Park HC, Ryu H, Kim K, Kim HS, Oh K-H, et al. Clinical correlates of mass effect in autosomal-dominant polycystic kidney disease. PLoS One. 2015;10(12):e0144526.
46. Barbier L, Ronot M, Aussilhou B, Cauchy F, Francoz C, Vilgrain V, et al. Polycystic liver disease: hepatic venous outflow obstruction lesions of the noncystic parenchyma have major consequences. Hepatology. 2018;68(2):652–62.
47. Timio M, Monarca C, Pede S, Gentili S, Verdura C, Lolli S. The spectrum of cardiovascular abnormalities in autosomal-dominant polycystic kidney disease: a 10-year follow-up in a five-generation kindred. Clin Nephrol. 1992;37(5):245–51.
48. Luciano RL, Dahl NK. Extra-renal manifestations of autosomal-dominant polycystic kidney disease (ADPKD): considerations for routine screening and management. Nephrol Dial Transplant. 2014;29(2):247–54.
49. Harris T, Sandford R, EAF members, Roundtable participants. European ADPKD Forum multidisciplinary position statement on autosomal-dominant polycystic kidney disease care: European ADPKD Forum and Multispecialist Roundtable participants. Nephrol Dial Transplant. 2018;33(4):563–73.
50. Bae KT, Zhu F, Chapman AB, Torres VE, Grantham JJ, Guay-Woodford LM, et al. Magnetic resonance imaging evaluation of hepatic cysts in early autosomal-dominant polycystic kidney disease: the consortium for radiologic imaging studies of polycystic kidney disease cohort. Clin J Am Soc Nephrol. 2006;1(1):64–9.
51. Gigot JF, Jadoul P, Que F, Van Beers BE, Etienne J, Horsmans Y, et al. Adult polycystic liver disease: is fenestration the most adequate operation for long-term management? Ann Surg. 1997;225(3):286–94.
52. Schnelldorfer T, Torres VE, Zakaria S, Rosen CB, Nagorney DM. Polycystic liver disease: a critical appraisal of hepatic resection, cyst fenestration, and liver transplantation. Ann Surg. 2009;250(1):112–8.
53. Temmerman F, Dobbels F, Ho TA, Pirson Y, Vanslembrouck R, Coudyzer W, et al. Development and validation of a polycystic liver disease complaint-specific assessment (POLCA). J Hepatol. 2014;61(5):1143–50.
54. Neijenhuis MK, Gevers TJG, Hogan MC, Kamath PS, Wijnands TFM, van den Ouweland RCPM, et al. Development and validation of a disease-specific questionnaire to assess patient-reported symptoms in polycystic liver disease. Hepatology. 2016;64(1):151–60.
55. Fong ZV, Wolf AM, Doria C, Berger AC, Rosato EL, Palazzo F. Hemorrhagic hepatic cyst: report of a case and review of the literature with emphasis on clinical approach and management. J Gastrointest Surg. 2012;16(9):1782–9.
56. Lantinga MA, Drenth JPH, Gevers TJG. Diagnostic criteria in renal and hepatic cyst infection. Nephrol Dial Transplant. 2015;30(5):744–51.
57. Marion Y, Brevartt C, Plard L, Chiche L. Hemorrhagic liver cyst rupture: an unusual life-threatening complication of hepatic cyst and literature review. Ann Hepatol. 2013;12(2):336–9.
58. Macutkiewicz C, Plastow R, Chrispijn M, Filobbos R, Ammori BA, Sherlock DJ, et al. Complications arising in simple and polycystic liver cysts. World J Hepatol. 2012;4(12):406–11.
59. Masyuk TV, Masyuk AI, LaRusso NF. Therapeutic targets in polycystic liver disease. CDT. 2017;18(8):950–7.

60. Wijnands TFM, Görtjes APM, Gevers TJG, Jenniskens SFM, Kool LJS, Potthoff A, et al. Efficacy and safety of aspiration sclerotherapy of simple hepatic cysts: a systematic review. AJR Am J Roentgenol. 2017;208(1):201–7.

61. Drenth JPH, Chrispijn M, Nagorney DM, Kamath PS, Torres VE. Medical and surgical treatment options for polycystic liver disease. Hepatology. 2010;52(6):2223–30.

62. Chebib FT, Harmon A, Irazabal Mira MV, Jung YS, Edwards ME, Hogan MC, et al. Outcomes and durability of hepatic reduction after combined partial hepatectomy and cyst fenestration for massive polycystic liver disease. J Am Coll Surg. 2016;223(1):118–126.e1.

63. van Keimpema L, Nevens F, Adam R, Porte RJ, Fikatas P, Becker T, et al. Excellent survival after liver transplantation for isolated polycystic liver disease: an European Liver Transplant Registry study. Transpl Int. 2011;24(12):1239–45.

64. Freeman RB, Gish RG, Harper A, Davis GL, Vierling J, Lieblein L, et al. Model for end-stage liver disease (MELD) exception guidelines: results and recommendations from the MELD Exception Study Group and Conference (MESSAGE) for the approval of patients who need liver transplantation with diseases not considered by the standard MELD formula. Liver Transpl. 2006;12(12 Suppl 3):S128–36.

65. Coquillard C, Berger J, Daily M, Shah M, Mei X, Marti F, et al. Combined liver-kidney transplantation for polycystic liver and kidney disease: analysis from the United Network for Organ Sharing dataset. Liver Int. 2016;36(7):1018–25.

66. Adeva M, El-Youssef M, Rossetti S, Kamath PS, Kubly V, Consugar MB, et al. Clinical and molecular characterization defines a broadened spectrum of autosomal-recessive polycystic kidney disease (ARPKD). Medicine (Baltimore). 2006;85(1):1–21.

67. de Tommaso AMA, Santos DSM, Hessel G. Caroli's disease: 6 case studies. Acta Gastroenterol Latinoam. 2003;33(1):47–51.

68. Zerres K, Rudnik-Schöneborn S, Deget F, Holtkamp U, Brodehl J, Geisert J, et al. Autosomal-recessive polycystic kidney disease in 115 children: clinical presentation, course and influence of gender. *Arbeitsgemeinschaft für Pädiatrische, Nephrologie*. Acta Paediatr. 1996;85(4):437–45.

69. Roy S, Dillon MJ, Trompeter RS, Barratt TM. Autosomal-recessive polycystic kidney disease: long-term outcome of neonatal survivors. Pediatr Nephrol. 1997;11(3):302–6.

70. Guay-Woodford LM, Desmond RA. Autosomal-recessive polycystic kidney disease: the clinical experience in North America. Pediatrics. 2003;111(5 Pt 1):1072–80.

71. Telega G, Cronin D, Avner ED. New approaches to the autosomal-recessive polycystic kidney disease patient with dual kidney-liver complications. Pediatr Transplant. 2013;17(4):328–35.

72. Bergmann C, Senderek J, Windelen E, Küpper F, Middeldorf I, Schneider F, et al. Clinical consequences of PKHD1 mutations in 164 patients with autosomal-recessive polycystic kidney disease (ARPKD). Kidney Int. 2005;67(3):829–48.

73. Cannella R, Giambelluca D, Diamarco M, Caruana G, Cutaia G, Midiri M, et al. Congenital cystic lesions of the bile ducts: imaging-based diagnosis. Curr Probl Diagn Radiol. 2020;49(4):285–93. https://doi.org/10.1067/j.cpradiol.2019.04.005. PMID: 31027922.

74. Kumar S, Rankin R. Renal insufficiency is a component of COACH syndrome. Am J Med Genet. 1996;61(2):122–6.

75. Parisi MA. The molecular genetics of Joubert syndrome and related ciliopathies: the challenges of genetic and phenotypic heterogeneity. Transl Sci Rare Dis. 2019;4(1–2):25–49.

76. Rivas A, Epelman M, Danzer E, Adzick NS, Victoria T. Prenatal MR imaging features of Caroli syndrome in association with autosomal-recessive polycystic kidney disease. Radiol Case Rep. 2019;14(2):265–8.

77. Hartung EA, Wen J, Poznick L, Furth SL, Darge K. Ultrasound elastography to quantify liver disease severity in autosomal-recessive polycystic kidney disease. J Pediatr. 2019;209:107–115.e5.

78. Alsomali MI, Yearsley MM, Levin DM, Chen W. Diagnosis of congenital hepatic fibrosis in adulthood. Am J Clin Pathol. 2020;153(1):119–25.

79. Angeli P, Bernardi M, Villanueva C, Francoz C, Mookerjee RP, Trebicka J, et al. EASL clinical practice guidelines for the management of patients with decompensated cirrhosis. J Hepatol. 2018;69(2):406–60.
80. Kruis T, Güse-Jaschuck S, Siegmund B, Adam T, Epple H-J. Use of microbiological and patient data for choice of empirical antibiotic therapy in acute cholangitis. BMC Gastroenterol. 2020;20(1):65.
81. Labib PL, Goodchild G, Pereira SP. Molecular pathogenesis of cholangiocarcinoma. BMC Cancer. 2019;19:185. https://www.ncbi.nlm.nih.gov/pmc/articles/PMC6394015/.
82. Srinath A, Shneider BL. Congenital hepatic fibrosis and autosomal-recessive polycystic kidney disease. J Pediatr Gastroenterol Nutr. 2012;54(5):580–7.
83. Shneider BL, Bosch J, de Franchis R, Emre SH, Groszmann RJ, Ling SC, et al. Portal hypertension in children: expert pediatric opinion on the report of the Baveno V Consensus Workshop on Methodology of Diagnosis and Therapy in Portal Hypertension. Pediatr Transplant. 2012;16(5):426–37.
84. Tsimaratos M, Cloarec S, Roquelaure B, Retornaz K, Picon G, Chabrol B, et al. Chronic renal failure and portal hypertension—is portosystemic shunt indicated? Pediatr Nephrol. 2000;14(8–9):856–8.
85. Verbeeck S, Mekhali D, Cassiman D, Maleux G, Witters P. Long-term outcome of transjugular intrahepatic portosystemic shunt for portal hypertension in autosomal-recessive polycystic kidney disease. Dig Liver Dis. 2018;50(7):707–12.
86. Guay-Woodford LM, Bissler JJ, Braun MC, Bockenhauer D, Cadnapaphornchai MA, Dell KM, et al. Consensus expert recommendations for the diagnosis and management of autosomal-recessive polycystic kidney disease: report of an international conference. J Pediatr. 2014;165(3):611–7.
87. Ros E, Navarro S, Bru C, Gilabert R, Bianchi L, Bruguera M. Ursodeoxycholic acid treatment of primary hepatolithiasis in Caroli's syndrome. Lancet. 1993;342(8868):404–6.
88. Dayton MT, Longmire WP, Tompkins RK. Caroli's disease: a premalignant condition? Am J Surg. 1983;145(1):41–8.
89. Mabrut J-Y, Kianmanesh R, Nuzzo G, Castaing D, Boudjema K, Létoublon C, et al. Surgical management of congenital intrahepatic bile duct dilatation, Caroli's disease and syndrome: long-term results of the French Association of Surgery Multicenter Study. Ann Surg. 2013;258(5):713–21; discussion 721.
90. Jang MH, Lee YJ, Kim H. Intrahepatic cholangiocarcinoma arising in Caroli's disease. Clin Mol Hepatol. 2014;20(4):402–5.
91. Rosen CB, Heimbach JK, Gores GJ. Liver transplantation for cholangiocarcinoma. Transpl Int. 2010;23(7):692–7.
92. Yamaguchi T, Cristaudi A, Kokudo T, Uldry E, Demartines N, Halkic N. Surgical treatment for monolobular Caroli's disease—report of a 30-year single center case series. BioSci Trends. 2018;12:426–31.
93. Mabrut J-Y, Partensky C, Jaeck D, Oussoultzoglou E, Baulieux J, Boillot O, et al. Congenital intrahepatic bile duct dilatation is a potentially curable disease: long-term results of a multi-institutional study. Ann Surg. 2007;246(2):236–45.
94. Fahrner R, Dennler SGC, Dondorf F, Ardelt M, Rauchfuss F, Settmacher U. Liver resection and transplantation in Caroli's disease and syndrome. J Visc Surg. 2019;156(2):91–5.
95. Lai Q, Lerut J. Proposal for an algorithm for liver transplantation in Caroli's disease and syndrome: putting an uncommon effort into a common task. Clin Transpl. 2016;30(1):3–9.
96. Harring TR, Nguyen NTT, Liu H, Goss JA, O'Mahony CA. Caroli's disease patients have excellent survival after liver transplant. J Surg Res. 2012;177(2):365–72.
97. Habib S, Shakil O, Couto OF, Demetris AJ, Fung JJ, Marcos A, et al. Caroli's disease and orthotopic liver transplantation. Liver Transpl. 2006;12(3):416–21.
98. Wen JW, Furth SL, Ruebner RL. Kidney and liver transplantation in children with fibrocystic liver-kidney disease: data from the US Scientific Registry of Transplant Recipients: 1990-2010. Pediatr Transplant. 2014;18(7):726–32.

99. Büscher R, Büscher AK, Cetiner M, Treckmann JW, Paul A, Vester U, et al. Combined liver and kidney transplantation and kidney after liver transplantation in children: indication, postoperative outcome, and long-term results. Pediatr Transplant. 2015;19(8):858–65.
100. Kitajima K, Ogawa Y, Miki K, Kai K, Sannomiya A, Iwadoh K, et al. Long-term renal allograft survival after sequential liver-kidney transplantation from a single living donor. Liver Transpl. 2017;23(3):315–23.
101. Rogers J, Bueno J, Shapiro R, Scantlebury V, Mazariegos G, Fung J, et al. Results of simultaneous and sequential pediatric liver and kidney transplantation. Transplantation. 2001;72(10):1666–70.
102. Astarcioglu I, Egeli T, Unek T, Akarsu M, Sagol O, Obuz F, et al. Liver transplant in patients with primary sclerosing cholangitis: long-term experience of a single center. Exp Clin Transplant. 2018;16(4):434–8.
103. Todani T, Watanabe Y, Narusue M, Tabuchi K, Okajima K. Congenital bile duct cysts: classification, operative procedures, and review of thirty-seven cases including cancer arising from choledochal cyst. Am J Surg. 1977;134(2):263–9.
104. Todani T, Watanabe Y, Toki A, Morotomi Y. Classification of congenital biliary cystic disease: special reference to type Ic and IVA cysts with primary ductal stricture. J Hepato-Biliary-Pancreat Surg. 2003;10(5):340–4.
105. Friedmacher F, Ford KE, Davenport M. Choledochal malformations: global research, scientific advances and key controversies. Pediatr Surg Int. 2019;35(3):273–82.
106. Wiseman K, Buczkowski AK, Chung SW, Francoeur J, Schaeffer D, Scudamore CH. Epidemiology, presentation, diagnosis, and outcomes of choledochal cysts in adults in an urban environment. Am J Surg. 2005;189(5):527–31; discussion 531.
107. Yamaguchi M. Congenital choledochal cyst. Analysis of 1433 patients in the Japanese literature. Am J Surg. 1980;140(5):653–7.
108. Söreide K, Körner H, Havnen J, Söreide JA. Bile duct cysts in adults. Br J Surg. 2004;91(12):1538–48.
109. Baison GN, Bonds MM, Helton WS, Kozarek RA. Choledochal cysts: similarities and differences between Asian and Western countries. World J Gastroenterol. 2019;25(26):3334–43.
110. Han SJ, Hwang EH, Chung KS, Kim MJ, Kim H. Acquired choledochal cyst from anomalous pancreatiobiliary duct union. J Pediatr Surg. 1997;32(12):1735–8.
111. Davenport M, Basu R. Under pressure: choledochal malformation manometry. J Pediatr Surg. 2005;40(2):331–5.
112. Soares KC, Kim Y, Spolverato G, Maithel S, Bauer TW, Marques H, et al. Presentation and clinical outcomes of choledochal cysts in children and adults: a multi-institutional analysis. JAMA Surg. 2015;150(6):577–84.
113. Fitoz S, Erden A, Boruban S. Magnetic resonance cholangiopancreatography of biliary system abnormalities in children. Clin Imaging. 2007;31(2):93–101.
114. Kim SH, Lim JH, Yoon HK, Han BK, Lee SK, Kim YI. Choledochal cyst: comparison of MR and conventional cholangiography. Clin Radiol. 2000;55(5):378–83.
115. Oduyebo I, Law JK, Zaheer A, Weiss MJ, Wolfgang C, Lennon AM. Choledochal or pancreatic cyst? Role of endoscopic ultrasound as an adjunct for diagnosis: a case series. Surg Endosc. 2015;29(9):2832–6.
116. Hiramatsu K, Paye F, Kianmanesh AR, Sauvanet A, Terris B, Belghiti J. Choledochal cyst and benign stenosis of the main pancreatic duct. J Hepato-Biliary-Pancreat Surg. 2001;8(1):92–4.
117. Li M-J, Feng J-X, Jin Q-F. Early complications after excision with hepaticoenterostomy for infants and children with choledochal cysts. HBPD INT. 2002;1(2):281–4.
118. Ramos A, Castelló J, Pinto I. Intestinal intussusception as a presenting feature of choledochocele. Gastrointest Radiol. 1990;15(3):211–4.
119. Arda IS, Tuzun M, Aliefendioglu D, Hicsonmez A. Spontaneous rupture of extrahepatic choledochal cyst: two pediatric cases and literature review. Eur J Pediatr Surg. 2005;15(5):361–3.
120. Diao M, Li L, Cheng W. Timing of choledochal cyst perforation. Hepatology. [cited 2020 Jan 28]. http://aasldpubs.onlinelibrary.wiley.com/doi/abs/10.1002/hep.30902.

121. Stain SC, Guthrie CR, Yellin AE, Donovan AJ. Choledochal cyst in the adult. Ann Surg. 1995;222(2):128–33.
122. ten Hove A, de Meijer VE, Hulscher JBF, de Kleine RHJ. Meta-analysis of risk of developing malignancy in congenital choledochal malformation. Br J Surg. 2018;105(5):482–90.
123. Chaudhary A, Dhar P, Sachdev A, Kumar N, Vij JC, Sarin SK, et al. Choledochal cysts—differences in children and adults. Br J Surg. 1996;83(2):186–8.
124. Fabris L, Perugorria MJ, Mertens J, Björkström NK, Cramer T, Lleo A, et al. The tumour microenvironment and immune milieu of cholangiocarcinoma. Liver Int. 2019;39(S1):63–78.
125. He X-D, Wang L, Liu W, Liu Q, Qu Q, Li B-L, et al. The risk of carcinogenesis in congenital choledochal cyst patients: an analysis of 214 cases. Ann Hepatol. 2014;13(6):819–26.
126. Okada T, Sasaki F, Ueki S, Hirokata G, Okuyama K, Cho K, et al. Postnatal management for prenatally diagnosed choledochal cysts. J Pediatr Surg. 2004;39(7):1055–8.
127. Lee J-H, Kim S-H, Kim H-Y, Choi YH, Jung S-E, Park K-W. Early experience of laparoscopic choledochal cyst excision in children. J Korean Surg Soc. 2013;85(5):225–9.
128. Shimotakahara A, Yamataka A, Yanai T, Kobayashi H, Okazaki T, Lane GJ, et al. Roux-en-Y hepaticojejunostomy or hepaticoduodenostomy for biliary reconstruction during the surgical treatment of choledochal cyst: which is better? Pediatr Surg Int. 2005;21(1):5–7.
129. Zhen C, Xia Z, Long L, Lishuang M, Pu Y, Wenjuan Z, et al. Laparoscopic excision versus open excision for the treatment of choledochal cysts: a systematic review and meta-analysis. Int Surg. 2015;100(1):115–22.
130. Han JH, Lee JH, Hwang DW, Song KB, Shin SH, Kwon JW, et al. Robot resection of a choledochal cyst with Roux-en-y hepaticojejunostomy in adults: initial experiences with 22 cases and a comparison with laparoscopic approaches. Ann Hepatobiliary Pancreat Surg. 2018;22(4):359–66.
131. Acker SN, Bruny JL, Narkewicz MR, Roach JP, Rogers A, Karrer FM. Preoperative imaging does not predict intrahepatic involvement in choledochal cysts. J Pediatr Surg. 2013;48(12):2378–82.
132. Saeki I, Takahashi Y, Matsuura T, Takahata S, Tanaka M, Taguchi T. Successful endoscopic unroofing for a pediatric choledochocele. J Pediatr Surg. 2009;44(8):1643–5.
133. Fujishiro J, Masumoto K, Urita Y, Shinkai T, Gotoh C. Pancreatic complications in pediatric choledochal cysts. J Pediatr Surg. 2013;48(9):1897–902.
134. Miyano T, Yamataka A, Kato Y, Segawa O, Lane G, Takamizawa S, et al. Hepaticoenterostomy after excision of choledochal cyst in children: a 30-year experience with 180 cases. J Pediatr Surg. 1996;31(10):1417–21.
135. Todani T, Watanabe Y, Urushihara N, Noda T, Morotomi Y. Biliary complications after excisional procedure for choledochal cyst. J Pediatr Surg. 1995;30(3):478–81.
136. de Vries JS, de Vries S, Aronson DC, Bosman DK, Rauws E. a. J, Bosma a, et al. Choledochal cysts: age of presentation, symptoms, and late complications related to Todani's classification. J Pediatr Surg. 2002;37(11):1568–73.
137. Masyuk TV, Radtke BN, Stroope AJ, Banales JM, Gradilone SA, Huang B, et al. Pasireotide is more effective than octreotide in reducing hepatorenal cystogenesis in rodents with polycystic kidney and liver diseases. Hepatology. 2013;58(1):409–21.
138. Masyuk TV, Masyuk AI, Torres VE, Harris PC, Larusso NF. Octreotide inhibits hepatic cystogenesis in a rodent model of polycystic liver disease by reducing cholangiocyte adenosine 3′,5′-cyclic monophosphate. Gastroenterology. 2007;132(3):1104–16.
139. Spirli C, Okolicsanyi S, Fiorotto R, Fabris L, Cadamuro M, Lecchi S, et al. Mammalian target of rapamycin regulates vascular endothelial growth factor–dependent liver cyst growth in polycystin-2–defective mice. Hepatology. 2010;51(5):1778–88.
140. Munoz-Garrido P, Marin JJG, Perugorria MJ, Urribarri AD, Erice O, Sáez E, et al. Ursodeoxycholic acid inhibits hepatic cystogenesis in experimental models of polycystic liver disease. J Hepatol. 2015;63(4):952–61.
141. Gradilone SA, Masyuk TV, Huang BQ, Banales JM, Lehmann GL, Radtke BN, et al. Activation of Trpv4 reduces the hyperproliferative phenotype of cystic cholangiocytes from an animal model of ARPKD. Gastroenterology. 2010;139(1):304–314.e2.

142. Urribarri AD, Munoz-Garrido P, Perugorria MJ, Erice O, Merino-Azpitarte M, Arbelaiz A, et al. Inhibition of metalloprotease hyperactivity in cystic cholangiocytes halts the development of polycystic liver diseases. Gut. 2014;63(10):1658–67.
143. Yoshihara D, Kurahashi H, Morita M, Kugita M, Hiki Y, Aukema HM, et al. PPAR-gamma agonist ameliorates kidney and liver disease in an orthologous rat model of human autosomal-recessive polycystic kidney disease. Am J Physiol Renal Physiol. 2011;300(2):F465–74.
144. Yoshihara D, Kugita M, Sasaki M, Horie S, Nakanishi K, Abe T, et al. Telmisartan ameliorates fibrocystic liver disease in an orthologous rat model of human autosomal-recessive polycystic kidney disease. PLoS One. 2013;8(12):e81480.

Biliary Hamartomas

3

Raffaella Motta, Andrea Pirazzini, Amalia Lupi,
Paolo Marchesi, Chiara Giraudo, and Annarosa Floreani

3.1 Introduction

Biliary amartomas, also called von Meyenburg complexes (VMCs), were firstly described by von Meyenburg in 1918 as "isolated groups of complex intrahepatic bile ducts in patients with cystic livers" [1]. Subsequently, several synonyms described this condition, including congenital hyperplasia of the interlobular ducts, multiple bile duct hamartomas, adenomata, and fibroadenomata [2]. The incidence is low, with a reported range from 0.35% in liver biopsy specimens [3] to 5.6% on autopsy series [4].

3.2 Embryogenesis

The biliary tree originates from the ductal plate, a transient structure, which begins to form in the first 7 days of the embryologic life and is formed by a layer of epithelial cells that surround each portal vein branch forming a cylindrical sleeve. The cells of ductal plate originate from progenitor cells that can differentiate to hepatocytes or cholangiocytes [5]. The extrahepatic biliary tract originates from a portion of ventral endoderm that is positioned immediately rostral to the ventral pancreatic

R. Motta (✉) · A. Pirazzini · A. Lupi · C. Giraudo
Institute of Radiology, Azienda Ospedale Università di Padova, University of Padova,
Padova, Italy
e-mail: raffaella.motta@unipd.it

P. Marchesi
Radiology Unit, Ospedale S. Antonio, Azienda Ospedale Università di Padova, Padova, Italy

A. Floreani
Scientific Consultant, Scientific Institute for Research, Hospitalization and Healthcare
(IRCCS) Negrar, Verona, Italy

Senior Scholar University of Padova, Padova, Italy

© Springer Nature Switzerland AG 2021
A. Floreani (ed.), *Diseases of the Liver and Biliary Tree*,
https://doi.org/10.1007/978-3-030-65908-0_3

bud, while cholangiocytes that line the intrahepatic bile ducts arise from hepato-blasts [6]. VMCs derive from a malformation of the ductal plate. This hypothesis is supported by the fact that VMCs are frequently associated with various defects of ductal plate formation, including Caroli disease, polycystic liver disease, and congenital hepatic fibrosis. These conditions may involve both the intra and extrahepatic bile ducts and may exist as individual conditions or in combination, which suggest their common origin [7].

3.3   Clinical Characteristics

VMCs are generally benign and asymptomatic. They are generally observed as an incidental finding on imaging exams performed for other reasons.

Histologically, VMCs present as multiple, small, greyish nodules, usually between 1 and 15 mm in size, unless they can reach up to 3 cm [8]. Microscopically, VMCs appear as groups of rounded biliary channels, lined by cuboid epithelium and often containing bile-stained granular material. VMCs do not communicate with the biliary tree, which looks normal [3].

Sporadic reports in the literature suggest that VMCs may transform into cholangiocarcinoma, similarly to other defects of plate duct malformation (i.e., Caroli disease and congenital hepatic fibrosis) [9–11]. In two cases of progression to cholangiocarcinoma, it has been observed that histologic progression was accompanied by sequential genetic alterations, that is, an allelic imbalance characterized by loss of heterozygosity [12].

3.4   Imaging

They usually present as cystic lesions with sharp margins and round or irregular shape, scattered throughout the liver parenchyma (mostly in the subcapsular region), usually between 1 and 15 mm in size. They do not increase in size over time.

At ultrasound (US) examination, VMCs are anechoic or hyperechoic: smaller lesions tend to be hyperechoic and produce "comet tail artefact," while larger lesions appear anechoic like cysts (Fig. 3.1). Parenchymal echotexture may appear heterogeneous due to the small, scattered lesions [13].

On computed tomography (CT), biliary hamartomas appear as hypoattenuating lesions with irregular or oval shapes that do not enhance after contrast medium administration (Fig. 3.2). Compressed liver parenchyma or inflammatory cell infiltration can produce a thin homogenous rim of enhancement around some lesions in portal and delayed phases [14].

The recommended diagnostic imaging modality to study VMCs is magnetic resonance with cholangiopancreatography (MRCP). They appear as well-delineated, round or irregularly shaped lesions, hypointense on T1-weighted and hyperintense on T2-weighted images [15]. With heavily T2-weighted images, such as MRCP, the signal intensity of these lesions increases, approaching the signal intensity of

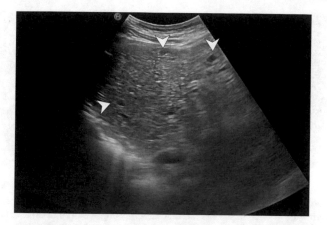

Fig. 3.1 US examination of the liver demonstrating many well-defined anechoic cystic lesions (arrowheads) along with innumerable hyperechoic lesions of 1–2 mm

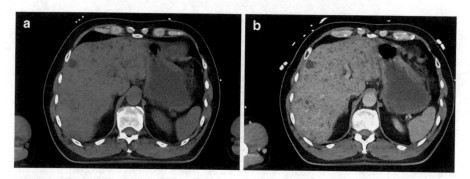

Fig. 3.2 The same patient of Fig. 3.1 underwent CT for further evaluation. (**a**) Transverse CT scan shows multiple hypoattenuating lesions in the liver. (**b**) Transverse CT scan acquired after contrast media administration in portal phase demonstrating no enhancement of the lesions and allowing for a better evaluation of their size, ranging from 2–4 up to 15 mm

cerebrospinal fluid. MRCP demonstrates normal intra and extrahepatic bile ducts and no connection between the hamartomas and the biliary tree. It can also depict the pathognomonic "starry-sky" appearance: small innumerable hyperintense lesions (biliary hamartomas) scattered throughout the hypointense hepatic parenchyma, resembling bright stars scattered throughout a dark sky (Fig. 3.3). On diffusion-weighted images (DWI), VMCs mimic the signal intensity of cystic lesions with free diffusion pattern. On T1-weighted images obtained after injection of gadoxetic acid, there will be no enhancement or thin, smooth-rim enhancement persistent in portal and delayed phase; the images acquired in hepatobiliary phase will confirm no connection with the biliary tree (Fig. 3.4) [16]. A small mural nodule of 1–2 mm can be observed in larger hamartomas; it has intermediate signal intensity on T1-weighted and T2-weighted images and enhances after contrast media administration [17].

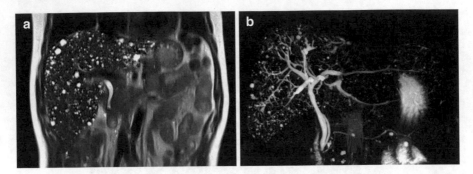

Fig. 3.3 To confirm the suspect of VMCs, the same patient of Figs. 3.1 and 3.2 underwent MRCP. (**a**) Coronal T2-weighted image and (**b**) coronal thick-slab MR cholangiogram show innumerable hyperintense lesions in the liver, not communicating with the normal intra and extrahepatic biliary system (the patient underwent cholecystectomy), and the pathognomonic appearance of "starry sky"

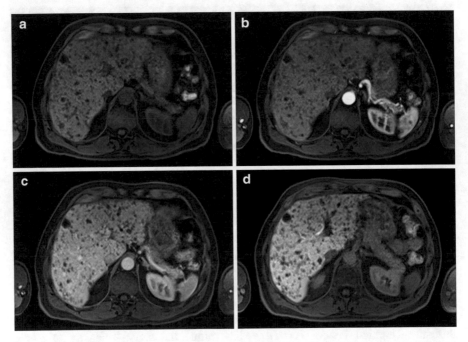

Fig. 3.4 To confirm the suspect of VMCs, the same patient of Figs. 3.1 and 3.2 underwent MRCP. T1-weighted images before (**a**) and after injection of gadoxetic acid in arterial phase (**b**), portal phase, (**c**) and hepatobiliary phase (**d**). The lesions appear hypointense in all images, including hepatobiliary phase, confirming the absence of communication with the biliary tree

3.5   Differential Diagnosis

Differential diagnosis includes a wide range of pathologies with cystic appearance: malignancies, benign cystic lesions, abscesses.

The main condition to be excluded concerns multiple small liver metastases, especially when staging patient with a known extrahepatic malignancy. The correct diagnosis may be challenging on US and usually requires CT and/or MR. Metastases tend to be more heterogeneous in size (including lesions larger than 15 mm), in distribution, and in attenuation (CT) or signal intensity (MR). They are usually less hyperintense on T2-weighted images, such as MRCP, and show restriction of diffusion on DWI. Metastatic lesions tend to have ill-defined margins and a certain amount of enhancement after contrast media administration. When a rim enhancement is visible, it's usually larger and more heterogeneous than what can be seen in VMCs. If metastases are not possible to be ruled out with enough confidence, short-term follow-up should settle any uncertainty since VMCs do not increase in size over time [18].

Hepatic lymphomas are more heterogeneous in size and in attenuation/signal intensity than biliary hamartomas, but are less frequent than metastases.

Diffuse primary hepatocellular carcinoma typically occurs in cirrhotic patients and rarely present as cystic lesions.

Simple hepatic cysts are usually round-shaped and can be extremely variable in size, number, and distribution. However, they can coexist with VMCs, and the differential diagnosis can be based on the size criteria.

Peribiliary cysts are small cystic dilatations of peribiliary glands located in the hepatic hilum and along the proximal portal tract that can increase in size and number. They do not communicate with the biliary tree and do not enhance, similar to VMCs. They are usually associated with chronic liver disease, cirrhosis, autosomal-dominant polycystic kidney disease (ADPKD), and portal hypertension [19].

Autosomal-dominant polycystic disease of the liver produces cysts that are usually larger and more numerous with only small areas of liver parenchyma intersperse between the cysts. The liver is often enlarged [20].

Clinical history of immunosuppression, recent fever, infection, or gastric pain helps differentiate microabscesses of the liver from VMCs. CT can be helpful if the abscesses appear loculated. Larger lesions on US can have a "target" appearance (i.e., hyperechoic rim between a hypoechoic center and a hypoechoic outer rim). On MR, microabscesses usually have restricted diffusion and perilesional edema visible as hyperintensity halo on T2-weighted images [21].

At US, VMCs may appear as multiple hyperechoic spots with comet-tail artifacts that can be misinterpreted for pneumobilia or intrahepatic stones. Pneumobilia is usually seen as linear branches or spots of gas attenuation on CT (very dark) and of gas signal intensity on MR (hypointense on T1-weighted and T2-weighted images). Intrahepatic stones are usually hyperintense on T1-weighted images and hypointense on T2-weighted MR images [22].

Biliary hamartomas can coexist with other fibropolycystic liver disease, such as Caroli disease.

References

1. von Meyenburg H. Über die cystenleber. Beitr Path Anat. 1918;64:477–532.
2. Chung EB. Multiple bile-duct hamartomas. Cancer. 1970;26(2):287–96. https://doi.org/10.1002/1097-0142(197008)26:2<287::aid-cncr2820260207>3.0.co;2-v.
3. Lin S, Weng Z, Xu J, Wang MF, Zhu YY, Jiang JJ. A study of multiple biliary hamartomas based on 1697 liver biopsies. Eur J Gastroenterol Hepatol. 2013;25(8):948–52. https://doi.org/10.1097/MEG.0b013e32835fb9ee.
4. Redston MS, Wanless IR. The hepatic von Meyenburg complex: prevalence and association with hepatic and renal cysts among 2843 autopsies [corrected]. Mod Pathol. 1996;9(3):233–7.
5. Kenney BJD. Ductal plate malformations. In: Ferrell L, Kakar S, editors. Liver pathology. New York: Demos Medical Publishing; 2011.
6. Si-Tayeb K, Lemaigre FP, Duncan SA. Organogenesis and development of the liver. Dev Cell. 2010;18(2):175–89. https://doi.org/10.1016/j.devcel.2010.01.011.
7. Cannella R, Giambelluca D, Diamarco M, Caruana G, Cutaia G, Midiri M, Salvaggio G. Congenital cystic lesions of the bile ducts: imaging-based diagnosis. Curr Probl Diagn Radiol. 2019;49:285. https://doi.org/10.1067/j.cpradiol.2019.04.005.
8. Drenth JP, Chrispijn M, Bergmann C. Congenital fibrocystic liver diseases. Best Pract Res Clin Gastroenterol. 2010;24(5):573–84. https://doi.org/10.1016/j.bpg.2010.08.007.
9. Bornfors M. The development of cholangiocarcinoma from multiple bile-duct adenomas. Report of a case and review of the literature. Acta Pathol Microbiol Immunol Scand A. 1984;92(4):285–9. https://doi.org/10.1111/j.1699-0463.1984.tb04405.x.
10. Burns CD, Kuhns JG, Wieman TJ. Cholangiocarcinoma in association with multiple biliary microhamartomas. Arch Pathol Lab Med. 1990;114(12):1287–9.
11. Honda N, Cobb C, Lechago J. Bile duct carcinoma associated with multiple von Meyenburg complexes in the liver. Hum Pathol. 1986;17(12):1287–90. https://doi.org/10.1016/s0046-8177(86)80575-5.
12. Jain D, Ahrens W, Finkelstein S. Molecular evidence for the neoplastic potential of hepatic von Meyenburg complexes. Appl Immunohistochem Mol Morphol. 2010;18(2):166–71. https://doi.org/10.1097/PAI.0b013e3181b94fd8.
13. Merkel D, Wiens D, Kammer J. The "dirty liver" as a coincidental finding on sonography: sonographic criteria for biliary microhamartomas of the liver. J Ultrasound Med. 2016;35(10):2139–45. https://doi.org/10.7863/ultra.15.11081.
14. Liu S, Zhao B, Ma J, Li J, Li X. Lesions of biliary hamartomas can be diagnosed by ultrasonography, computed tomography and magnetic resonance imaging. Int J Clin Exp Med. 2014;7(10):3370–7.
15. Pech L, Favelier S, Falcoz MT, Loffroy R, Krause D, Cercueil JP. Imaging of von Meyenburg complexes. Diagn Interv Imaging. 2016;97(4):401–9. https://doi.org/10.1016/j.diii.2015.05.012.
16. Zheng RQ, Zhang B, Kudo M, Onda H, Inoue T. Imaging findings of biliary hamartomas. World J Gastroenterol. 2005;11(40):6354–9. https://doi.org/10.3748/wjg.v11.i40.6354.
17. Tohme-Noun C, Cazals D, Noun R, Menassa L, Valla D, Vilgrain V. Multiple biliary hamartomas: magnetic resonance features with histopathologic correlation. Eur Radiol. 2008;18(3):493–9. https://doi.org/10.1007/s00330-007-0790-z.
18. Mortele KJ, Ros PR. Cystic focal liver lesions in the adult: differential CT and MR imaging features. Radiographics. 2001;21(4):895–910. https://doi.org/10.1148/radiographics.21.4.g01jl16895.
19. Kudo M. Hepatic peribiliary cysts: clinically harmless disease with potential risk due to gradual increase in size and number. J Gastroenterol. 2001;36(4):286–8. https://doi.org/10.1007/s005350170119.
20. Mamone G, Carollo V, Cortis K, Aquilina S, Liotta R, Miraglia R. Magnetic resonance imaging of fibropolycystic liver disease: the spectrum of ductal plate malformations. Abdom Radiol (NY). 2019;44(6):2156–71. https://doi.org/10.1007/s00261-019-01966-9.

21. Bachler P, Baladron MJ, Menias C, Beddings I, Loch R, Zalaquett E, Vargas M, Connolly S, Bhalla S, Huete A. Multimodality imaging of liver infections: differential diagnosis and potential pitfalls. Radiographics. 2016;36(4):1001–23. https://doi.org/10.1148/rg.2016150196.
22. Bricault I. Biliary obstruction: not always simple! Diagn Interv Imaging. 2013;94(7–8):729–40. https://doi.org/10.1016/j.diii.2013.03.011.

Part II

Genetic Cholangiopathies

Alagille Syndrome

4

Paola Gaio, Elena Reffo, Claudia Mescoli, and Mara Cananzi

Abbreviations

ALGS   Alagille syndrome
LT   Liver transplantation

4.1   Introduction

Alagille syndrome (ALGS) is a rare, autosomal dominant disorder caused by defects in genes (*JAG1* or *NOTCH2*) involved in the Notch signaling pathway, and characterized by multisystem anomalies resulting from the abnormal development of intrahepatic bile ducts, heart, kidneys, bones, eyes, and vessels [1].

The disorder was firstly described in 1969 by the French hepatologist Daniel Alagille who reported a small number of patients with paucity of the interlobular bile ducts and concomitant extra-hepatic features (heart murmur, peculiar facies, embryotoxon, and butterfly vertebrae) [2]. Soon after (1973), the association between neonatal liver disease and congenital heart malformations was

P. Gaio · M. Cananzi (✉)
Unit of Pediatric Gastroenterology, Digestive Endoscopy, Hepatology and Care of the Child with Liver Transplantation, Department for Woman's and Child's Health, University Hospital of Padova, Padova, Italy
e-mail: mara.cananzi@aopd.veneto.it

E. Reffo
Unit of Pediatric Cardiology, Department for Woman's and Child's Health, University Hospital of Padova, Padova, Italy

C. Mescoli
Surgical Pathology and Cytopathology Unit, Department of Medicine (DIMED), University Hospital of Padova, Padova, Italy

© Springer Nature Switzerland AG 2021
A. Floreani (ed.), *Diseases of the Liver and Biliary Tree*,
https://doi.org/10.1007/978-3-030-65908-0_4

independently described by Watson and Miller [3]. Along the years, different terminologies were employed to identify the disease, including "intrahepatic biliary atresia," "syndromic bile duct paucity," "arteriohepatic dysplasia," and "Alagille-Watson syndrome." The term "Alagille syndrome" (ORPHA: 52) was ultimately assigned as the official nomenclature to provide a tribute to the observations of Daniel Alagille and to appreciate the multisystem nature of the disorder reducing emphasis on hepatic and cardiac manifestations [4].

The following sections will comprehensively review the epidemiology, genetic basis, pathogenesis, clinical manifestations, diagnostic modalities, and management strategies of ALGS.

4.2　Epidemiology

ALGS is a rare disease with cases reported worldwide in multiple ethnic groups [5–7]. Prior to the advent of genetic testing for ALGS, disease incidence was solely established based on the presence of neonatal liver disease and reported at 1:70,000 live births [8]. Nowadays, molecular diagnostics has led to an estimate of 1:30,000–50,000 live births. Indeed, genetic tests allow for the identification of those individuals (mainly relatives of known ALGS patients) that would escape clinical diagnosis. Notwithstanding, the existence of individuals without an obvious familial history and with isolated signs of ALGS (such as isolated heart disease or facial features) suggests that ALGS frequency is still underestimated and supports the utility of wider epidemiological and genetic studies in unselected subjects [9, 10].

4.3　Pathogenesis

ALGS is an autosomal dominant disease caused by pathogenic variants in genes involved in the Notch signaling pathway.

4.3.1　Notch Signaling Pathway and Bile Duct Development

Notch pathway is a highly evolutionarily conserved intercellular signaling mechanism involved in cell fate determination and tissue differentiation processes during development and postnatal life. To date, five canonical ligands (DLL1, DLL3, DLL4, JAGGED-1, and JAGGED-2) and four NOTCH [1–4] receptors have been attributed to the mammalian Notch pathway. Although there is some degree of functional redundancy among Notch receptors and ligands, each component of the pathway is endowed with a unique function, wherein the JAGGED-1/NOTCH2 signaling axis plays a major role in biliary specification and morphogenesis [11].

JAGGED-1 is a transmembrane protein composed by 1218 amino acids that serves as a ligand for the four NOTCH receptors (NOTCH1–4). It is encoded by *JAG1*, a 26 exon-containing gene located on chromosome 20p12.2. During embryonic development, the expression of *JAG1* is concentrated in pulmonary and systemic arteries, mesocardium, metanephros, branchial arches, pancreas, liver (portal mesenchymal cells, portal endothelial cells, biliary epithelial cells), and otocyst [11, 12]. Postnatally, *JAG1* continues to be expressed in multiple tissues including pancreas, heart, lung, kidney, liver, thymus, and leucocytes.

NOTCH2 is a transmembrane protein composed by 2471 amino acids which acts as receptor for three membrane-bound ligands: JAGGED-1, JAGGED-2, and DLL1. It is encoded by *NOTCH2*, a 34 exon-containing gene located on chromosome 1p12. During development, Notch2 signaling is mainly relevant for the development of heart, liver, kidneys, and bones, while after birth it is mainly involved in immune function, tissue repair, and bone remodeling.

Communication between JAGGED-1 and NOTCH2 is accomplished through the direct interaction of their extracellular domains. Once the receptor–ligand interaction has occurred, the NOTCH2 intracellular domain is cleaved from the inner surface of the membrane and translocates into the nucleus, where it regulates the transcription of different downstream target genes.

The exact mechanism whereby *JAG1* and *NOTCH2* mutations lead to paucity of intrahepatic bile ducts in ALGS is not fully elucidated. Substantial experimental evidences, however, support that Notch signaling pathway is critical for the morphogenesis and the maturation of the intrahepatic biliary system: (1) NOTCH2 drives the differentiation of bipotential hepatoblasts towards a biliary fate, enhances biliary cell survival and promotes tubulogenesis [13]; (2) inactivation of JAGGED-1 in the portal vein mesenchyme during liver development leads to bile duct paucity [14]; (3) Notch signaling regulates the density of biliary tree branches in a dosage-dependent manner [15]; (4) pharmacological inhibition of Notch signaling in early postnatal life results in impaired elongation of the biliary tree [16].

4.3.2 Genetics

ALGS is caused by monoallelic mutations in either *JAG1* (ALGS type 1; OMIM #118450) or *NOTCH2* (ALGS type 2; OMIM #610205) that are transmitted via an autosomal dominant mode of inheritance. Collectively, *JAG1* and *NOTCH2* pathogenic variants account for up to 96% of ALGS cases (*JAG1* 92–94%; *NOTCH2* 2–4%) (see Sect. 4.5.3 for more details on mutations). As the vast majority of ALGS patients (>85%) carry protein-truncating mutations or gene deletions, haploinsufficiency (i.e., loss of an allele resulting in insufficient protein levels to support Notch signaling) is considered the main pathogenetic mechanism underlying ALGS. Few studies, however, also support the possibility of a dominant negative effect of mutant transcripts. Among these, Guan et al. reported that induced pluripotent stem cells (iPSCs) containing heterozygous *JAG1* mutations have a reduced efficiency in forming liver organoids in comparison to iPSCs with heterozygous *JAG1* knockout, thus suggesting that the presence of a mutated JAG1 protein is more deleterious than the absence of one *JAG1* allele [17].

ALGS is characterized by a high penetrance (94%) and a significant phenotypical variability. Many studies have attempted, without success, to identify genotype-phenotype correlations able to predict disease prognosis [18]. Conversely, an extremely variable clinical expressivity has been observed among subjects carrying the same pathogenic variant, including monozygotic twins [1, 19–23]. Based on these observations, many studies have investigated the potential role of modifier genes in ALGS pathogenesis. Variants in genes encoding for Fringe proteins (LFNG, RFNG, and MFNG), Thrombospondin2 (THBS2), and SOX9 have been recognized as risk factors for the development of a more severe liver disease [11, 24, 25]. Further studies are needed to unravel the genetic bases of ALGS phenotypic variability, identify novel prognostic factors and recognize potential therapeutic targets.

4.4　Clinical Manifestations and Prognosis

As the Notch signaling pathway operates in many tissues and cell types at various developmental stages, ALGS is characterized by multisystem structural and functional anomalies resulting from the abnormal development of intrahepatic bile ducts, heart, kidneys, craniofacial structures, eyes, bones, and vessels (Figs. 4.1 and 4.2). The clinical manifestations of the disease are extremely variable with

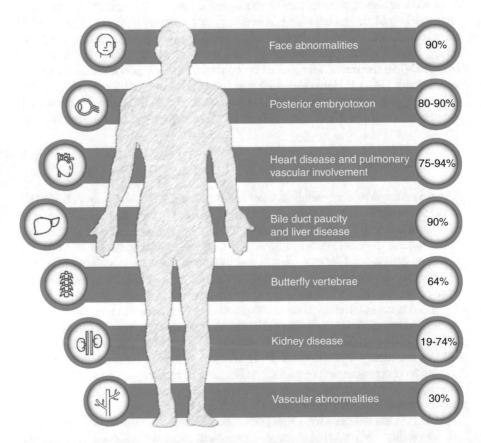

Fig. 4.1 Schematic of organ involvement in ALGS with related prevalences

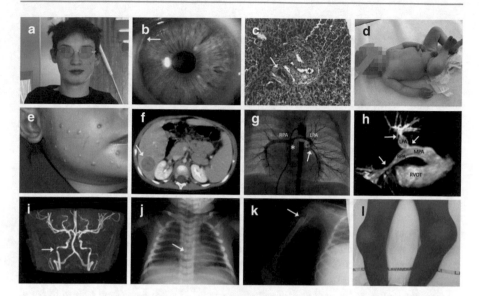

Fig. 4.2 Representative clinical features of ALGS. (**a**) 15-year-old male showing the typical ALGS facial appearance. (**b**) Slit-lamp examination showing posterior embryotoxon (arrow) consisting of thickening and displacement of the Schwalbe line. (**c**) Liver biopsy of a 2-month-old infant with bile duct paucity showing a portal tract with preserved artery (arrow) and portal vein branch (asterisk) along with loss of native bile duct (hematoxylin-eosin, ×200). (**d**) 7-month-old infant with jaundice and pruritus due to cholestatic liver disease and with acrocyanosis due to congenital heart disease. (**e**) Facial xanthomata. (**f**) Abdominal CT scan of a 2-year-old child showing a 3 × 3 cm hepatocellular carcinoma of the right hepatic lobe (arrow). (**g**) Selective thoracic aortography of a 8-month-old child affected by Tetralogy of Fallot (TOF) with pulmonary atresia (asterisk) and a major aorta-pulmonary collateral artery (MAPCA; arrow) supplying retrogradely a hypoplastic pulmonary circulation. RPA: right pulmonary artery, LPA: left pulmonary artery. (**h**) Cardiac angio-MRI of an 18-year-old patient showing pulmonary artery arborization with proximal LPA stenosis and bilateral distal stenoses (arrows). RVOT: right ventricular outflow tract, MPA main pulmonary artery, RPA right pulmonary artery, LPA left pulmonary artery. (**i**) Brain MRI showing a severe stenosis of both internal carotid arteries (arrow). (**j**) Thorax X-ray of a 2-month-old girl showing a sagittal cleft of the thoracic vertebral bodies (i.e., "butterfly vertebrae") (arrow). (**k**) Pathologic fracture of the right humerus in a 13-year-old girl with severe osteodystrophy. (**l**) Chronic arthritis with swelling of both knees in a 13-year-old girl. (**a–l**) All images have been obtained from ALGS patients cared at the Unit of Pediatric Gastroenterology and Hepatology of the University Hospital of Padova. The patient represented in (**a**) gave informed consent to the publication of his image (including face)

regard to both the organs involved and the severity of the accompanying organ damage, thereby resulting in heterogeneous clinical phenotypes even in relatives with identical mutations [1, 19–22]. Several phenotypical differences have also been observed in relation to the molecular etiology of ALGS. These include: (1) a minor prevalence of cardiac involvement (60% vs. 90%), vertebral anomalies (10% vs. 64%), and facial features (10–20% vs. 90%) in subjects carrying *NOTCH2* vs. *JAG1* pathogenic variants [26]; (2) the presence of additional phenotypic features not usually associated with ALGS, such as developmental delay and hearing loss, in patients carrying large deletions in chromosome 20p [27].

The clinical presentation of ALGS was recently described in a systematic review [1]. The age at presentation ranges from less than 16 weeks to up to 10 years of age with the majority of patients being diagnosed within the first year of life. Common presenting features include signs of cholestatic liver disease (e.g., jaundice, hepatomegaly, pruritus), cardiovascular malformations, failure to thrive, xanthomas, abnormal facies, and renal disease [1].

Few publications have examined ALGS prognosis in the long term. Among these publications mortality ranges from 11% to 35% with a median age of death around 2 and 4 years of age (range 2 months - 31 years) [1, 28–30]. In patients with a severe disease phenotype, death mainly results from vascular accidents, cardiac malformations or liver disease [1]. Non-cardiac vascular complications are the leading cause of death accounting for up to the 34% of mortality [28, 31]. Heart disease is responsible for nearly all early deaths [32]. Childhood mortality due to liver disease has benefit from liver transplantation, which, however, carries a significant risks, including surgical complications, nephropathy, and immune dysregulation [33]. Available data support that ALGS can be a devastating, life-shortening disease of childhood associated with multiple morbidities [1].

The typical patterns of organ involvement in ALGS are described below in separated sections.

4.4.1   Liver Disease

Although it is now clear that many individuals with ALGS can have no clinical overt hepatic disease, the liver is the most commonly and potentially most severely affected organ in subjects carrying either *JAG1* or *NOTCH2* mutations [20, 34]. When present, hepatic involvement may be highly heterogeneous in terms of initial presentation and long-term prognosis ranging from mild liver test abnormalities to end-stage liver disease requiring LT [35].

4.4.1.1 Presentation
The vast majority of patients with hepatic involvement (80–90%) presents in the first 6–12 months of life with cholestatic liver disease, while the minority of patients presenting later in life are usually referred to the hepatologist for a family history or for extra-hepatic manifestations of ALGS [31, 36].

Symptomatic infants typically present with jaundice, hyperchromic urine, and hepatomegaly (Fig. 4.2). Stool color is variable in relation to the degree of cholestasis but acholic stools, mimicking biliary atresia, may be observed in a significant proportion of patients [37]. Splenomegaly is not typically present during the early course of disease, but may develop overtime as a consequence of progressive hepatic fibrosis (35–70% of patients). Pruritus is more relevant than in other cholestatic liver disorders and affects 60–90% of children with ALGS. It usually becomes apparent after the first 3–6 months of life (Fig. 4.2), is disproportionately more intense than expected from hyperbilirubinemia and can persist despite the resolution of jaundice. Commonly affected areas include ears, trunk, and feet, although itching can be anywhere. Pruritus is often severe and may be debilitating in up to 45% of the patients in whom it may cause skin lesions, sleep problems, mood disturbances, and quality of life impairment [1, 35, 38, 39]. When blood cholesterol levels exceed 500 mg/dL, xanthomas emerge on the skin as yellow papules or plaques (30–40% of patients) [1]. They usually appear in the first 2 years of life and preferably locate on fingers, palms, knees, groin, and skin creases (Fig. 4.2) [1]. Xanthomas are not painful but can interfere with fine motor skills or vision (if on the eye lids) and may be disfiguring [1, 35]. They can regress or disappear if the hypercholesterolemia improves or if the patient undergoes LT. Persistent cholestasis can cause fat malabsorption with poor growth, fat-soluble vitamin deficiencies (vitamin A, D, E, and K), and increased bone fracture risk [1, 31, 35].

4.4.1.2 Prognosis

The natural history of liver disease in ALGS has a unique course. Children without cholestasis are unlikely to develop a significant hepatic impairment later in life. Conversely, infants with cholestasis generally suffer from a more severe course of hepatic disease during their first 5 years of life. Thereafter, some children experience a clinical improvement that in few cases may lead to the resolution of jaundice and pruritus, while others (40% by 20 years of age) suffer from the complications of persistent cholestasis (i.e., pruritus, malnutrition, growth failure, bone fractures) and/or develop clinically evident portal hypertension (i.e., ascites treated by diuretics, esophageal/gastric varices, gastrointestinal bleeding, splenomegaly with thrombocytopenia). While older studies reported that 15–50% of individuals with ALGS require LT [29–31, 40, 41], a recent longitudinal study showed that only a quarter of children with cholestatic liver disease survive to early adulthood with their native liver [35].

The possibility of a spontaneous liver improvement during childhood is well documented but it is not clear if this phenomenon is due to a true amelioration of hepatic function or to a survival selection bias [42]. Anyway, at present there is no genotypic, histologic, or radiologic marker able to prognosticate which cholestatic infant will spontaneously improve or will eventually require LT along life. A retrospective review of laboratory data from a small population of patients showed that high levels of bilirubin (total >6.5 mg/dL, conjugated >4.5 mg/dL) and cholesterol (>520 mg/dL) in children younger than 5 years of age are associated with severe liver disease in later life [43]. A larger multicenter retrospective study ($n = 144$) showed that patients who have total bilirubin >3.8 mg/dL between 12 and 24 months of life, fibrosis on liver biopsy before 5 years of age, and xanthomata on clinical examination are more likely to have a "severe" liver disease outcome defined by death, listing for LT, or significant morbidity [44]. Other than these prognostic factors, Kaye et al. reported that children with ALGS who underwent Kasai portoenterostomy for misdiagnosed biliary atresia had a worse outcome, probably reflecting a severe hypoplasia of the biliary tree or possibly resulting from an exacerbated liver disease after surgical intervention [45–47].

Hepatocellular carcinoma (HCC) has been reported in adults and children (as young as 1.5 years of age) affected by ALGS with or without cirrhosis [48, 49]. Albeit the exact incidence of HCC in ALGS is unknown, tumor screening with alpha-fetoprotein measurement and liver imaging should be warranted independently from patient age and liver disease severity at least every 6–12 months [40, 48]. Other hepatic focal lesions have been more rarely described in association to ALGS such as focal nodular hyperplasia, regenerative nodules, and adenomas [50–52].

4.4.1.3 Liver Biochemical Profile

Findings related to cholestasis and biliary damage are the most relevant hepatic laboratory abnormalities seen in ALGS. Serum bilirubin and bile salts can be elevated 30 and 100 times normal, respectively. On average serum bilirubin is higher during childhood (median of 6.9 mg/dL in the first year of age) and lower in subjects ≥13 years surviving with native liver (median of 1.3 mg/dL). Serum bile salts tend to remain elevated even if hyperbilirubinemia resolves. Cholesterol levels are usually increased and may exceed 1000–2000 mg/dL. Markers of bile duct damage are commonly increased especially during childhood. The median level of GGT is higher in infants (median 612 U/L) and lower in patients ≥13 years surviving with native liver (median 268 U/L). Serum aminotransferases are usually elevated from 3 to 10 times the normal value but tend to fluctuate overtime [35]. Normal levels of liver enzymes have also been observed and should not preclude the diagnosis of ALGS [36]. Markers of hepatic synthetic function are typically normal at presentation but may deteriorate with the progression of liver disease [40]. Similarly, platelet count is normal during infancy but progressively declines <150,000 per mL over childhood for a cumulative incidence of 33% by 20 years of age [35].

4.4.1.4 Liver Histopathology

Bile duct paucity is the hallmark histological feature of ALGS reported in the vast majority of cases (75–100%) [1]. Bile duct to portal space ratio normally ranges between 0.9 and 1.8. Bile duct paucity is defined as an absence or a marked reduction of interlobular bile ducts within portal tracts when at least six portal tracts are examined. As paucity typically progresses with age, the bile duct to portal space ratio is considered pathologically reduced when <0.9 in neonates or young infants and <0.5–0.75 in older subjects [40, 42]. Indeed, Emerick et al. showed that bile duct paucity was present in the 60% of liver biopsies performed before 6 months of age and in the 95% of those undertaken at later ages [31]. Furthermore, histopathologic signs consistent with biliary obstruction, such as ductular proliferation and giant cell hepatitis, have also been described in a small proportion of young infants with ALGS and severe biliary tree hypoplasia. In these cases, when also the interpretation of an intraoperative cholangiogram may be misleading, the differential diagnosis between ALGS and biliary atresia is challenging and early *JAG1/NOTCH2* genetic testing should be considered prior to Kasai portoenterostomy [45, 46].

Table 4.1 Causes of congenital and acquired non-syndromic bile duct paucity that can be considered in the differential diagnosis of ALGS syndrome

Chromosomal defects	Trisomy 17, 18, 21
	Turner syndrome
Congenital infections	Cytomegalovirus
	Rubella
	Syphilis
Endocrinological disorders	Hypopituitarism
Genetic and metabolic disorders	Alpha-1 antitrypsin deficiency
	Arthrogryposis-renal dysfunction-cholestasis (ARC) syndrome
	Cystic fibrosis
	HNF1β deficiency
	Niemann-Pick type C
	Progressive familial intrahepatic cholestasis type 1 and 2
	Williams syndrome
	Zellweger syndrome and other peroxisomal disorders
Immunological disorders	Graft vs. host disease
	Chronic hepatic rejection
	Primary sclerosing cholangitis
Idiopathic	

Of note, bile duct paucity is not universally associated to ALGS but may be observed in a broad group of disorders including congenital infections, chromosomal defects, genetic, metabolic, endocrinological and immunological disorders (see Table 4.1 for causes of non-syndromic bile duct paucity) [53, 54].

4.4.2   Heart Disease and Pulmonary Vascular Involvement

Cardiac involvement is present in a high proportion of individuals with ALGS (75–94%), an observation in support of the relevance of the Notch signaling pathway in ventricular and atrioventricular septation as well as in outflow tract and arterial development [35, 55–57]. Peripheral pulmonary arterial hypoplasia and/or stenosis of the branch pulmonary arteries are the most common cardiovascular congenital anomalies (60–75%) (Fig. 4.2) [58]. Their presence, either as an isolated finding or in association with other cardiac defects, should always prompt a clinical suspicion of ALGS. Also, patients may present with right-sided or left-sided congenital heart disease as well as with septal defects. Right-sided congenital heart disease, mainly presenting as tetralogy of Fallot, pulmonary valve stenosis, and pulmonary atresia, has been documented in up to 25% of patients (Fig. 4.2). Left-sided congenital heart disease, most commonly constituted by aortic valve stenosis, supravalvular aortic stenosis, and aortic coarctation, has been described in up to 10% of patients [31, 58]. The combination of right- and left-sided heart disease has also been observed in a small subset of ALGS patients [58, 59]. Accordingly, patients with tetralogy of Fallot or congenital pulmonary abnormalities with congenital aortic or aortic valve disease should be evaluated for ALGS. Septal defects (atrial or ventricular) may be present in up to 10–15% of patients either alone or, more commonly, in association with the aforementioned anomalies.

Cardiac involvement is a major independent determinant of prognosis in ALGS [32]. Up to 10–25% of patients require cardiac surgery [29, 31, 41, 60]. Subjects with complex cardiac defects have a significantly worse survival with respect to those without cardiac involvement (40% vs. 96% 6-year survival) [31]. Also, survival of ALGS patients with either unrepaired or repaired congenital heart disease is significantly worse than that of non-syndromic patients with similar cardiac conditions. This higher mortality is likely related to the pulmonary vascular abnormalities and to the multiorgan involvement that typically characterize ALGS.

4.4.3 Bone Disease and Skeletal Involvement

Patients with ALGS may present with a spectrum of skeletal anomalies. These include abnormalities of craniofacial development (ALGS-distinct facies), bone developmental defects (e.g., butterfly vertebrae), and bone mass reduction (osteoporosis and increased risk of bone fractures).

4.4.3.1 ALGS-Distinct Facies
Subjects with ALGS have a typical facial appearance consisting of prominent forehead, moderate hypertelorism with deep-set eyes, upslanting palpebral fissures, depressed nasal bridge, straight nose with a bulbous tip, large ears, prominent mandible, and pointed chin [61, 62]. This characteristic facial phenotype varies along life. It can be difficult to identify during infancy, usually becomes clinically evident throughout childhood, and may attenuate during adulthood when the development of a square jaw can temper the typical triangular appearance of the face (Fig. 4.2) [62]. Of note, facial features may be more difficult to recognize in patients of non-Caucasian ethnicity [26, 63, 64].

4.4.3.2 Skeletal Developmental Defects
Butterfly vertebrae (or anterior rachischisis) are the skeletal hallmark of ALGS [65]. They consist of a sagittal cleft in the vertebral body, usually at the D6-9 level, caused by an incomplete fusion of the anterior vertebral arch during embryogenesis. The name is based on the radiological appearance of the two hemivertebrae emerging as butterfly wings from the central cleft (Fig. 4.2). Remarkably, butterfly vertebrae may occur in normal individuals and may be also seen in other conditions, such as 22q deletion syndrome and VACTERL association [42].

Other congenital skeletal anomalies, usually not associated with any functional impairment, have been reported in ALGS such as fusion of adjacent vertebrae, hemivertebrae, absence of the 12th rib, radioulnar synostosis, square shaped proximal phalange, and shortened distal phalanges. Recently, structural defects of the middle ear bones causing hearing loss have also been observed [66].

4.4.3.3 Metabolic Bone Disease

Subjects with ALGS are prone to develop osteoporosis and pathologic bone fractures (Fig. 4.2) [67–69]. The pathogenesis of osteopenia is likely to be multifactorial. While chronic cholestatic liver disease may predispose to hepatic osteodystrophy (secondary to malabsorption, fat-soluble vitamin deficiencies, and alterations of calcium homeostasis), increasing evidences support that NOTCH signaling disruption may cause bone fragility *per se* [67, 68, 70]. A recent longitudinal study including 293 patients with cholestasis reported a 26% cumulative incidence of fracture by the age of 20 years with most fractures occurring during childhood [35]. In some cases, recurrent fractures and osteoporosis have been such severe to constitute an indication for LT [30, 31].

4.4.4 Ophthalmologic Features

The most common ocular finding in ALGS is posterior embryotoxon, a congenital corneal anomaly consisting of thickening and displacement of the Schwalbe line (Fig. 4.2). It does not affect visual acuity and can be easily identified by slit-lamp evaluation as an irregular, thin, grey-white line concentric and anterior to the limbus. Posterior embryotoxon is highly prevalent in ALGS (80–90% both in patients with *JAG1* and *NOTCH2* mutations) but can also be detected in healthy subjects (10–30%) or in patients with other ocular anomalies (e.g., Axenfeld–Rieger syndrome) or genetic disorders (e.g., velocardiofacial syndrome) [26, 71].

Other ocular features have been associated to ALGS such as pupil abnormalities, retinal pigmentary anomalies, and optic disc drusen [72].

4.4.5 Kidney Disease

Kidney abnormalities have been described in a variable proportion of patients (19–74%) and are considered as the sixth major disease-defining feature of ALGS [35, 73]. Renal disease may be the predominant symptom of ALGS and can present at any age including adulthood [22, 74]. Many different structural and functional conditions have been reported, which collectively recall the various roles of Notch signaling in glomerular, tubular, and renal vascular development. These included glomerular mesangiolipidosis (3–69%), renal hypoplasia/dysplasia with or without cysts (4–59%), congenital anomalies of the urinary tract (e.g., vesico-ureteral reflux, ureteropelvic obstruction, hydronephrosis, duplex collecting systems) (2–32%), renal tubular acidosis (8–59%), and renovascular hypertension due to midaortic syndrome or renal artery stenosis (2–8%) [1, 74, 75]. The occurrence of kidney failure in ALGS has not been prospectively evaluated. In a large retrospective study, end-stage renal disease was described in a small proportion of ALGS patients affected by congenital renal anomalies [73]. Case studies have also described the need for renal replacement therapy and kidney transplantation [1, 74].

The impact of renal dysfunction in the long term is not known. Secondary kidney injuries can complicate advancing heart and liver disease. After LT, renal complications are common (9.9%) and children with pre-existing kidney failure do not generally experience improvement of renal function [33]. These observations support the presence of an intrinsic renal disease not correctable by LT.

4.4.6   Extra-Cardiac/Extra-Pulmonary Vascular Involvement

Up to 30% of ALGS patients are affected by extra-cardiac/extra-pulmonary vascular anomalies, presentations in line with the relevance of Notch signaling in vascular morphogenesis, angiogenesis, and homeostasis [28, 76, 77]. Many arterial abnormalities (hypoplasia, stenosis, aneurysm) have been reported in both intracranial and systemic circulation and are currently considered as the seventh disease-defining feature of ALGS in support of the original definition of the disease as *"arteriohepatic dysplasia"* [3, 78].

The prevalence of cerebrovascular disease in ALGS has been reported as low as 4% to as high as 38% in asymptomatic patients undergoing neuroimaging (Fig. 4.2) [28, 31, 79]. Three main cerebrovascular phenotypes have been described: cerebral aneurysms (mainly occurring in the posterior circulation), Moyamoya syndrome, and dolichoectasia of the internal carotid arteries. Cerebral aneurysms constitute the most common cause of hemorrhagic stroke in adults, while Moyamoya typically presents with ischemic stroke during the first decade of life. Although to a lesser extent than intracranial defects, many vascular systemic abnormalities have been described in ALGS such as aneurysms or stenosis of the aorta and the renal, celiac, mesenteric, and subclavian arteries [28, 31, 78].

A bleeding tendency has also been observed in ALGS and episodes of bleeding unrelated to structural vascular anomalies or coagulation defects have been reported in up to 15% of patients. An underlying pathogenetic hypothesis is that the intrinsic impaired integrity of blood vessels in ALGS may predispose to vascular injury. Hemorrhage may arise spontaneously, after minor traumas or during invasive procedures. Bleeding has principally been observed in the intracranial circulation as subarachnoid, subdural, epidural, or intra-parenchymal hemorrhage [31, 34, 78, 80].

Vascular abnormalities constitute a significant cause of morbidity with vascular accidents and spontaneous bleeding episodes accounting for 34% of the overall mortality in ALGS [28, 31]. Also, patients with ALGS who undergo LT have a higher incidence of vascular complications [56].

4.4.7   Additional Features

4.4.7.1 Growth Impairment

Short stature and failure to thrive are described in 50–90% of patients with ALGS [81]. The pathogenesis is considered to be multifactorial in relation to inadequate caloric intake, fat malabsorption secondary to cholestatic liver disease, increased energy expenditure due to heart disease, and growth hormone resistance in the context of chronic kidney disease [82]. A recent longitudinal study including 293 ALGS patients with cholestasis showed that hyperbilirubinemia has a negative, although modest, effect on height and weight z-scores, and did not observe any association between congenital heart defects and growth impairment [35]. These results support that growth impairment may be intrinsic to ALGS genetic determinants rather than to heart or liver disease [32]. Indeed, notwithstanding a larger degree of post-transplant catch-up growth in comparison to other cholestatic liver disorders [33], children with ALGS retain a deficit in linear growth even after LT [83].

4.4.7.2 Developmental Delay

Impaired gross motor skills and intellectual disability has been reported in approximately 10% of ALGS patients [31]. Before LT severe pruritus, xanthomas, and low weight/height z-scores have been recognized as significant predictors of intellectual disability [84]. After LT children with ALGS have lower school performance and higher prevalence of intellectual disability (10%) in comparison to children transplanted for biliary atresia [33]. Almost half of ALGS patients require a special education both before and after LT [33, 39].

4.4.7.3 Immune Dysregulation

An "immunological phenotype" characterized by recurrent otitis media and respiratory infections has been described in up to a third of ALGS patients [41, 85]. Moreover, few patients have been reported with chronic inflammatory conditions (i.e., inflammatory bowel disease, vasculitis, granulomatous disease) [31, 86–88]. Very recently the association between ALGS and rheumatologic disorders has been highlighted by a multicentric survey showing a 5% prevalence of chronic arthritis in a population of almost 200 ALGS patients (Fig. 4.2). Arthritis was generally difficult to treat and resistant to the conventional drugs used for juvenile idiopathic arthritis [89]. The pathogenic mechanism underlying the immunological features of ALGS is still undetermined but may involve local anatomical anomalies/dysmorphisms compromising the drainage of airway secretions as well as an immune dysregulation caused by failure of the JAGGED-1/Notch/CD46 system [88, 90].

4.5 Diagnosis

4.5.1 Diagnostic Criteria

ALGS was historically a purely clinical and histologically based diagnosis requiring the demonstration of bile duct paucity on liver biopsy in addition to at least three out of five major clinical features: cholestasis, cardiac defects, characteristic facial appearance, posterior embryotoxon, and butterfly shaped vertebrae. In recent years, not only the phenotypic criteria of ALGS have been expanded to include kidney and vascular abnormalities, but also the presence/absence of genetic mutations in *JAG1* or *NOTCH2* and a family history of disease have been added into the diagnostic criteria of ALGS (see Table 4.2 for the revised diagnostic criteria of ALGS by Kamath et al. [42]).

4.5.2 Clinical Evaluation

As ALGS is a multisystem disease, a thorough clinical assessment should be performed. The main biochemical tests and imaging studies needed for the initial evaluation of subjects with suspected ALGS are summarized in Table 4.3. If the patient fulfills ALGS diagnostic criteria, liver biopsy is no longer mandatory to confirm diagnosis [91]. However, it may be considered when other liver disorders

Table 4.2 Revised diagnostic criteria for ALGS adapted from Kamath et al. [42]

Pathogenic variant in *JAG1* or *NOTCH2*	Family history of ALGS	Number of clinical criteria required	Clinical criteria of ALGS
Identified	None (proband)	At least 1[a]	1. **Liver:** bile duct paucity, cholestasis 2. **Heart:** peripheral pulmonary stenosis, tetralogy of Fallot 3. **Face:** typical facial appearance 4. **Eye:** posterior embryotoxon 5. **Skeleton:** butterfly vertebrae 6. **Kidney:** renal hypoplasia/dysplasia with or w/o cysts, CAKUT[b], renal tubular acidosis 7. **Vessels:** aneurysms/stenosis of intracranial vessels, Moyamoya disease, aneurysms/stenosis of systemic arteries
Identified	Present	Any or none	
Not identified[c]	None (proband)	3 or more	
Not identified[c]	Present	2 or more	

[a]The exact terminology regarding an individual with a disease-causing variant but no clinical features of ALGS remains to be determined. This individual cannot be described as "affected" by ALGS but still has a 50% chance of disease transmission to offspring. For the purposes of making the diagnosis of ALGS in a proband, at least one clinical feature is required in addition to a pathogenic genetic variant
[b]*CAKUT* Congenital Anomalies of the Kidneys and of the Urinary Tract
[c]"Not identified" should be intended as genetic test not done or performed employing molecular diagnostic techniques with low mutation detection rates. If after adequate genetic tests no pathogenic variants are identified in the *JAG1* or *NOTCH2* gene and chromosomal defects are excluded, the likelihood of ALGS is very low, particularly if clinical manifestations are not cardinal features

Table 4.3 Main biochemical tests and imaging studies performed during the initial evaluation of subjects with suspected ALGS

Liver	Assessment of liver function tests, bile acids, cholesterol, clotting parameters, fat-soluble vitamins.
	Liver ultrasound. Liver biopsy (if indicated).
Face	Dysmorphological evaluation.
Heart	Cardiac evaluation, electrocardiogram, echocardiogram.
Skeleton	Spinal or A-P chest X-ray.
Eye	Ophthalmologic assessment.
Kidney	Assessment of renal function tests and kidney ultrasound.

are suspected (for example during the diagnostic evaluation of infant cholestasis), when genetic testing is unavailable, or when the diagnosis of ALGS is uncertain [40, 42].

4.5.3 Genetic Testing

Pathogenic variants in *JAG1* (ALGS type 1; OMIM #118450) and *NOTCH2* (ALGS type 2; OMIM #610205) account for up to 96% of cases of ALGS (*JAG1*, 92–94%; *NOTCH2*, 2–4%) [92]. The majority of *JAG1* variants (85%) consists of nonsense, missense, and splice site mutations, while the minority (around 10%) is constituted by large deletions in chromosome 20p. *NOTCH2* disease-causing variants are predominantly missense, but also include splice site and nonsense pathogenic mutations [18, 92].

Based on the above, genetic testing for ALGS requires both sequencing and copy number analyses, which can be carried out by Sanger sequencing and chromosomal deletion/duplication analysis, or next generation sequencing (NGS) with copy number variation (CNV) analysis. The usual current approach is to sequence all exons and adjacent intronic regions of *JAG1*. If CNV analysis is not carried out simultaneously with sequencing, second tier diagnostics involves large deletion/duplication analysis through array comparative genomic hybridization (aCGH), multiplex ligation-dependent probe amplification (MLPA), or fluorescence in situ hybridization (FISH), which can identify an additional 10% of pathogenic variants. If no pathogenic variants are identified in *JAG1*, *NOTCH2* sequencing is performed to uncover an additional 2–4% of pathogenic variants. As no large deletions or duplications of *NOTCH2* have been described so far, the analysis of this gene does not typically include copy number analysis [18, 92]. However, thanks to the latest technological improvements, sequencing of the coding region of *JAG1* and *NOTCH2* together with *JAG1* CNV analysis can now be simultaneously performed employing the NGS technology coupled with CNV investigation. Once a *JAG1* or *NOTCH2* pathogenic variant is identified in a proband, parents should be tested to establish if the mutation has been inherited (30–50% of cases) or has occurred *de novo* (50–70% of cases) [42]. If no parental mutation is identified, the recurrence risk is limited to the chance of germline mosaicism, which is estimated around 1–3% [42].

In subjects (3–6%) with clinical features of ALGS but no pathogenic variants in *JAG1* or *NOTCH2* (after adequate genetic investigations), other diagnoses should be suspected and more comprehensive genetic investigations (such as whole exome sequencing, whole genome sequencing, or RNA sequencing) performed. Indeed, clinical features overlapping with those of ALGS have been observed in patients affected by other genetic disorders such as progressive familial intrahepatic cholestasis type 1 (*ATP8B1*) and 3 (*ABCB4*), hepatic-pancreatic-dysplasia 2 (*NEK8*), and *HFN1β* deficiency (HFN1β) [54, 92–95].

4.6   Management

ALGS is a multisystem disorder characterized by a highly variable disease severity ranging from trivial to life-threatening clinical manifestations. A multidisciplinary approach is required to define the degree of organ involvement and to establish an appropriate management tailored on the single patient phenotype. Although no treatment is available for the definitive cure of ALGS, several supportive and corrective treatments are available. These treatments vary depending on the type and severity of organ involvement and may involve extended hospitalizations, surgical operations, transplantations, and other costly interventions [1].

The cornerstones of ALGS management are described below in separated sections.

4.6.1   Liver Disease

There is currently no etiologic treatment for ALGS-related liver disease. Thus, its management is either constituted by supportive measures or by substitution of the liver with a healthy allograft. Other than those required for any kind of chronic liver disease, supportive measures mainly focus on controlling pruritus, supporting nutrition and fat-soluble vitamin deficiencies and managing cholesterol levels.

4.6.1.1 Pruritus

The management of pruritus in ALGS is challenging and often requires the employment of a combination of multiple pharmacological therapies and possibly surgical interventions. There are no specific therapeutic strategies, but a stepwise approach is usually preferred [40, 96]. If itching is intermittent and mild, antihistamines, such as hydroxyzine or diphenhydramine, can be used. Unfortunately, antihistamines are short lived and not typically effective in the long term. Patients with persistent and moderate to severe pruritus require a chronic treatment. Options for therapy include different drugs, usually employed in combination. First-line therapy is ursodeoxycholic acid (UDCA) which stimulates biliary secretion and reduces bile toxicity. It has an excellent safety profile but it is usually not sufficient to control pruritus as a mono-therapy [40, 96]. Cholestyramine and rifampin are used as second- and third-line treatments, respectively. Cholestyramine is a bile sequestrant that interrupts the enterohepatic circulation of bile acids. Its efficacy is hampered by poor palatability and by possible adverse effects (bloating, constipation, malabsorption of fat and fat-soluble vitamins) [40, 96]. Rifampicin is a pregnane-X receptor (PXR) agonist which induces the hydroxylation of bile acids promoting their urinary excretion. Treatment with rifampicin is very effective in controlling pruritus and, despite a potential risk of hepatotoxicity, presents a very low rate of adverse effects [40, 96]. Naltrexone, a μ-opioid receptor antagonist, constitutes a fourth line of treatment. It is similarly effective as rifampicin but less tolerated. In the largest reported study, almost a third of children with ALGS experienced side effects, mainly consisting of opioid with-drawal symptoms [40, 96]. As a fifth-line option, sertraline, a selective serotonin re-uptake inhibitor (SSRI), can be applied. Despite its mechanism of action remains elusive, sertraline has proven effective in controlling pruritus both in chil-dren and adults with ALGS. Non-severe behavior disorders have been reported in children with ALGS treated with sertraline, all of which resolved after discontinu-ation of treatment [97]. Newer pharmacological therapies for cholestatic pruritus, such as apical sodium-dependent bile acid transporter (ASBT) inhibitors (e.g., maralixibat, odevixibat), are currently being investigated and may be effective in ALGS [98].

Even with optimal medical management, pruritus may persist in up to 20% of patients [96]. In this case, surgery or LT have to be considered. Surgical interven-tions are performed in around 10% of patients with ALGS [35]. They aim to disrupt the enterohepatic circulation of bile acids and include partial external biliary diver-sion (PEBD), ileal exclusion, and internal biliary diversion. In patients without end-stage liver disease, these operations have proven to be effective in ameliorating pruritus and to carry lower morbidity and mortality than LT. They did not appear, however, to prevent the progression of liver disease [96, 99–101].

4.6.1.2 Nutrition

Malabsorption due to cholestasis can lead to growth failure, malnutrition, and fat-soluble vitamin (A, D, E, K) deficiencies. Nutritional care and constant monitoring of growth are thus mandatory in ALGS patients, especially during childhood. Adequate caloric and protein intake should be granted either by the oral or enteral route. Medium-chain triglycerides (MCT), which do not require micellar formation for absorption, are usually employed in cholestatic patients to increase lipid intesti-nal absorption. Fat-soluble vitamins should be periodically checked (2–3 times/year) and supplemented if deficient [40].

4.6.1.3 Hypercholesterolemia

Hypercholesterolemia is one of the hallmark features of ALGS. The increase in serum cholesterol is proportional to the degree of the cholestasis and is caused by multiple abnormalities in the hepatic metabolism of cholesterol. These include: (1) an overall augmented cholesterol production due to increased HMG CoA-reductase activity; (2) an augmented production of unesterified cholesterol due to inhibition of the lecithin/cholesterol acyltransferase (LCAT) activity; (3) the development of an abnormal lipoprotein (called lipoprotein X or LpX), formed as a complex of free unesterified cholesterol and albumin, that cannot be effectively cleared from the blood by the LDL receptor [102]. Apart from isolated case reports describing the presence of atheromatous plaques in subjects with ALGS [41, 103], the majority of the studies did not demonstrate an increased risk of atherosclerosis, possibly due to the protective effect of LpX and HDL elevation [104, 105]. Based on these observa-tions, at present there are no indications for the pharmacological treatment of hyper-cholesterolemia in ALGS.

4.6.1.4 Liver Transplantation

LT is a well-established therapy in ALGS and is required in a significant proportion of patients (see Sect. 4.4.1.2). ALGS represents approximately 5% of overall indications for LT in children with a median age at operation ranging from 2 to 6.5 years of age [83]. The reported indications for LT in ALGS are extremely heterogeneous and can be broadly classified into: (1) complications of chronic liver disease such as decompensation of hepatic synthetic function, uncontrolled portal hypertension, or chronic encephalopathy; (2) complications of chronic cholestasis such as intractable pruritus, failure to thrive, malnutrition, disfiguring xanthomas, severe hypercholesterolemia, bone fractures, or hepatic osteodystrophy [1]. The outcome of LT in ALGS is hampered by higher morbidity and mortality rates in comparison to other cholestatic liver disorders, especially in children. The largest multicenter retrospective study, reporting data from the UNOS (United Network for Organ Sharing) database, examined the outcome of 461 children with ALGS over a 21-year period (1987–2008). Patient survival was 82.9% and 78.4% at 1 years and 5 years after LT, respectively [106]. Another study, reporting data from the SPLIT (Studies in Pediatric Liver Transplantation) registry, examined the outcome of 91 children with ALGS over a 14-year period (1995–2009). One- and 5-year patient survival were similar at 87% and 86% [33]. A single study of 44 adults (mean age 30 years, UNOS database) found that 1- and 5-year patient survival (95.5% and 90.9%, respectively) are superior in adults than in children [107]. The higher mortality in ALGS mainly occurs in the first 30 days after LT due to post-transplant surgical problems such as vascular (20%) and biliary tract complications (15%) [1, 33]. Renal complications are also common (9.9%) both in the short- and long term after LT due to the underlying ALGS kidney disease and to the exposure to nephrotoxic drugs such as calcineurin inhibitors (see also Sects. 4.4.5 and 4.6.4) [1, 33]. Pre-transplant heart disease has been identified as an independent predictor of early post-transplant mortality [31]. Based on these data, the indication(s) for LT should be carefully considered in ALGS. Moreover, a thorough evaluation of all comorbidities, with particular attention to the cardiovascular and renal involvement, is mandatory before LT to estimate surgical risks [83].

4.6.2   Heart Disease and Pulmonary Vascular Involvement

Given the high prevalence of congenital heart disease, all subjects with or suspected with ALGS should undergo a full cardiac evaluation. In case of peripheral pulmonary arterial hypoplasia and/or stenosis, Tc-99 lung perfusion scan and pulmonary angiography can provide information regarding the relative distribution of blood flow to the lungs and the anatomy of the pulmonary arterial vessels, respectively. Cardiovascular involvement should be fully investigated and potentially treated prior to any consideration for LT [56]. Right ventricular hypertrophy and pulmonary hypertension complicating pulmonary vascular involvement may decrease cardiac vascular reserve [108, 109]. In fact, the inability to increase right ventricular output in the early post-transplant period may cause fluid overload, acute heart failure, and graft loss. In addition to standard procedures, an invasive dynamic stress test evaluating cardiac performance has been proposed: an increase $\geq 40\%$ of cardiac output during continuous infusion of dobutamine is indicative of a cardiac reserve adequate for LT [108].

No specific indications or guidelines exist for the treatment of congenital heart defects in ALGS, which can be managed according to standard practice. Cardiac surgery as well as non-surgical strategies (e.g., vasal stenting, valvuloplasty) and combined surgical-transcatheter interventions have all been successfully employed in ALGS patients [91, 110–112]. A single case of combined heart-lung-liver transplant has been reported in a child with ALGS [113].

4.6.3 Bone Disease

The presence of osteopenia/osteoporosis should be investigated through dual-energy X-ray absorptiometry especially in patients with severe cholestasis and/or bone fractures. Vitamin D and calcium supplementations are recommended in order to optimize bone health [67, 91]. No specific guidelines exist for the treatment of bone disease secondary to ALGS and/or chronic cholestasis, although if a patient has recurrent fractures, treatment with bisphosphonates and LT have to be considered.

4.6.4 Kidney Disease

Any patient diagnosed with ALGS should undergo an initial nephrological evaluation including blood pressure management, renal laboratory tests, urinalysis, and kidney ultrasound. If arterial hypertension is present, additional evaluations of the abdominal aorta and renal arteries are warranted to look for causes of renovascular hypertension (e.g., abdominal CT or magnetic resonance angiography). Serial nephrological assessments are also indicated as renal disease can manifest at any age and renal function may be negatively affected by concomitant heart and/or liver disease(s) [22, 74]. Management of ALGS-related nephro-urological disorders should be tailored on the specific phenotype according to standard practice.

Given the risk of renal damage after LT, a thorough nephrological assessment should be conducted in all patients undergoing evaluation for transplantation and renal function should be regularly supervised in the post-transplant period [114, 115]. Although there is no established specific immunosuppression regimen, careful monitoring, minimization, or avoidance of potentially nephrotoxic immunosuppressive therapy should be strongly considered [73, 74]. In some institutions, ALGS patients receive a tailored immunosuppression using early introduction of mycophenolate mofetil and reduced tacrolimus levels from 3 months or earlier because of risk of renal dysfunction (particularly renal tubular acidosis) exacerbated by tacrolimus [109].

4.6.5   Extra-Cardiac/Extra-Pulmonary Vascular Involvement

Given the high prevalence of cerebral vasculopathies in ALGS, a prompt neuroimaging should be provided to all patients with neurological concerns. As no specific treatment exists for ALGS-related vascular disease, eventual treatment approaches should follow standard strategies.

Due to limited data regarding the natural history of vasculopathy in ALGS, the role of routine neuroimaging in asymptomatic patients remains controversial. Several authors recommend that all ALGS patients undergo a screening magnetic resonance angiography at an age at which they do not require sedation and/or prior to any major surgerical intervention including LT [28, 78, 79].

4.7   Conclusions

After 50 years from the first description of the disease by the French hepatologist Daniel Alagille, the comprehensive knowledge about ALGS has grown incredibly. The genetic basis as well as the clinical complexity of ALGS are now well acknowledged. Next generation sequencing technologies currently allow for a timely, efficient and inexpensive diagnosis of ALGS and for reliable genetic counseling. Nowadays, LT constitutes the standard of care for the treatment of ALGS patients affected by end-stage liver disease or overwhelmed by the complications of chronic cholestasis.

Still, many biological questions and clinical challenges remain to be solved. The pathogenic mechanisms by which *JAG1* and *NOTCH2* mutations lead to bile duct paucity remain to be elucidated. The molecular determinants of the broad phenotypic variability and of the unique course of liver disease in ALGS are mostly unrecognized. Novel treatments are needed to control pruritus, which still constitutes an extremely burdensome symptom for many patients. Specific therapeutic strategies allowing for a definite cure of ALGS are lacking. Future studies will surely aim to provide answers to these questions and solutions to these unmet needs.

4.8   Highlights

1. ALGS is a rare, autosomal dominant disorder caused by defects in genes (*JAG1* or *NOTCH2*) involved in the Notch signaling pathway and characterized by multisystem anomalies resulting from the abnormal development of intrahepatic bile ducts, heart, kidneys, bones, eyes, and vessels.
2. ALGS is characterized by a highly variable severity ranging from trivial to life-threatening clinical manifestations. The overall mortality rate ranges from 10% to 35% with main causes of death consisting of vascular accidents, cardiac malformations, and liver disease.

3. The liver is the most commonly affected organ with bile duct paucity being the hallmark histological feature of ALGS. Most patients (80–90%) present in the first year of life with cholestatic liver disease. Almost half (40%) suffer from the complications of persistent cholestasis and/or present clinically evident portal hypertension by 20 years of age. A significant, albeit variable, proportion of affected individuals (15–75%) require LT along life.
4. The diagnosis relies on the demonstration of *JAG1* or *NOTCH2* pathogenic variants, on the presence of a family history of disease and on the identification of one or more clinical features of ALGS. Liver biopsy is no longer mandatory if diagnostic criteria are fulfilled.
5. No curative treatment is available for ALGS. The management of liver disease is either constituted by supportive measures (mainly focused on controlling pruritus and supporting nutrition) or by substitution of the liver with a healthy allograft.
6. The outcome of LT in ALGS is hampered by higher morbidity and mortality rates in comparison to other cholestatic liver disorders, especially in children.

References

1. Kamath BM, Baker A, Houwen R, Todorova L, Kerkar N. Systematic review: the epidemiology, natural history, and burden of Alagille syndrome. J Pediatr Gastroenterol Nutr. 2018;67(2):148–56.
2. Alagille D, Borde J, Habib EC, Thomassin N. Tentatives chirurgicales au cours des atrésies des voies biliaires intra-hépatiques avec voie biliaire extra-hépatique perméable. Etude de 14 observations chez l'enfant. Arch Fr Pediatr. 1969;26(1):51–71.
3. Watson GH, Miller V. Arteriohepatic dysplasia. Familial pulmonary arterial stenosis with neonatal liver disease. Arch Dis Child. 1973;48(6):459–66.
4. Piccoli DA. Alagille syndrome: overview and introduction. In:Alagille syndrome: pathogenesis and clinical management. Cham: Springer International Publishing; 2018. p. 1–9.
5. Valamparampil JJ, Reddy MS, Shanmugam N, Vij M, Kanagavelu RG, Rela M. Living donor liver transplantation in Alagille syndrome—single center experience from south Asia. Pediatr Transplant. 2019;23(8):e13579.
6. Heritage ML, MacMillan JC, Colliton RP, Genin A, Spinner NB, Anderson GJ. Jagged1 (JAG1) mutation detection in an Australian Alagille syndrome population. Hum Mutat. 2000;16(5):408–16.
7. Li L, Dong J, Wang X, Guo H, Wang H, Zhao J, et al. JAG1 mutation spectrum and origin in chinese children with clinical features of Alagille syndrome. PLoS One. 2015;10(6):e0130355.
8. Danks DM, Campbell PE, Jack I, Rogers J, Smith AL. Studies of the aetiology of neonatal hepatitis and biliary atresia. Arch Dis Child. 1977;52(5):360–7.
9. Eldadah ZA. Familial tetralogy of fallot caused by mutation in the jagged1 gene. Hum Mol Genet. 2001;10(2):163–9.
10. Le Caignec C, Lefevre M, Schott JJ, Chaventre A, Gayet M, Calais C, et al. Familial deafness, congenital heart defects, and posterior embryotoxon caused by cysteine substitution in the first epidermal-growth-factor-like domain of Jagged 1. Am J Hum Genet. 2002;71(1):180–6.
11. Adams JM, Jafar-Nejad H. The roles of notch signaling in liver development and disease. Biomolecules. 2019;9:608.
12. Jones EA, Clement-Jones M, Wilson DI. JAGGED1 expression in human embryos: correlation with the Alagille syndrome phenotype. J Med Genet. 2000;37(9):658–62.

13. Tchorz JS, Kinter J, Müller M, Tornillo L, Heim MH, Bettler B. Notch2 signaling promotes biliary epithelial cell fate specification and tubulogenesis during bile duct development in mice. Hepatology. 2009;50(3):871–9.

14. Hofmann JJ, Zovein AC, Koh H, Radtke F, Weinmaster G, Iruela-Arispe ML. Jagged1 in the portal vein mesenchyme regulates intrahepatic bile duct development: insights into Alagille syndrome. Development. 2010;137(23):4061–72.

15. Sparks EE, Perrien DS, Huppert KA, Peterson TE, Huppert SS. Defects in hepatic Notch signaling result in disruption of the communicating intrahepatic bile duct network in mice. Dis Model Mech. 2011;4(3):359–67.

16. Tanimizu N, Kaneko K, Itoh T, Ichinohe N, Ishii M, Mizuguchi T, et al. Intrahepatic bile ducts are developed through formation of homogeneous continuous luminal network and its dynamic rearrangement in mice. Hepatology. 2016;64(1):175–88.

17. Guan Y, Xu D, Garfin PM, Ehmer U, Hurwitz M, Enns G, et al. Human hepatic organoids for the analysis of human genetic diseases. JCI Insight. 2017;2(17):e94954.

18. Gilbert MA, Spinner NB. Genetics of Alagille syndrome. In:Alagille syndrome: pathogenesis and clinical management. Cham: Springer International Publishing; 2018. p. 33–48.

19. Dhorne-Pollet S, Deleuze JF, Hadchouel M, Bonaïti-Pellié C. Segregation analysis of Alagille syndrome. J Med Genet. 1994;31(6):453–7.

20. Kamath BM, Bason L, Piccoli DA, Krantz ID, Spinner NB. Consequences of JAG1 mutations. J Med Genet. 2003;40(12):891–5.

21. Bauer RC, Laney AO, Smith R, Gerfen J, Morrissette JJD, Woyciechowski S, et al. Jagged1 (JAG1) mutations in patients with tetralogy of fallot or pulmonic stenosis. Hum Mutat. 2010;31(5):594–601.

22. Jacquet A, Guiochon-Mantel A, Noël LH, Sqalli T, Bedossa P, Hadchouel M, et al. Alagille syndrome in adult patients: it is never too late. Am J Kidney Dis. 2007;49(5):705–9.

23. Izumi K, Hayashi D, Grochowski CM, Kubota N, Nishi E, Arakawa M, et al. Discordant clinical phenotype in monozygotic twins with Alagille syndrome: possible influence of non-genetic factors. Am J Med Genet A. 2016;170(2):471–5.

24. Tsai EA, Gilbert MA, Grochowski CM, Underkoffler LA, Meng H, Zhang X, et al. THBS2 is a candidate modifier of liver disease severity in Alagille syndrome. Cell Mol Gastroenterol Hepatol. 2016;2(5):663–675.e2.

25. Adams JM, Huppert KA, Castro EC, Lopez MF, Niknejad N, Subramanian S, et al. Sox9 is a modifier of the liver disease severity in a mouse model of Alagille syndrome. Hepatology. 2020;71(4):1331–49.

26. Kamath BM, Hutchinson A, Bauer R, Gerfen J, Krantz ID, Piccoli DA, et al. 26 Notch2 mutations in Alagille syndrome. J Hepatol. 2011;54(2):S12–3.

27. Kamath BM, Thiel BD, Gai X, Conlin LK, Munoz PS, Glessner J, et al. SNP array mapping of chromosome 20p deletions: genotypes, phenotypes, and copy number variation. Hum Mutat. 2009;30(3):371–8.

28. Kamath BM, Spinner NB, Emerick KM, Chudley AE, Booth C, Piccoli DA, et al. Vascular anomalies in Alagille syndrome: a significant cause of morbidity and mortality. Circulation. 2004;109(11):1354–8.

29. Lykavieris P, Hadchouel M, Chardot C, Bernard O. Outcome of liver disease in children with Alagille syndrome: a study of 163 patients. Gut. 2001;49(3):431–5.

30. Hoffenberg EJ, Narkewicz MR, Sondheimer JM, Smith DJ, Silverman A, Sokol RJ. Outcome of syndromic paucity of interlobular bile ducts (Alagille syndrome) with onset of cholestasis in infancy. J Pediatr. 1995;127(2):220–4.

31. Emerick KM, Rand EB, Goldmuntz E, Krantz ID, Spinner NB, Piccoli DA. Features of Alagille syndrome in 92 patients: frequency and relation to prognosis. Hepatology. 1999;29(3):822–9.

32. Mitchell E, Gilbert M, Loomes KM. Alagille syndrome. Clin Liver Dis. 2018;22(4):625–41.

33. Kamath BM, Yin W, Miller H, Anand R, Rand EB, Alonso E, et al. Outcomes of liver transplantation for patients with Alagille syndrome: the studies of pediatric liver transplantation experience. Liver Transpl. 2012;18(8):940–8.

34. Kamath BM, Loomes KM. Alagille syndrome: pathogenesis and clinical management. Cham: Springer International Publishing; 2018.
35. Kamath BM, Ye W, Goodrich NP, Loomes KM, Romero R, Heubi JE, et al. Outcomes of childhood cholestasis in Alagille syndrome: results of a multicenter observational study. Hepatol Commun. 2020;4(3):387–98.
36. Subramaniam P, Knisely A, Portmann B, Qureshi S, Aclimandos W, Karani J, et al. Diagnosis of Alagille syndrome-25 years of experience at King's College Hospital. J Pediatr Gastroenterol Nutr. 2011;52(1):84–9.
37. Wang JS, Wang XH, Zhu QR, Wang ZL, Hu XQ, Zheng S. Clinical and pathological characteristics of Alagille syndrome in Chinese children. World J Pediatr. 2008;4(4):283–8.
38. Kamath BM, Abetz-Webb L, Kennedy C, Hepburn B, Gauthier M, Johnson N, et al. Development of a novel tool to assess the impact of itching in pediatric cholestasis. Patient. 2018;11(1):69–82.
39. Elisofon SA, Emerick KM, Sinacore JM, Alonso EM. Health status of patients with Alagille syndrome. J Pediatr Gastroenterol Nutr. 2010;51(6):759–65.
40. Kriegermeier A, Wehrman A, Kamath BM, Loomes KM. Liver disease in Alagille syndrome. In:Alagille syndrome: pathogenesis and clinical management. Cham: Springer International Publishing; 2018. p. 49–65.
41. Quiros-Tejeira RE, Ament ME, Heyman MB, Martin MG, Rosenthal P, Hall TR, et al. Variable morbidity in Alagille syndrome: a review of 43 cases. J Pediatr Gastroenterol Nutr. 1999;29(4):431–7.
42. Kamath BM, Spinner NB, Piccoli DA. Alagille syndrome. Liver disease in children. 4th ed. New York, NY: Cambridge University Press; 2011. p. 216–33.
43. Kamath BM, Munoz PS, Bab N, Baker A, Chen Z, Spinner NB, et al. A longitudinal study to identify laboratory predictors of liver disease outcome in Alagille syndrome. J Pediatr Gastroenterol Nutr. 2010;50(5):526–30.
44. Mouzaki M, Bass LM, Sokol RJ, Piccoli DA, Quammie C, Loomes KM, et al. Early life predictive markers of liver disease outcome in an international, multicentre cohort of children with Alagille syndrome. Liver Int. 2016;36(5):755–60.
45. Gunadi, Kaneshiro M, Okamoto T, Sonoda M, Ogawa E, Okajima H, et al. Outcomes of liver transplantation for Alagille syndrome after Kasai portoenterostomy: Alagille syndrome with agenesis of extrahepatic bile ducts at porta hepatis. J Pediatr Surg. 2019;54(11):2387–91.
46. Fujishiro J, Suzuki K, Watanabe M, Uotani C, Takezoe T, Takamoto N, et al. Outcomes of Alagille syndrome following the Kasai operation: a systematic review and meta-analysis. Pediatr Surg Int. 2018;34(10):1073–7.
47. Kaye AJ, Rand EB, Munoz PS, Spinner NB, Flake AW, Kamath BM. Effect of Kasai procedure on hepatic outcome in Alagille syndrome. J Pediatr Gastroenterol Nutr. 2010;51(3):319–21.
48. Valamparampil JJ, Shanmugam N, Vij M, Reddy MS, Rela M. Hepatocellular carcinoma in paediatric patients with Alagille syndrome: case series and review of literature. J Gastrointest Cancer. 2020;51(3):1047.
49. Tsai S, Gurakar A, Anders R, Lam-Himlin D, Boitnott J, Pawlik TM. Management of large hepatocellular carcinoma in adult patients with Alagille syndrome: a case report and review of literature. Dig Dis Sci. 2010;55:3052–8.
50. Pacheco MC, Monroe EJ, Horslen SP. Hepatic adenoma arising in a patient with Alagille syndrome: a case report. Pediatr Dev Pathol. 2018;21(6):585–9.
51. Ennaifer R, Ben Farhat L, Cheikh M, Romdhane H, Marzouk I, Belhadj N. Focal liver hyperplasia in a patient with Alagille syndrome: diagnostic difficulties. A case report. Int J Surg Case Rep. 2016;25:55–61.
52. Rapp JB, Bellah RD, Maya C, Pawel BR, Anupindi SA. Giant hepatic regenerative nodules in Alagille syndrome. Pediatr Radiol. 2017;47(2):197–204.
53. Yehezkely-Schildkraut V, Munichor M, Mandel H, Berkowitz D, Hartman C, Eshach-Adiv O, et al. Nonsyndromic paucity of interlobular bile ducts: report of 10 patients. J Pediatr Gastroenterol Nutr. 2003;37:546–9.

54. Pinon M, Carboni M, Colavito D, Cisarò F, Peruzzi L, Pizzol A, et al. Not only Alagille syndrome. Syndromic paucity of interlobular bile ducts secondary to HNF1β deficiency: a case report and literature review. Ital J Pediatr. 2019;45(1):27.
55. Niessen K, Karsan A. Notch signaling in cardiac development. Circ Res. 2008;102:1169–81.
56. Tretter JT, McElhinney DB. Cardiac, aortic, and pulmonary vascular involvement in Alagille syndrome. In:Alagille syndrome: pathogenesis and clinical management. Cham: Springer International Publishing; 2018. p. 77–90.
57. Hofmann JJ, Briot A, Enciso J, Zovein AC, Ren S, Zhang ZW, et al. Endothelial deletion of murine Jag1 leads to valve calcification and congenital heart defects associated with Alagille syndrome. Development. 2012;139(23):4449–60.
58. McElhinney DB, Krantz ID, Bason L, Piccoli DA, Emerick KM, Spinner NB, et al. Analysis of cardiovascular phenotype and genotype-phenotype correlation in individuals with a JAG1 mutation and/or Alagille syndrome. Circulation. 2002;106(20):2567–74.
59. Fattouh AM, Mogahed EA, Hamid NA, Sobhy R, Saber N, El-Karaksy H. The prevalence of congenital heart defects in infants with cholestatic disorders of infancy: a single-centre study. Arch Dis Child. 2016;101(9):803–7.
60. Alagille D, Estrada A, Hadchouel M, Gautler M, Odièvre M, Dommergues JP. Syndromic paucity of interlobular bile ducts (Alagille syndrome or arteriohepatic dysplasia): review of 80 cases. J Pediatr. 1987;110(2):195–200.
61. Turnpenny PD, Ellard S. Alagille syndrome: pathogenesis, diagnosis and management. Eur J Hum Genet. 2012;20(3):251–7.
62. Kamath BM, Loomes KM, Oakey RJ, Emerick KEM, Conversano T, Spinner NB, et al. Facial features in Alagille syndrome: specific or cholestasis facies? Am J Med Genet. 2002;112(2):163–70.
63. Lin HC, Le Hoang P, Hutchinson A, Chao G, Gerfen J, Loomes KM, et al. Alagille syndrome in a Vietnamese cohort: mutation analysis and assessment of facial features. Am J Med Genet A. 2012;158 A(5):1005–13.
64. Humphreys R, Zheng W, Prince LS, Qu X, Brown C, Loomes K, et al. Cranial neural crest ablation of Jagged1 recapitulates the craniofacial phenotype of Alagille syndrome patients. Hum Mol Genet. 2012;21(6):1374–83.
65. Katsuura Y, Kim HJ. Butterfly vertebrae: a systematic review of the literature and analysis. Glob Spine J. 2019;9:666–79.
66. Teng CS, Yen HY, Barske L, Llamas J, Segil N, Go J, et al. Requirement for Jagged1-Notch2 signaling in patterning the bones of the mouse and human middle ear. Sci Rep. 2017;7(1):1–11.
67. Bales CB, Kamath BM, Munoz PS, Nguyen A, Piccoli DA, Spinner NB, et al. Pathologic lower extremity fractures in children with Alagille syndrome. J Pediatr Gastroenterol Nutr. 2010;51(1):66–70.
68. Wang C, Inzana JA, Mirando AJ, Ren Y, Liu Z, Shen J, et al. NOTCH signaling in skeletal progenitors is critical for fracture repair. J Clin Invest. 2016;126(4):1471–81.
69. Loomes KM, Spino C, Goodrich NP, Hangartner TN, Marker AE, Heubi JE, et al. Bone density in children with chronic liver disease correlates with growth and cholestasis. Hepatology. 2019;69(1):245–57.
70. Hilton MJ, Tu X, Wu X, Bai S, Zhao H, Kobayashi T, et al. Notch signaling maintains bone marrow mesenchymal progenitors by suppressing osteoblast differentiation. Nat Med. 2008;14(3):306–14.
71. Rennie CA, Chowdhury S, Khan J, Rajan F, Jordan K, Lamb RJ, et al. The prevalence and associated features of posterior embryotoxon in the general ophthalmic clinic. Eye. 2005;19(4):396–9.
72. Hingorani M, Nischal KK, Davies A, Bentley C, Vivian A, Baker AJ, et al. Ocular abnormalities in Alagille syndrome. Ophthalmology. 1999;106(2):330–7.
73. Kamath BM, Podkameni G, Hutchinson AL, Leonard LD, Gerfen J, Krantz ID, et al. Renal anomalies in Alagille syndrome: a disease-defining feature. Am J Med Genet A. 2012;158 A(1):85–9.

74. Kamath BM, Spinner NB, Rosenblum ND. Renal involvement and the role of notch signalling in Alagille syndrome. Nat Rev Nephrol. 2013;9(7):409–18.
75. Romero R. The renal sequelae of Alagille syndrome as a product of altered notch signaling during kidney development. In:Alagille syndrome: pathogenesis and clinical management. Cham: Springer International Publishing; 2018. p. 103–20.
76. Pitulescu ME, Schmidt I, Giaimo BD, Antoine T, Berkenfeld F, Ferrante F, et al. Dll4 and notch signalling couples sprouting angiogenesis and artery formation. Nat Cell Biol. 2017;19(8):915–27.
77. Krebs LT, Xue Y, Norton CR, Shutter JR, Maguire M, Sundberg JP, et al. Notch signaling is essential for vascular morphogenesis in mice. Genes Dev. 2000;14(11):1343–52.
78. Vandriel SM, Ichord RN, Kamath BM. Vascular manifestations in Alagille syndrome. In:Alagille syndrome: pathogenesis and clinical management. Cham: Springer International Publishing; 2018. p. 91–102.
79. Carpenter CD, Linscott LL, Leach JL, Vadivelu S, Abruzzo T. Spectrum of cerebral arterial and venous abnormalities in Alagille syndrome. Pediatr Radiol. 2018;48(4):602–8.
80. Lykavieris P, Crosnier C, Trichet C, Meunier-Rotival M, Hadchouel M. Bleeding tendency in children with Alagille syndrome. Pediatrics. 2003;111(1):167–70.
81. Arvay JL, Zemel BS, Gallagher PR, Rovner AJ, Mulberg AE, Stallings VA, et al. Body composition of children aged 1 to 12 years with biliary atresia or Alagille syndrome. J Pediatr Gastroenterol Nutr. 2005;40(2):146–50.
82. Bucuvalas JC, Horn JA, Carlsson L, Balistreri WF, Chernausek SD. Growth hormone insensitivity associated with elevated circulating growth hormone-binding protein in children with Alagille syndrome and short stature. J Clin Endocrinol Metab. 1993;76(6):1477–82.
83. Hsu E, Rand E. Transplant considerations in Alagille syndrome. In:Alagille syndrome: pathogenesis and clinical management. Cham: Springer International Publishing; 2018. p. 67–76.
84. Mohammad S, Alonso EM. Health-related quality of life and neurocognition in Alagille syndrome. In:Alagille syndrome: pathogenesis and clinical management. Cham: Springer International Publishing; 2018. p. 159–65.
85. Tilib Shamoun S, Le Friec G, Spinner N, Kemper C, Baker AJ. Immune dysregulation in Alagille syndrome: a new feature of the evolving phenotype. Clin Res Hepatol Gastroenterol. 2015;39(5):566–9.
86. Mannion M, Zolak M, Kelly DR, Beukelman T, Cron RQ. Sarcoidosis in a young child with Alagille syndrome: a case report. Pediatr Rheumatol. 2012;10(1):32.
87. Kavukçu S, Demir K, Soylu A, Anal Ö, Saatçi O, Göktay Y. A case of Takayasu disease with findings of incomplete Alagille syndrome. Rheumatol Int. 2005;25(7):555–7.
88. Baker A. Immune dysregulation in Alagille syndrome: a feature of the evolving phenotype. In:Alagille syndrome: pathogenesis and clinical management. Cham: Springer International Publishing; 2018. p. 137–57.
89. Ferrara G, Giani T, Lieberman SM, Kremer C, Hong S, Indolfi G, et al. Alagille syndrome and chronic arthritis: an international case series. J Pediatr. 2020;218:228–230.e1.
90. Cardone J, Le Friec G, Vantourout P, Roberts A, Fuchs A, Jackson I, et al. Complement regulator CD46 temporally regulates cytokine production by conventional and unconventional T cells. Nat Immunol. 2010;11(9):862–71.
91. Kamath BM, Loomes KM, Piccoli DA. Medical management of Alagille syndrome. J Pediatr Gastroenterol Nutr. 2010;50(6):580–6.
92. Gilbert MA, Bauer RC, Rajagopalan R, Grochowski CM, Chao G, McEldrew D, et al. Alagille syndrome mutation update: comprehensive overview of JAG1 and NOTCH2 mutation frequencies and insight into missense variant classification. Hum Mutat. 2019;40(12):2197–220.
93. Grochowski CM, Loomes KM, Spinner NB. Jagged1 (JAG1): structure, expression, and disease associations. Gene. 2016;576(1):381–4.
94. Rajagopalan R, Grochowski CM, Gilbert MA, Falsey AM, Coleman K, Romero R, et al. Compound heterozygous mutations in NEK8 in siblings with end-stage renal disease with hepatic and cardiac anomalies. Am J Med Genet A. 2016;170(3):750–3.

95. Schatz SB, Jüngst C, Keitel-Anselmo V, Kubitz R, Becker C, Gerner P, et al. Phenotypic spectrum and diagnostic pitfalls of ABCB4 deficiency depending on age of onset. Hepatol Commun. 2018;2(5):504–14.

96. Kronsten V, Fitzpatrick E, Baker A. Management of cholestatic pruritus in paediatric patients with Alagille syndrome: the King's College Hospital experience. J Pediatr Gastroenterol Nutr. 2013;57(2):149–54.

97. Thébaut A, Habes D, Gottrand F, Rivet C, Cohen J, Debray D, et al. Sertraline as an additional treatment for cholestatic pruritus in children. J Pediatr Gastroenterol Nutr. 2017;64(3):431–5.

98. Shneider BL, Spino C, Kamath BM, Magee JC, Bass LM, Setchell KD, et al. Placebo-controlled randomized trial of an intestinal bile salt transport inhibitor for pruritus in Alagille syndrome. Hepatol Commun. 2018;2(10):1184–98.

99. Mattei P, Von Allmen D, Piccoli D, Rand E. Relief of intractable pruritis in Alagille syndrome by partial external biliary diversion. J Pediatr Surg. 2006;41(1):104–7.

100. Sheflin-Findling S, Arnon R, Lee S, Chu J, Henderling F, Kerkar N, et al. Partial internal biliary diversion for Alagille syndrome: case report and review of the literature. J Pediatr Surg. 2012;47(7):1453–6.

101. Neimark E, Shneider B. Novel surgical and pharmacological approaches to chronic cholestasis in children: partial external biliary diversion for intractable pruritus and xanthomas in Alagille syndrome. J Pediatr Gastroenterol Nutr. 2003;36(2):296–7.

102. Hannoush ZC, Puerta H, Bauer MS, Goldberg RB. New JAG1 mutation causing Alagille syndrome presenting with severe hypercholesterolemia: case report with emphasis on genetics and lipid abnormalities. J Clin Endocrinol Metab. 2017;102(2):350–3.

103. Pombo F, Isla C, Gayol A, Bargiela A. Aortic calcification and renal cysts demonstrated by CT in a teenager with Alagille syndrome. Pediatr Radiol. 1995;25(4):314–5.

104. Nagasaka H, Yorifuji T, Egawa H, Yanai H, Fujisawa T, Kosugiyama K, et al. Evaluation of risk for atherosclerosis in Alagille syndrome and progressive familial intrahepatic cholestasis: two congenital cholestatic diseases with different lipoprotein metabolisms. J Pediatr. 2005;146(3):329–35.

105. Ijichi S, Kusaka T, Okada H, Tada S, Isobe K, Itoh S. Cellular cholesterol levels in platelets before and after liver transplantation in Alagille syndrome complicated by severe hypercholesterolemia. J Pediatr Gastroenterol Nutr. 2014;58(1):e9–10.

106. Arnon R, Annunziato R, Miloh T, Suchy F, Sakworawich A, Hiroshi S, et al. Orthotopic liver transplantation for children with Alagille syndrome. Pediatr Transplant. 2010;14(5):622–8.

107. Arnon R, Annunziato R, Schiano T, Miloh T, Baisley M, Sogawa H, et al. Orthotopic liver transplantation for adults with Alagille syndrome. Clin Transpl. 2012;26(2):E94.

108. Razavi RS, Baker A, Qureshi SA, Rosenthal E, Marsh MJ, Leech SC, et al. Hemodynamic response to continuous infusion of dobutamine in Alagille's syndrome. Transplantation. 2001;72(5):823–8.

109. Kamath BM, Schwarz KB, Hadžić N. Alagille syndrome and liver transplantation. J Pediatr Gastroenterol Nutr. 2010;50(1):11–5.

110. Zussman M, Hirsch R, Beekman RH, Goldstein BH. Impact of percutaneous interventions for pulmonary artery stenosis in Alagille syndrome. Congenit Heart Dis. 2015;10(4):310–6.

111. Bauser-Heaton H, Borquez A, Han B, Ladd M, Asija R, Downey L, et al. Programmatic approach to management of tetralogy of fallot with major aortopulmonary collateral arteries. Circ Cardiovasc Interv. 2017;10(4):e004952.

112. Cunningham JW, McElhinney DB, Gauvreau K, Bergersen L, Lacro RV, Marshall AC, et al. Outcomes after primary transcatheter therapy in infants and young children with severe bilateral peripheral pulmonary artery stenosis. Circ Cardiovasc Interv. 2013;6(4):460–7.

113. Gandhi SK, Reyes J, Webber SA, Siewers RD, Pigula FA. Case report of combined pediatric heart-lung-liver transplantation. Transplantation. 2002;73(12):1968–9.

114. Kelly DA, Bucuvalas JC, Alonso EM, Karpen SJ, Allen U, Green M, et al. Long-term medical management of the pediatric patient after liver transplantation: 2013 practice guideline by the American Association for the Study of Liver Diseases and the American Society of Transplantation. Liver Transpl. 2013;19(8):798–825.
115. Squires RH, Ng V, Romero R, Ekong U, Hardikar W, Emre S, et al. Evaluation of the pediatric patient for liver transplantation: 2014 practice guideline by the american association for the study of liver diseases, american society of transplantation and the north american society for pediatric gastroenterology, hepatology and nutrition. Hepatology. 2014;60(1):362–98.

Caroli's Disease

5

Raffaella Motta, Amalia Lupi, Andrea Pirazzini,
Chiara Giraudo, and Paolo Marchesi

5.1 Introduction

Caroli's disease was described for the first time in 1958 by a French gastroenterologist, Jacques Caroli. It is an autosomal recessive congenital disease, with an estimated incidence of 1:1,000,000 and higher prevalence in females.

Among biliary system non-neoplastic pathology, cystic disease represents a rare congenital condition. Todani's classification of bile duct cysts describes five main groups of cysts depending on intra- and/or extrahepatic bile ducts involvement. Caroli's disease is also referred to as type V bile duct cysts according to this classification.

The five main groups of Todani's classification are:

- **Type I**, choledochal cyst. It is the most frequent form (80–90%) and is thought to be due to an anomalous pancreatic-biliary junction, which results in a reflux of pancreatic secretion into the bile duct. The dilatation may extend to the entire extrahepatic duct (Ia) or be segmental (Ib) or fusiform (Ic).
- **Type II**, supraduodenal extrahepatic bile duct diverticulum. It accounts for 3% of all bile duct cysts.
- **Type III**, choledochocele, intramural segment dilatation, observed in 5% of cases and responsible of recurrent biliary colic or pancreatitis.

R. Motta (✉) · A. Lupi · A. Pirazzini · C. Giraudo
Institute of Radiology, Azienda Ospedale Università di Padova, University of Padova,
Padova, Italy
e-mail: raffaella.motta@unipd.it

P. Marchesi
Radiology Unit, Ospedale S. Antonio, Azienda Ospedale Università di Padova, Padova, Italy

© Springer Nature Switzerland AG 2021
A. Floreani (ed.), *Diseases of the Liver and Biliary Tree*,
https://doi.org/10.1007/978-3-030-65908-0_5

- **Type IV**, consists of intra- and extrahepatic (IVa) or extrahepatic only (IVb) bile ducts multiple dilatations, present in 10% of cases.
- **Type V**, known as Caroli Disease (CD) and characterized by multiple intrahepatic cystic dilatation.

5.2   Pathogenesis

CD is the result of an abnormal development of the ductal plate, a transient structure that appears at the sixth week of fetal life. From the 12th week to the end of the gestation or the very first postnatal period, the remodeling and partial involution of the ductal plate forms the biliary tree. The remodeling of the ductal plate starts from the hepatic hilum and progresses toward the periphery: the partial or complete interruption of this process may cause congenital cystic lesion formation, with different phenotypes depending on the stage in which the defect occurs (Fig. 5.1). The so-called *fibro-polycystic liver diseases* include:

1. Large bile ducts involvement: *Caroli's disease* (intrahepatic bile ducts involvement) or *choledochal cyst* (extrahepatic bile ducts involvement)
2. Medium bile ducts involvement: *autosomal dominant polycystic liver disease* (ARPKD)
3. Small bile ducts involvement: *biliary hamartomas* or *congenital hepatic fibrosis*

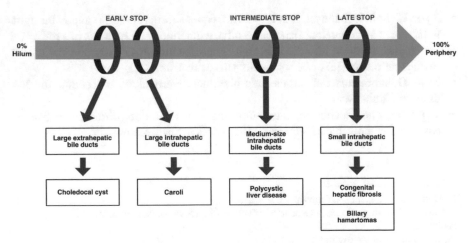

Fig. 5.1 Schematic representation of biliary system malformations. The remodeling and partial involution of the ductal plate starts at the hilum around the 12th week and progresses peripherally until it is completed by the end of the gestation. The phenotype of the fibro-polycystic liver disease depends on the stage of the embryological development in which the defect occurs

5.3   Clinical Characteristics

The onset of symptoms occurs during childhood or young adulthood, with intermittent abdominal pain (at the right upper quadrant), jaundice, and pruritus related to recurrent cholangitis episodes. Possible complications are related to bile stasis: intrahepatic stone formation, bacteremia, sepsis, hepatic abscesses, recurrent cholangitis, and secondary biliary cirrhosis. Cholangitis and abscesses are typically characterized by fever and malaise. An increased risk of cholangiocarcinoma is reported with a prevalence of 7%; chronic inflammation of the biliary epithelium may play an important role.

When both early and late stage anomalies of the ductal plate development occur, the CD coexists with another fibro-polycystic liver disease, typically congenital hepatic fibrosis. This condition is called Caroli's syndrome and it's more frequent than Caroli's disease. The association with congenital hepatic fibrosis can lead eventually to the development of portal hypertension, with subsequent ascites and variceal hemorrhages.

ARPKD and other fibro-polycystic liver diseases can occur in association with CD and congenital hepatic fibrosis.

5.4   Diagnosis

Imaging techniques well demonstrate diffuse, lobar, or segmental involvement of intrahepatic biliary ducts, as non-obstructive saccular or fusiform dilatations, usually up to about 5 cm in diameter, often containing calculi or sludge. Ultrasound (US) shows intraductal bridging, as echogenic septa traversing the dilated lumen, and stones, if present. The appearance of echogenic portal vein branches surrounded by hypoechoic dilated bile ducts is better seen on axial Computed Tomography (CT) scans examination as "central dot sign," in which the dot is represented by the portal branch cross-sectional view and become more evident after contrast media administration, in portal phase enhancement (Fig. 5.2). The "central dot sign" occasionally occurs in other pathologies (e.g., peribiliary cysts, periportal lymphedema, and jaundice due to biliary obstruction).

Magnetic Resonance Imaging (MRI) with cholangiopancreatography (MRCP) is the most efficient method to visualize non-invasively the biliary and pancreatic duct system. Dilated biliary tracts appear hypointense on T1-weighted images and hyperintense on T2w ones; signs of cholangitis (i.e., thickening of the walls with irregular margins and enhancement, due to fibrosis and edema) can also be recognized; furthermore, MRCP well demonstrates the associated stenoses (Fig. 5.3) and the continuity between cystic dilatations and the biliary tree. The T1-weighted images acquired after contrast media administration may reveal the "central dot sign" (Fig. 5.4), whereas the administration of hepatobiliary contrast agent (gadoxetic acid) may also prove communication of the cystic dilatations with the biliary tree (Fig. 5.5).

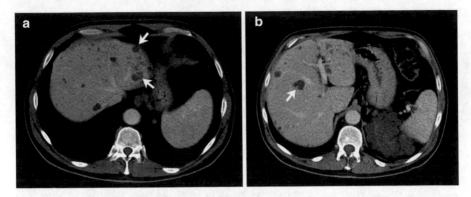

Fig. 5.2 Transverse CT scans obtained after contrast media injection in portal phase (**a**, **b**) showing multiple hypoattenuating liver lesions of different sizes scattered throughout the parenchyma. Some of them have a central hyperattenuating small vessel that creates the "central dot sign" (arrows). If the vessel is parallel to the plane of the image, the dot becomes a line

Fig. 5.3 Magnetic resonance T2-weighted transverse image showing a hyperintense cystic dilatation of the biliary tree that contains an intrahepatic stone, seen as a darker formation inside it (arrow)

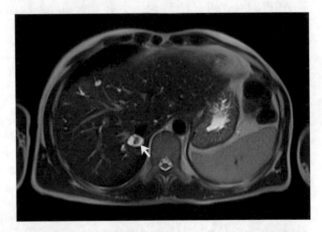

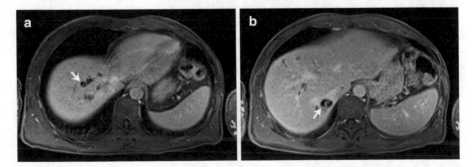

Fig. 5.4 Magnetic resonance T1-weighted transverse images after non-specific contrast agent injection: "central dot sign" due to the cross-sectional view of the vessel (arrow) (**a**); the vessel is parallel to the plane of the image, appearing as a line within the hypointense formation (**b**)

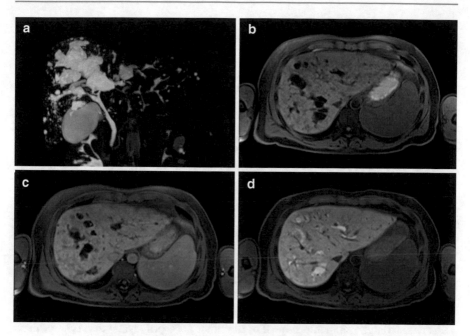

Fig. 5.5 T2-weighted MRCP image showing hyperintense cystic dilatation of the biliary tree (**a**). T1-weighted transverse images acquired before (**b**) and after the administration of hepatobiliary contrast agent (gadoxetic acid), depicting "central dot sign" in portal venous phase (**c**) and lumen contrast enhancement in hepatobiliary phase (**d**), confirming the communication of the cystic dilatations with the biliary tree

An older technique for confirmation of biliary dilatation is represented by the "HIDA scan," hepatic cholescintigraphy that uses radiotracers called TC^{99m}-IDA (iminodiacetic acid) analogs.

In case of hepatic abscess, a plain abdominal radiograph may show indirect signs like pneumobilia, gas beneath the diaphragm, and right-sided pleural effusion. US demonstrates poorly demarcated collections with variable appearance (i.e., hypo- to hyperechoic) and gas bubbles; no perfusion is observed in the central—necrotic—portion at Color Doppler. Contrast enhancement of the walls may be useful to measure the size of the lesion and to depict internal septation. Similarly, at CT scan "double target sign" is observed, with central low attenuation, a high attenuation inner rim (i.e., abscess membrane) that enhances early, and a low attenuation outer ring (i.e., parenchymal edema) that enhances on delayed phase. MRI identifies centrally hypointense lesions on T1-weighted and hyperintense signal on T2-weighted images, with enhancement of the capsule and septations, and signal restriction on diffusion weighted images (DWI).

The association between CD and cholangiocarcinoma requires a regular follow-up, usually performed with CT or MR (Fig. 5.6).

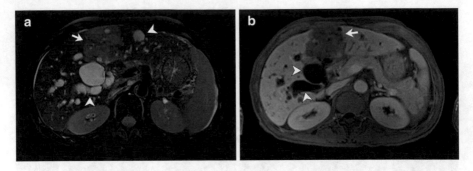

Fig. 5.6 Magnetic resonance of a patient with Caroli's disease who developed an intrahepatic cholangiocarcinoma. T2-weighted (**a**) and T1-weighted (**b**) transverse images showing an irregular mass slightly hyperintense in T2, with poor and inhomogeneous contrast enhancement in T1 that turned out to be a cholangiocarcinoma (arrow). It compressed the biliary tree, causing dilation of the biliary tree, that coexisted with the dilation caused by CD

5.5   Differential Diagnosis

Differential diagnosis includes most of the other fibro-polycystic diseases, primary sclerosing cholangitis, pyogenic cholangitis, and obstructive biliary dilatation.

- *Polycystic liver disease*: hereditary condition that occur in up to 90% of patients with *autosomal dominant polycystic kidney disease*. No biliary duct dilatation or communication with biliary ducts are generally observed. They are usually more numerous and may bleed, causing a fluid-fluid level inside.
- *Primary sclerosing cholangitis*: inflammatory condition associated with *inflammatory bowel disease* in 70% of patients. Dilatations are typically smaller, fusiform and paired with strictures resulting in a "beaded appearance" of the biliary tree. Suggestive hepatic morphology changes are enlargement of the caudate and left lobe hypertrophy. If elevated serum IgG-4 is found along with other IgG-4 related conditions, an IgG-4 related sclerosing cholangitis should be considered.
- *Pyogenic cholangitis*: should be suspected in patients with fever and septicemia. Imaging demonstrates biliary strictures and dilatations of both intra- and extrahepatic bile ducts that usually contain stones.
- *Obstructive biliary dilatation*: a mechanical obstruction of the biliary tree is demonstrated.

CD can coexist with *other fibro-polycystic liver disease*, such as biliary hamartomas (Fig. 5.7).

Fig. 5.7 The same patient of Fig. 5.2 underwent MRCP, for further evaluation, showing the cystic dilatation of the biliary tree already depicted by CT and multiple small hyperintense lesions scattered throughout the liver without communication with the biliary tree, pathognomonic of biliary hamartomas. CD coexists with biliary hamartomas

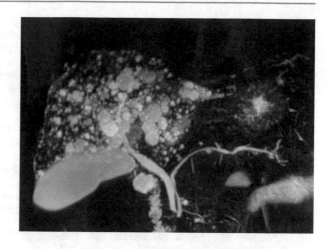

5.6 Treatment

If CD is not diffuse, segmentectomy or lobectomy may be performed; otherwise, conservative management is generally applied (i.e., ursodeoxycholic acid), and liver transplantation could be considered. For cholangitis and hepatic abscesses, antibiotic therapy is required. Interventional radiology percutaneous drainage, under US or CT guidance, plays a role for bigger abscess, if no septations are present [1–27].

References

1. Ahmadi T, Itai Y, Minami M. Central dot sign in entities other than Caroli disease. Radiat Med. 1997;15(6):381–4.
2. Bachler P, Baladron MJ, Menias C, Beddings I, Loch R, Zalaquett E, Vargas M, Connolly S, Bhalla S, Huete A. Multimodality imaging of liver infections: differential diagnosis and potential pitfalls. Radiographics. 2016;36(4):1001–23. https://doi.org/10.1148/rg.2016150196.
3. Brancatelli G, Federle MP, Vilgrain V, Vullierme MP, Marin D, Lagalla R. Fibropolycystic liver disease: CT and MR imaging findings. Radiographics. 2005;25(3):659–70. https://doi.org/10.1148/rg.253045114.
4. Caroli J, Couinaud R. Une affection nouvelle, des voies biliares. La dilatation kystique unilobulaire des canaux hepatiques. In: Seminar Hopitales Paris; 1958. p. 496–502.
5. Chan JH, Tsui EY, Luk SH, Fung AS, Yuen MK, Szeto ML, Cheung YK, Wong KP. Diffusion-weighted MR imaging of the liver: distinguishing hepatic abscess from cystic or necrotic tumor. Abdom Imaging. 2001;26(2):161–5. https://doi.org/10.1007/s002610000122.
6. Choi BI, Yeon KM, Kim SH, Han MC. Caroli disease: central dot sign in CT. Radiology. 1990;174(1):161–3. https://doi.org/10.1148/radiology.174.1.2294544.
7. Desmet VJ. Ludwig symposium on biliary disorders--Part I. Pathogenesis of ductal plate abnormalities. Mayo Clin Proc. 1998;73(1):80–9. https://doi.org/10.4065/73.1.80.
8. Gebel M. Ultrasound in gastroenterology and hepatology. Berlin: Blackwell Science; 2000.
9. Griffin N, Charles-Edwards G, Grant LA. Magnetic resonance cholangiopancreatography: the ABC of MRCP. Insights Imag. 2012;3(1):11–21. https://doi.org/10.1007/s13244-011-0129-9.

10. Hintze RE, Adler A, Veltzke W, Abou-Rebyeh H, Hammerstingl R, Vogl T, Felix R. Clinical significance of magnetic resonance cholangiopancreatography (MRCP) compared to endoscopic retrograde cholangiopancreatography (ERCP). Endoscopy. 1997;29(3):182–7. https://doi.org/10.1055/s-2007-1004160.
11. Joshi G, Crawford KA, Hanna TN, Herr KD, Dahiya N, Menias CO. US of right upper quadrant pain in the emergency department: diagnosing beyond gallbladder and biliary disease. Radiographics. 2018;38(3):766–93. https://doi.org/10.1148/rg.2018170149.
12. Khalefa AA, Alrasheed M, Saeedan MB. Central dot sign. Abdom Radiol (NY). 2016;41(11):2289–90. https://doi.org/10.1007/s00261-016-0836-2.
13. Krige J, Beckingham I. ABC of diseases of liver, pancreas, and biliary system: liver abscesses and hydatid disease. BMJ. 2001;322(7285):537.
14. Lall NU, Hogan MJ. Caroli disease and the central dot sign. Pediatr Radiol. 2009;39(7):754. https://doi.org/10.1007/s00247-009-1147-3.
15. Levy AD, Rohrmann CA Jr, Murakata LA, Lonergan GJ. Caroli's disease: radiologic spectrum with pathologic correlation. AJR Am J Roentgenol. 2002;179(4):1053–7. https://doi.org/10.2214/ajr.179.4.1791053.
16. Leyendecker JR, Brown JJ, Merkle EM. Practical guide to abdominal and pelvic MRI. Philadelphia, PA: Wolters Kluwer Health; 2014.
17. Maccioni F, Martinelli M, Al Ansari N, Kagarmanova A, De Marco V, Zippi M, Marini M. Magnetic resonance cholangiography: past, present and future: a review. Eur Rev Med Pharmacol Sci. 2010;14(8):721–5.
18. Martin RF. Biliary cysts: a review and simplified classification scheme. Surg Clin North Am. 2014;94(2):219–32. https://doi.org/10.1016/j.suc.2014.01.011.
19. Mathieu D, Vasile N, Fagniez PL, Segui S, Grably D, Larde D. Dynamic CT features of hepatic abscesses. Radiology. 1985;154(3):749–52. https://doi.org/10.1148/radiology.154.3.3969480.
20. Mendez RJ, Schiebler ML, Outwater EK, Kressel HY. Hepatic abscesses: MR imaging findings. Radiology. 1994;190(2):431–6. https://doi.org/10.1148/radiology.190.2.8284394.
21. Park HJ, Kim SH, Jang KM, Lee SJ, Park MJ, Choi D. Differentiating hepatic abscess from malignant mimickers: value of diffusion-weighted imaging with an emphasis on the periphery of the lesion. J Magn Reson Imaging. 2013;38(6):1333–41.
22. Riordan R, Khonsari M, Jeffries J, Maskell G, Cook P. Pineapple juice as a negative oral contrast agent in magnetic resonance cholangiopancreatography: a preliminary evaluation. Br J Radiol. 2004;77(924):991–9.
23. Skucas J. Advanced imaging of the abdomen. London: Springer; 2017.
24. Taylor AC, Little AF, Hennessy OF, Banting SW, Smith PJ, Desmond PV. Prospective assessment of magnetic resonance cholangiopancreatography for noninvasive imaging of the biliary tree. Gastrointest Endosc. 2002;55(1):17–22. https://doi.org/10.1067/mge.2002.120324.
25. Visser BC, Suh I, Way LW, Kang SM. Congenital choledochal cysts in adults. Arch Surg. 2004;139(8):855–60. https://doi.org/10.1001/archsurg.139.8.855; discussion 860–2.
26. Yonem O, Bayraktar Y. Clinical characteristics of Caroli's disease. World J Gastroenterol. 2007;13(13):1930.
27. Yu J, Turner MA, Fulcher AS, Halvorsen RA. Congenital anomalies and normal variants of the pancreaticobiliary tract and the pancreas in adults: part 2, Pancreatic duct and pancreas. AJR Am J Roentgenol. 2006;187(6):1544–53. https://doi.org/10.2214/AJR.05.0774.

Liver Disease in Cystic Fibrosis

6

Carla Colombo, Laura Zazzeron, Chiara Lanfranchi, and Valeria Daccò

6.1 Introduction

Cystic fibrosis (CF) is a severe autosomal recessive genetic disorder caused by mutations of the CF Transmembrane Conductance Regulator (CFTR) gene, which encodes for the CFTR protein, a chloride channel located at the apical membrane of epithelial cells. CF is a multiorgan disease affecting mostly the lungs, the pancreas, liver, intestine and sweat glands. With advances in medical care, a remarkable increase in survival has occurred, from 16 years in 1970 to 47.7 years in 2016. Further improvements are predicted in the near future due to the recent availability of an increasing number of innovative drugs targeting the CF basic defect (CFTR modulators) [1].

As a result of prolonged survival, the extrapulmonary comorbidities have become more frequent. With regard to the hepatobiliary system, a large spectrum of clinical manifestations have been described, with different pathogenetic mechanisms, including those related to specific alterations induced by the CFTR protein defect, lesions of iatrogenic origin, or those related to a disease process that occurs outside the liver [2] (Table 6.1). Liver disease in CF (LD) is one of the main comorbidity of the disease and has been identified as the third most frequent cause of death in CF patients after respiratory failure and transplantation related complications, accounting for 3.4% of overall mortality in the USA in 2018 [3]. In this chapter, the clinical manifestations of the characteristic LD associated with CF will be described with particular attention to the phenotypic expression in adult patients.

C. Colombo (✉) · L. Zazzeron · C. Lanfranchi · V. Daccò
Cystic Fibrosis Center, Fondazione IRCCS Ca' Granda Ospedale Maggiore Policlinico, Department of Pathophysiology and Transplantation, Università degli Studi di Milano, Milan, Italy
e-mail: carla.colombo@unimi.it

Table 6.1 Liver and biliary tract problems in cystic fibrosis

Clinical manifestation	Frequency	Notes
Isolated abnormalities in serum liver enzymes	Quite common, particularly during the first years of life	Frequently iatrogenic (drug hepatotoxicity)
		Exclusion of other causes of LD needed (viral infections, drugs, metabolic and structural conditions)
Focal biliary cirrhosis	20–30%	Mostly related to the CFTR defect in cholangiocytes
Multilobular biliary cirrhosis	5–10%	Treatment with UDCA (20 mg/kg/die) probably beneficial in early stages
Portal hypertension	2–5%	Most relevant hepatic complication of CF
		Not necessarily associated with cirrhosis
		Requires careful monitoring of complications and primary prophylaxis of GI bleeding
Non-cirrhotic portal hypertension	Undefined	Vascular rather than biliary-related pathogenesis
		May include nodular regenerative hyperplasia due to chronic drug-induced liver injury
		More frequent in adulthood
		Hepatic venous pressure gradient is generally normal
		Ultrasonography, transient elastography and even biopsy may be normal
Liver failure	<1% Rare	Indication for liver transplantation
Liver steatosis	23–67%	Essential fatty acid and/or other nutritional deficiencies relevant in the pathogenesis
Gallbladder involvement	24–50%	Microgallbladder, gallbladder distention, and/or dysfunction generally asymptomatic
Cholelithiasis	15%	Most commonly calcium bilirubinate stones
		Often asymptomatic
		UDCA treatment uneffective
		Cholecystectomy in symptomatic patients
Cholangiopathy	69%	Frequently detected by NMR in a high proportion of CF patients with and without other signs of LD
Cholangitis		Generally asymptomatic
Neonatal cholestasis	<2%	Due to obstruction by inspissated biliary secretions
		Differential diagnosis with biliary atresia

6.2   Pathogenesis

The basic defect of CF has been considered to play a major role in the pathogenesis. In the liver and biliary tract, the CFTR protein is specifically expressed at the apical membrane of the epithelial cells lining the biliary epithelium (cholangiocytes) [4], and its main role is to regulate the level of bile hydration and alkalization. This is achieved by maintaining chloride ion (Cl^-) gradient that drives the secretion into the bile of bicarbonate by anion exchanger (AE2/SLC4A2) expressed either in the canaliculi or in the luminal membrane of bile duct epithelial cells [5].

Therefore, focal biliary cirrhosis, the typical hepatic lesion of CF has been considered the direct consequence of lack or dysfunction of CFTR protein in cholangiocytes, leading to inspissated biliary secretions, bile duct plugging, hepatocyte damage, inflammation and progressive periportal fibrosis [6]. The fact that only one-third of CF patients develops LD has been explained by the three alternative Cl^- secretory cholangiocyte's mechanisms that may in part bypass CFTR defect [7].

However, other pathogenetic factors are likely to be involved. For example, recent studies suggest that the gut-liver axis may play a role in the development of cirrhosis in CF [8, 9]. CF patients often present increased intestinal permeability [10], small intestinal bacterial overgrowth [11] and evidence of intestinal inflammation at capsule endoscopy [12]. In addition, alterations in gut microbiota CF have been documented, in terms of both number and type of bacteria [13, 14] which may have important consequences within and beyond the CF gut. This dysbiosis may in turn further increase gut permeability and promote translocation of bacterial factors into the portal circulation, exposing the liver to gut-derived endotoxins. Indeed, compared to CF patients without LD faecal microbiome was shown to be significantly different in CF patients with cirrhosis, who also showed more macroscopic intestinal inflammatory lesions as well as slower bowel transit time [15].

Finally, in a subset of CF patients the pathogenesis may be related to a vascular rather than to a biliary disease. A condition of idiopathic non-cirrhotic portal hypertension (INCPH) has been increasingly identified over the last few years, particularly in adult patients with CF (Table 6.2), which is histologically characterized by presinusoidal portal hypertension due to obliterative venopathy with fibrosis within the portal vein branches [16–19].

Biopsies from CF patients with LD have also shown evidence of nodular regenerative hyperplasia which is a type of INCPH and may be related to recurrent vascular and infectious complications and possibly drug-induced liver injury [16].

6.3   Presentation of Liver Disease

LD in CF may present at any age. Presentation in infancy, although uncommon, may occur with a picture of neonatal cholestasis generally associated with meconium ileus and total parenteral nutrition. Cholestasis usually resolves spontaneously within the first few months of life, and only in a few cases, progression to fibrosis and cirrhosis may occur.

Table 6.2 Idiopathic non-cirrhotic portal hypertension (INCPH) in CF patients

Author	No of patients with liver disease and PH	No of patients with INCPH	Median age of INCPH diagnosis (years)	Liver disease clinical and laboratory features	Histology and/or hepatic venous portal gradient (HVPG)	Outcome
Witters 2017 [17]	8	8	21	6/8 oesophageal varices	0/8 cirrhosis (F4)	5/8 liver transplantations
				2/8 oesophageal bleeding without oesophageal varices at biopsy	2/8 incomplete septal cirrhosis	
				3/8 ascites	6/8 fibrosis (2 F0-1F1-1F2-4F3)	
				7/8 splenomegaly and thrombocytopenia	7/8 vascular changes with obliterative venopathy	
					4/8 HVPG[a] (4–9 mmHg)	
Witters 2011 [74]	12	7	N.A.	10/12 oesophageal varices	5/12 cirrhosis at biopsy	4/7 liver transplantation
				11/12 splenomegaly and thrombocytopenia	7/12 fibrosis (1F0-1F1-1F2-4F3) and portal branch venopathy	
					2/7 HVPG[a] (5–9 mmHg)	
Lewindon 2011 [43]	17	15	13.3	11/17 splenomegaly	14/17 fibrosis (1 F1-4 F2-9 F3)	1/17 heart + lung transplantation
				14/17 hepatomegaly	2/17 cirrhosis (F4)	1/17 liver transplantation
				14/17 abnormal US hepatic pattern		6/17 deaths
Hillaire 2017 [16]	10	8	25.6	9/10 oesophageal varices (8 ligations and 1 TIPS) and thrombocytopenia, no bleeding	8/10 nodular regeneration and obliterative venopathy	9/10 lung + liver transplantation
				10/10 splenomegaly	6/10 ductopenia	2/10 deaths
				2/10 cirrhosis	10/10 fibrosis	1/10 liver transplantation
					3/10 biliary fibrosis	
					4/10 portal inflammation	

Wu 2019 [75]	17	17	15	15/17 splenomegaly with thrombocytopenia and oesophageal varices (94% confirmed endoscopically)	17/17 no cirrhosis	17/17 liver transplantation for portal hypertension
				13/17 US diffuse capsular surfaces nodularity (56,3% confirmed at liver explants)	11/17 obliterative venopathy 16/17 nodular regenerative hyperplasia (NRH) no signs of biliary obstruction	
Lupi 2020 [58]	1	1	30	Portal hypertension with preserved liver function	HVPG^a:14 mmHg	Successful TIPS with decreasing of portal pressure gradient
				Recurrent variceal bleeding		No bleeding after TIPS
				Prior bilateral lung transplant		
				Fibroscan: stiffness 7 kPa		

N.A. not available

[a]*HVPG* hepatic venous portal gradient

In older children, liver involvement may manifest as hepatic steatosis (often associated to malnutrition and/or essential fatty acid deficiency), and with the pathognomonic form of LD in CF, focal biliary cirrhosis, which may progress to multilobular cirrhosis.

A few long-term prospective studies with careful monitoring of hepatic status carried out two decades ago consistently indicated that LD develops generally before puberty in around one-third of CF patients, it is often asymptomatic with a mean age at diagnosis ranging between 7 [20] and 12 years [21], and rarely after the age of 18 years [20–22]. Thus, LD has been considered a paediatric complication of the disease and progression to cirrhosis and portal hypertension was described in no more than 10% of patients, with long-term preservation of liver synthetic function [20, 21]. In these studies, LD was defined by a variable combination of criteria (presence of hepatomegaly on clinical examination, persistent abnormalities in liver biochemistry as well as at ultrasonography), leading to inclusion of both early and advanced LD with cirrhosis and portal hypertension, but excluding steatosis [20–22].

CF patients with pancreatic insufficiency and carry mutations associated with a severe genotype are at increased risk to develop liver disease [20, 23]. Others risk factors are still debated, such as male sex and a history of meconium ileus [19, 20, 22, 24], a severe neonatal intestinal obstruction involving about 15% of CF newborns [25]. Finally, the role of genetic modifiers has been explored by a large international study in CF patients with extreme hepatic phenotype, showing that CF patients heterozygous for the SERPINA 1 allele of alpha-1 antitrypsin are at increased risk of developing severe LD [26]. The role of this gene has been recently confirmed by data provided by the French CF Modifier Gene Study showing that the cumulative incidence of severe LD by age 25 was extremely high among patients heterozygous for the SERPINA 1 allele (47%) [19].

In contrast, LD in adult patients with CF has not been adequately characterized, thereby resulting in high variability in the reported prevalence (ranging from 2% to 37%), age at onset and outcome [27].

A few cross-sectional studies have addressed prevalence, natural history and the impact of LD on CF patients surviving into adulthood [24, 27, 28] and the main available data are summarized in Table 6.3.

Development of significant liver disease seems to be infrequent in adulthood, and most of the hepatic complications were manly observed in CF patients with LD diagnosed in childhood. Nash et al. documented the presence of LD in about 37% of adult patients; however, the age at diagnosis of LD was not reported; a relatively benign course was reported in the majority of patients, probably resulting from active and regular screening of LD with early detection of "mild" phenotypes and no further progression due to early treatment with UDCA [27]. In the study by Desmond et al. [28], prevalence of LD was much lower (10%), diagnosis occurred more frequently in adulthood at a mean age of 23 years (ranging 8–47 years) and severe liver complications were observed in more than 20% of cases.

A higher risk of liver decompensation (39%) was reported by Chryssostalis et al. who carried out a retrospective analysis of 285 adult CF patients regularly followed:

Table 6.3 Liver disease in adult CF patients

Author	No of adult patients	No of adult patients with liver abnormalities	Age at diagnosis of liver disease	Follow up (median years)	Characteristic of liver disease population	Outcome
Nash 2008 [27]	154 (>16 years)	57 (37%)	N.A.	5	43 (28%) cirrhosis	1 liver decompensation
					5 (3%) steatosis	1 lung-liver transplantation (died)
					9 (6%) splenomegaly alone	7 deaths, none for liver-related causes
					97 (63%) normal	No deterioration in lung function
						No deterioration in nutritional status
Desmond 2007 [28]	278 (>18 years)	27 (10%)	23 years (8–47)	7	18 (67%) cirrhosis with portal hypertension	2 (7%) variceal haemorrhage
			17 (6%) in adulthood		12 (44%) oesophageal varices	3 (11%) ascites
			10 (4%) in childhood		25 (93%) US abnormalities	6 (22%) hepatic decompensation
					8 (30%) hepatomegaly	9 (33%) deaths, none liver-related
					251 (90%) normal	No liver transplantation
						5 (19%) lung transplantation

(continued)

Table 6.3 (continued)

Author	No of adult patients	No of adult patients with liver abnormalities	Age at diagnosis of liver disease	Follow-up (median years)	Characteristic of liver disease population	Outcome
Chryssostalis 2011 [24]	285	90 (32%)	Onset unusual in adulthood (n = 6; 7%)	N.A.	23 (25%) cirrhosis	17 (74%) PH with oesophageal varices
					67 (75%) no cirrhosis	9 (39%) liver decompensation and variceal bleeding
					195 (68%) normal	3 (3%) liver transplantation
						3 (3%) combined liver-lung transplantation
						No liver-related death
						No progression of liver disease in patients without cirrhosis at first observation at the adult centre
Koh 2017 [18]	36	17 (47%) [a]	36.6 years	24,5	In adults liver disease is more prevalent than previously described, with a second wave in incident and impact on mortality	1 (6%) cirrhosis with PH, variceal bleeding and nodular hyperplasia
						11 (65%) deaths, 2 for liver decompensation

Boëlle 2019 [19]	3328 (multicentre study)	605 (18%)	1% increase in incidence every year, reaching 32.2% by age of 25	13	431 (71%) liver involvement without cirrhosis	97 (16%) cirrhosis
					174 (29%) severe LD (cirrhosis and/or portal hypertension/ oesophageal varices)	71 (12%) portal hypertension
						6 (1%) oesophageal varices
						Severe LD incidence increases only after age 5, reaching 10% by age 30
Scott-Jupp 1991 [76]	328 (>16 years; multicentre study)	32 (10%)	10.5 years	N.A.	Among 46/1100 (4%) patients with clinical liver disease (not only adult):	6 (13%) deaths: 2 for variceal bleeding and 4 for liver decompensation
					11 (24%) oesophageal varices and splenomegaly	
					4 (9%) splenomegaly	Prevalence of LD peaks during adolescence and a fall in prevalence over age 20
					6 (13%) alteration liver function	Liver disease seems to be associated with earlier death
					11 (24%) hepatomegaly only	
					3 (6%) splenomegaly only	
					32 (69%) hepatosplenomegaly	

N.A. not available

[a]Diagnostic tools included transient elastography, APRI and FIB-4

LD was already present at first observation at the adult centre in one-third of cases and the presence of advanced cirrhosis was identified as an independent factor associated with liver decompensation, early mortality and lung transplantation [24].

More recently, two other studies reported incidence of significant LD in adulthood.

A large retrospective study by Boelle et al. evaluating 3328 CF patients born after 1985 and enrolled in the French CF Modifier Gene Study since 2004, reported that the cumulative incidence of liver involvement increases by approximately 1% every year, reaching 32.2% by the age of 25 [19]. The incidence of severe LD with cirrhosis and/or portal hypertension increased only after the age of 5, reaching 10% by age 30.

In contrast, incidence rates in childhood were found to be significantly lower than in prospective studies, probably due to the problematic detection of LD at an early stage in the context of a retrospective study [19].

Evidence of a second wave of LD incidence at an average age of 37 years in adult patients with no evidence of liver abnormalities in childhood was also provided by Koh et al. [18], using a new diagnostic algorithm which included non-invasive liver fibrosis biomarkers as the aspartate transaminase/platelets ratio-index (APRI), the fibrosis index based on the 4 factors (fibrosis 4 index, FIB-4) and transient elastography (fibroscan), in addition to serological and radiological tests [18].

This diagnostic algorithm was able to identify 25% more adult patients with LD, also suggesting that onset in adulthood may be more frequent than previously reported [18]. However, the pathogenesis of LD developing in adulthood may be different from that in childhood and, to some extent, unrelated to the CF basic defect. Adult patients may be affected by forms of the non-cirrhotic portal hypertension spectrum due to obliterative portal venopathy (Table 6.2) [19].

Moreover, Koh et al. reported cases of nodular regenerative hyperplasia possibly related to chronic drug-induced liver injury from long-standing antibiotic use [18].

6.4   Clinical Manifestations and Natural History of LD in CF

LD is frequently asymptomatic and diagnosis may be very difficult in the early phases. The most common presentation is the occasional detection of abnormalities of liver biochemistry, often associated to the finding of an enlarged liver. Progression from early asymptomatic stage (with focally distributed hepatic lesions) to cirrhosis and PH involves less than 10% of CF patients. However, this clinical course is difficult to predict. As in other forms of LD characterized by initial involvement of the bile ducts rather than hepatocytes liver failure, ascites and encephalopathy are rare and late events [29]. In contrast, the hemodynamic consequences of cirrhosis are characteristically prominent, favouring early development of PH. In patients with INCPH, progression to end-stage LD may be even more rapid and many of the reported cases required liver transplantation (Table 6.2).

In a recent longitudinal study, which retrospectively collected data on the occurrence of portal hypertension in 577 CF patients diagnosed by neonatal screening and followed up in two CF centres, cumulative incidence of severe liver disease was 8.8% [30].

This study showed a fourfold increase in mortality/transplant occurrence in those with severe liver disease with PH as compared with the non-PH subgroup [30].

In the advanced stages of the LD, the most frequent complication is bleeding from esophageal or gastric varices that may occur quite unexpectedly and lead to the diagnosis of cirrhosis. According to Cystic Fibrosis Foundation Patient Registry data, variceal bleeding occurred in 6.6% of 943 cirrhotic CF patients (at a mean age of 18.1 years) in the 10-year period after the diagnosis of cirrhosis [31], and there was a similarly low rate for other adverse liver outcomes (cumulative 10-year incidence rate: liver transplant 9.9%, liver-related death 6.9%).

In cirrhotic CF patients, hypersplenism may also develop, with thrombocytopenia, leukopenia and massive spleen enlargement, which may cause abdominal discomfort or pain.

With regard to the impact of cirrhosis and PH on CF disease, a progressive deterioration of pulmonary function and nutritional status may occur in affected patients.

Several factors may contribute to lung deterioration, including development of intrapulmonary vascular shunting, diaphragmatic splinting due to organomegaly and presence of ascites.

Hepatopulmonary syndrome, resulting from dilatation of intrapulmonary capillaries with consequent right to left shunt and hypoxemia, may be more frequent than so far reported and be underdiagnosed due to the confounding symptoms of the coexisting chronic CF lung disease [32]. Therefore, routine screening for this complication in CF patients with severe LD and PH should be accomplished. A significant decrease in oxygen saturation (>5%) when the patient moves from the supine to the upright position (orthodeoxia) is suggestive of the diagnosis. Proof of intrapulmonary capillary dilatation may be then obtained by means of contrast enhanced (bubble) echocardiography or technetium 99-labelled macro aggregated albumin scintigraphy [32, 33].

Deterioration of nutritional status occurs frequently in CF patients with advanced LD. The pathogenesis is multifactorial, resulting from increased resting energy expenditure, reduced caloric intake (due to anorexia and, in patients with encephalopathy, to protein restriction), intestinal malabsorption related to reduced bile flow, pancreatic insufficiency and abnormal nutrient metabolism. Hepatic osteodystrophy and osteoporosis may also develop [34]. In addition, CF patients with LD are at increased risk of developing diabetes due to hepatic induced insulin resistance [35].

All these factors may ultimately affect survival. Studies based on Registry data seem to confirm a higher risk for early mortality due to respiratory failure in CF patients with cirrhosis and an approximately 10-year lower median age at death [36].

6.5   Diagnosis of LD

As LD in CF is usually asymptomatic, a regular monitoring of hepatic status with accurate clinical examination, liver biochemistry and abdominal ultrasonography (US) is essential and should be included in the routine annual monitoring since the time of diagnosis of CF [33].

Evaluation of hepatomegaly should be carried out at each visit and should include liver span measurement at the mid-clavicular line; the presence of splenomegaly should also be carefully evaluated, as a first sign of PH.

A mild or intermittent increase in serum levels of transaminases and gamma-glutamyl transferase is frequent in CF patients, but may be due to drug hepatotoxicity (mostly induced by beta lactam antibiotics, quinolones and antifungal agents) or infections. Therefore, particularly as an isolated finding, abnormal liver biochemistry has low sensitivity and specificity in detecting LD, even in patients who have already developed cirrhosis.

Abnormal gamma-glutamyl transferase may be more common in cirrhotic patients and persistently high levels have been associated with a future diagnosis of cirrhosis within 2 years [37]. A significant drop in platelet count over time often reflects development of PH and when $<150 \times 10^3$ should require further evaluations [38]. Coagulopathy (INR > 1.2), not corrected by parenteral vitamin K administration, and reduced serum albumin (<3 g/dL) provide evidence of hepatic decompensation and, in case of a progressive deterioration, may lead to consider the option of liver transplantation (LT).

US is the most suitable standard imaging technique in order to differentiate the spectrum of hepatic abnormalities found in CF, including steatosis, fibrosis, cirrhosis, PH and biliary abnormalities (Fig. 6.1). Doppler ultrasound can provide complementary information by documenting the typical abnormal hepatofugal flow pattern of PH [39].

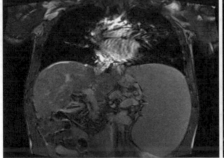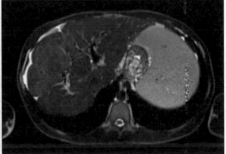

Fig. 6.1 Magnetic resonance imaging of a 12-year-old boy with cystic fibrosis. T2 weighted axial and coronal images in- (upper panel) and out- (lower panel) of phase show irregular margins of the liver with a pseudo-nodular structure, fibrotic bands crossing the liver parenchyma, and splenomegaly. (Kindly provided by Dr Irene Borzani, Paediatric Radiology, Fondazione IRCCS Ca' Granda; Ospedale Maggiore Policlinico)

Abnormal liver echogenicity may precede clinical and biochemical manifestations of LD. Furthermore, US seems to be correlated with biomarkers of severity of liver disease, such as platelet count, spleen size and non-invasive indices of liver fibrosis [40].

Computed tomography (CT) may play a role in accurate detection of different abdominal complications of CF; however, its employment is limited in order to avoid an excessive radiation exposure.

Hepatic and biliary Magnetic Resonance (MR) provides high quality imaging without radiation exposure and allows to document a variety of abnormalities that are not shown by other non-invasive techniques [41]. MR can reveal signs of liver dysmorphia (atrophy of hepatic lobes and/or hypertrophy of the caudate lobe, lobulation of the liver surface), portal hypertension and cholangitis (abnormalities of intra- and extrahepatic bile ducts with stenosis, rigidity, intrahepatic lithiasis). It is also useful to differentiate between steatosis and fibrosis and for assessing the nature of focal lesions documented by US [42].

Currently liver biopsy is not a standard practice in LD, although it may provide important information on the type of the predominant hepatic lesion (steatosis or focal biliary cirrhosis), the extent of portal fibrosis [43], the rate of progression of LD and the response to therapeutic interventions. Due to the patchy distribution of hepatic lesions, liver biopsy may underestimate its severity or even give false-negative results. Moreover, risks costs and impossibility to perform serial measurements still limit its use in CF patients. Therefore, the interest on non-invasive tools for assessing fibrosis has progressively increased over the last years, particularly APRI and FIB-4. In a liver biopsy-validated study involving paediatric patients, APRI was found to be superior to FIB-4 in predicting the presence of LD and severe fibrosis, with specific cut-off for lower stages and full agreement with histology [44]. In addition, in the international LD genetic modifier study that involved 497 CF patients with cirrhosis and PH, both indices could identify those patients who had developed secondary complications of PH [45].

Non-invasive diagnostic tools also include transient elastography (Fibroscan), Acoustic Radiation Force Impulse (ARFI), and magnetic resonance elastography that can assess the degree of fibrosis and might improve non-invasive identification of CF patients at risk for LD and its progression [42, 46, 47].

Fibroscan, an ultrasonographic technique to evaluate liver stiffness, can provide information on the extent of liver fibrosis and has replaced liver biopsy in several chronic liver diseases. It is a non-invasive, rapid and reproducible tool for the detection of LD also in CF [48] and may have a potential role for identifying patients with portal hypertension who generally have higher liver stiffness values [42].

ARFI imaging combines conventional ultrasonography with measurement of ultrasound guided liver stiffness and shear wave velocities and may have the advantage, compared to Fibroscan, not to be influenced by hepatic steatosis [46].

Finally, there is an increasing interest on serum miRNA biomarkers, i.e. short interfering RNAs that silence gene expression at a post-transcriptional level. Preliminary observations in 124 children with CF suggest that altered circulatory miR-122 expression is a possible early marker of liver injury and when used in combination with the platelet ratio (APRI index), seem to be able to predict LD severity [48]. However, all these procedures still need to be validated on larger number of patients.

Esophagogastroduodenoscopy is useful in detecting the presence of oesophageal varices and portal hypertensive gastropathy and should be performed at least annually in the follow-up in subjects with PH [33].

This complication is considered clinically significant when hepatic venous pressure gradient (HVPG), as an expression of intrahepatic resistance, is 10 mmHg or more. It should be noted that INCPH could be underdiagnosed by using HVPG because of presinusoidal aetiology of PH.

Finally, percutaneous transhepatic cholangiography and endoscopic retrograde cholangiography (ERCP) are invasive procedures, but are still used for the investigation and treatment of specific and rare conditions, such as sclerosing cholangitis, distal stenosis of the common bile duct and choledocholithiasis [33].

6.6   Treatment Options for LD

At present, medical treatments of proven efficacy to improve and delay progression of LD are not yet available. The only therapeutic option is the administration of UDCA, a hydrophilic bile acid with choleretic properties. UDCA seems to reduce bile viscosity, improve biliary secretion and modify the bile acid pool composition by decreasing the proportion of toxic hydrophobic bile acids. UDCA has been shown to improve liver biochemistry [49], biliary drainage at hepatobiliary scintigraphy [50], histopathological alterations [51], and to reduce liver stiffness in CF patients with mild liver disease [52].

The European guidelines for the clinical management of LD recommend the use of UDCA at a dose of 20 mg/kg/day as soon as the diagnosis is established [33].

However, the long-term effects of UDCA on clinically relevant endpoints such as survival or liver transplantation could not be assessed in the context of randomized controlled trials, due to the limited number of patients and the short follow-up of the studies so far carried out [53]. In addition data from the French CF Modifier Gene Study, although largely based on retrospective observations, have recently suggested that UDCA treatment may not influence the development of severe LD with cirrhosis and portal hypertension [19]. Further studies are therefore needed on the real utility of this therapy.

The management of CF patients with advanced LD does not substantially differ from other chronic hepatic conditions and includes nutritional support, treatment of PH complications, and liver transplantation (LT) [33, 38].

Special attention should be addressed to increasing energy intake in order to reach up to 150% of recommended dietary allowances [54], if necessary by means of enteral feeding, as severe malnutrition itself can also favour hepatic steatosis, whereas the use of gastrostomy is not recommended in patients with PH to avoid the risk of gastrointestinal bleeding. Liposoluble vitamin supplementation should be prescribed using doses and formulations effective in achieving the recommended ranges, whereas salt supplementation, when necessary, should be strictly monitored to avoid the development of ascites.

With respect to treatment of PH, the indications, optimal timing and benefits of the available treatment options have not been established. The use of beta blockers is generally contraindicated in CF patients as they may cause bronchospasm and oxygen desaturation.

With regard to variceal bleeding, oesophageal band ligation is preferable to sclerotherapy, as it does not require anaesthesia and repeated antibiotic prophylaxis. Primary prophylaxis of gastrointestinal bleeding should be considered in the presence of grade >2 (with red signs and subcardial extension) by means of band ligation [32].

Symptomatic PH may be also be treated with transjugular intrahepatic portosystemic shunt (TIPS) [55], even if this procedure should better be considered as a bridge to LT, in CF patients with advanced LD [56].

In the past, elective surgical portosystemic shunt was performed for refractory bleeding in CF patients without liver failure and with severe pulmonary disease, allowing prolonged post-operative survival [57]; complications included development of hepatic encephalopathy, shunt thrombosis, and this procedure is presently seldom performed. Portosystemic shunting might be preferable over transplantation given the absence of cirrhosis and the preserved liver function in NCPH [58].

In patients with hypersplenism, total or partial splenectomy has been proposed, alone or in association with splenorenal shunt [59, 60]; however, also these procedures are presently not recommended.

Isolated liver transplantation (LT) is a well-established therapeutic option for end-stage liver disease that confers a survival benefit in patients with cirrhosis and those with NCPH [61]. However, selection criteria and optimal timing for LT in CF are still debated. As previously mentioned, liver failure, the main indication for LT in other diseases, is a late event in CF patients, who generally show long-term preservation of synthetic function. In addition to hepatic synthetic dysfunction, indications in CF have included portal hypertension and associated complications (refractory ascites, recurrent variceal bleeding), hepatic encephalopathy, hepatorenal and hepatopulmonary syndrome, and portopulmonary hypertension [62]. Even if LT has been successfully performed in CF patients with deteriorating nutritional status [63], poor growth or nutrition secondary to liver disease are considered relatively weak indications [62]. It should be noted that a rapid decline in lung function is not considered an indication for isolated liver transplant, as a significant improvement in FEV 1 post liver transplant was not consistently obtained. Absolute contraindications to LT include extrahepatic malignancies, uncontrolled or systemic or pulmonary infection, active pulmonary exacerbations or venoarterial extracorporeal membrane oxygenation, severe portopulmonary hypertension nonresponsive to medical treatment, and multiorgan disease.

Overall, survival after isolated liver transplant in CF is lower than transplantation undertaken for other diseases, with a 5-year survival reported in 69–75% in adults and 74–86% in children [61]. Several complications may develop following LT, including chronic renal failure due to the immunosuppressive drugs that may require further graft [64], and vascular thrombosis that represents the main cause for retransplant [62]. Mortality is primary attributed to sepsis and progression of the respiratory disease, rather than allograft failure.

As CF is a multisystem disease, in the setting of evaluation for liver transplantation it is important to establish whether liver transplantation alone is required or if a multiorgan transplantation may be more appropriate, carefully evaluating the severity of pulmonary and pancreatic involvement.

It is reasonable offering an isolated liver transplant when lung disease is relatively mild, with a forced vital capacity greater than 75% predicted and FEV 1 greater than 60% predicted. Currently the outcome of combined liver and lung transplantations is becoming similar to liver transplantation alone, both in children and adults [62–69].

A few lung transplant centres have achieved successful outcome following lung transplantation without liver transplantation in patients with advanced LD including portal hypertension and known varices [66].

Double liver and pancreas transplantation has been also successfully carried out in CF patients with LD, CF-related diabetes and pancreatic insufficiency, with a 2-year survival of 88%. However, this intervention is rarely performed, despite the potential benefit it may provide on endocrine and exocrine pancreatic functions [70].

6.7   Novel Therapies for LD in CF

Recent advances in the understanding of pathological mechanisms of CF are paving the way to novel promising therapies. Since the pathogenetic mechanism of LD in CF is mainly related to the basic defect, the already available CFTR modulators as well as novel compounds under evaluation may prove to be effective in the treatment and prevention of this relevant complication of CF. However, the effects of these agents on the liver are not well characterized, since the presence of LD has been a consistent exclusion criteria for enrolment in clinical trials so far carried out, due to their potential hepatotoxicity [71].

Interestingly, a recent post-marketing multicentre observational study on 845 F508del homozygous patients has described the effects of treatment lumacaftor–ivacaftor (a combination of a corrector and a potentiator of the CFTR protein), including a subgroup of 42 CF patients (5%) with cirrhosis or portal hypertension [72]. Overall, 154 had to discontinue treatment, of whom eight had cirrhosis and PH. The reasons for discontinuation in cirrhotic patients were mostly extrahepatic; only one patient showed marked liver enzyme elevation (ALT 9xN, AST 7xN) and this also the case for another patient with biochemical liver abnormalities but no cirrhosis.

These data suggest that lumacaftor–ivacaftor could be well tolerated in most patients with CF-related liver disease and the effects of such treatment on LD progression could be explored [72].

Other potential treatments for CF-associated LD include novel therapeutic agents such as *nor*-ursodeoxycholic acid (a side chain-shortened homologue of UDCA, that does not undergo a full enterohepatic cycle but is passively absorbed from chol-angiocytes, generating a HCO_3-rich hypercholeresis), and obeticholic acid (a selective farnesoid-X-receptor agonist that is able to increase bile flow in cholestatic conditions), that may have potential clinical benefit [62]. No data are presently available for CF patients.

6.8 Conclusions

The interest for LD in CF has progressively increased over the last decades, and prospective studies have provided reliable information on the natural history, risk factors and outcome. However, its characteristics in adult patients should be further defined, the diagnostic definition remains controversial and alternative algorithms are under evaluation in order to ensure harmonized international data [73]. Another important issue relates to identification of risk factors and biomarkers for progression of this important comorbidity of CF.

One of the greatest challenges in the management of patients in the early stage of LD in CF is to prevent the progression of fibrosis and further evolution to cirrhosis. For these patients, UDCA has been so far the only available therapy; however, there is no evidence of its efficacy in halting the progression to more severe LD. Long-term prospective studies involving large number of patients with clinically relevant endpoints, such as occurrence of severe LD with PH, need of liver transplantation and survival, are required to draw definitive conclusions about the clinical benefits of UDCA as well as of any other novel treatments of LD in CF.

References

1. Bell SC, et al. The future of cystic fibrosis care: a global perspective. Lancet Respir Med. 2020;8(1):65–124.
2. Collawn JF, Matalon S. CFTR and lung homeostasis. Am J Phys Lung Cell Mol Phys. 2014;307(12):L917–23.
3. Cystic Fibrosis Foundation. Cystic Fibrosis Foundation patient registry. Annual data report 2018. Bethesda, MD: Cystic Fibrosis Foundation; 2018.
4. Cohn JA, Strong T, Picciotto MR, et al. Localization of the cystic fibrosis transmembrane conductance regulator in human bile duct epithelial cells. Gastroenterology. 1993;105(6):1857–64.
5. Martínez-Ansó E, Castillo JE, Díez J, Medina JF, Prieto J. Immunohistochemical detection of chloride/bicarbonate anion exchangers in human liver. Hepatology. 1994;19(6):1400–6.
6. Flass T, Narkewicz MR. Cirrhosis and other liver disease in cystic fibrosis. J Cyst Fibros. 2013;12(2):116–24.
7. Lazaridis KN, Strazzabosco M, Larusso N. The cholangiopathies: disorders of biliary epithelia. Gastroenterology. 2004;127:1565–77.
8. Staufer K, Halilbasic E, Trauner M, Kazemi-Shirazi L. Cystic fibrosis related liver disease--another black box in hepatology. Int J Mol Sci. 2014;15(8):13529–49.
9. Rogers GB, Narkewicz MR, Hoffman LR. The CF gastrointestinal microbiome: structure and clinical impact. Pediatr Pulmonol. 2016;51(S44):S35–44.
10. Hallberg K, Grzegorczyk A, Larson G, Strandvik B. Intestinal permeability in cystic fibrosis in relation to genotype. J Pediatr Gastroenterol Nutr. 1997;25(3):290–5.

11. Demeyer S, De Boeck K, Witters P, Cosaert K. Beyond pancreatic insufficiency and liver disease in cystic fibrosis. Eur J Pediatr. 2016;175(7):881–94.
12. Werlin SL, Benuri-Silbiger I, Kerem E, et al. Evidence of intestinal inflammation in patients with cystic fibrosis. J Pediatr Gastroenterol Nutr. 2010;51(3):304–8.
13. Manor O, Levy R, Pope C, et al. Metagenomic evidence for taxonomic dysbiosis and functional imbalance in the gastrointestinal tracts of children with cystic fibrosis. Sci Rep. 2016;6:22493.
14. Schippa S, Iebba V, Santangelo F, et al. Cystic fibrosis transmembrane conductance regulator (CFTR) allelic variants relate to shifts in faecal microbiota of cystic fibrosis patients. PLoS One. 2013;8:e61176.
15. Flass T, Tong S, Frank DN, et al. Intestinal lesions are associated with altered intestinal microbiome and are more frequent in children and young adults with cystic fibrosis and cirrhosis. PLoS One. 2015;10:e0116967.
16. Hillaire S, Cazals-Hatem D, Bruno O, de Miranda S, Grenet D, Poté N, Soubrane O, Erlinger S, Lacaille F, Mellot F, Vilgrain V, Paradis V. Liver transplantation in adult cystic fibrosis: clinical, imaging, and pathological evidence of obliterative portal venopathy. Liver Transpl. 2017;23(10):1342–7.
17. Witters P, Libbrecht L, Roskams T, et al. Liver disease in cystic fibrosis presents as non-cirrhotic portal hypertension. J Cyst Fibros. 2017;16:e11–3.
18. Koh C, Sakiani S, Surana P, Zhao X, Eccleston J, Kleiner DE, et al. Adult-onset cystic fibrosis liver disease: diagnosis and characterization of an underappreciated entity. Hepatology. 2017;66(2):591–601.
19. Boëlle PY, Debray D, Guillot L, Clement A, Corvol H, French CF, Modifier Gene Study Investigators. Cystic fibrosis liver disease: outcomes and risk factors in a large cohort of french patients. Hepatology. 2019;69(4):1648–56.
20. Colombo C, Battezzati PM, Crosignani A, et al. Liver disease in cystic fibrosis: a prospective study on incidence, risk factors, and outcome. Hepatology. 2002;36(6):1374–82.
21. Lindblad A, Glaumann H, Strandvik B. Natural history of liver disease in cystic fibrosis. Hepatology. 1999;30(5):1151–8.
22. Lamireau T, Monnereau S, Martin S, et al. Epidemiology of liver disease in cystic fibrosis: a longitudinal study. J Hepatol. 2004;41(6):920–5.
23. Wilschanski M, Rivlin J, Cohen S, et al. Clinical and genetic risk factors for cystic fibrosis-related liver disease. Pediatrics. 1999;103(1):52–7.
24. Chryssostalis A, Hubert D, Coste J, Kanaan R, Burgel PR, Desmazes-Dufeu N, Soubrane O, Dusser D, Sogni P. Liver disease in adult patients with cystic fibrosis: a frequent and independent prognostic factor associated with death or lung transplantation. J Hepatol. 2011;55(6):1377–82.
25. Norsa L, Nicastro E, Di Giorgio A, Lacaille F, D'Antiga L. Prevention and treatment of intestinal failure-associated liver disease in children. Nutrients. 2018;10(6):664.
26. Bartlett JR, Friedman KJ, Ling SC, Pace RG, Bell SC, Bourke B, Castaldo G, Castellani C, Cipolli M, Colombo C, et al. Gene Modifier Study Group. Genetic modifiers of liver disease in cystic fibrosis. JAMA. 2009;302(10):1076–83.
27. Nash KL, Allison ME, McKeon D, Lomas DJ, Haworth CS, Bilton D, Alexander GJ. A single centre experience of liver disease in adults with cystic fibrosis 1995-2006. J Cyst Fibros. 2008;7(3):252–7.
28. Desmond CP, Wilson J, Bailey M, Clark D, Roberts SK. The benign course of liver disease in adults with cystic fibrosis and the effect of ursodeoxycholic acid. Liver Int. 2007;27(10):1402–8.
29. Melzi ML, Kelly DA, Colombo C, et al. Liver transplant in cystic fibrosis: a poll among European centers. A study from the European Liver Transplant Registry. Transpl Int. 2006;19(9):726–31.
30. Cipolli M, Fethney J, Waters D, Zanolla L, Meneghelli I, Shoma D, Assael Baroukh M, Gaskin KJ. Occurrence, outcomes and predictors of portal hypertension in cystic fibrosis: a longitudinal prospective birth cohort study. J Cyst Fibros. 2020;19(3):455–9.
31. Ye W, Narkewicz MR, Leung DH, Karnsakul W, Murray KF, Alonso EM, Magee JC, Schwarzenberg SJ, Weymann A, Molleston JP, CFLD Net Research Group. Variceal hemorrage

and adverse liver outcomes in patients with Cystic Fibrosis cirrhosis. J Pediatr Gastroenterol Nutr. 2018;66:122–7.

32. Breuer O, Shteyer E, Wilschanski M, Perles Z, Cohen-Cymberknoh M, Kerem E, Shoseyov D. Hepatopulmonary syndrome in patients with Cystic Fibrosis and liver disease. Chest. 2016;149(2):e35–8.

33. Debray D, Kelly D, Houwen R, Strandvik B, Colombo C. Best practice guidance for the diagnosis and management of cystic fibrosis-associated liver disease. J Cyst Fibros. 2011;10(Suppl 2):S29–36.

34. Bianchi M, Romano G, Saraifoger S, Costantini D, Limonta C, Colombo C. BMD and body composition in children and young patients affected by cystic fibrosis. J Bone Miner Res. 2006;21(3):388–96.

35. Minicucci L, Lorini R, Giannattasio A, Colombo C, Iapichino L, Reali MF, Padoan R, Calevo MG, De Alessandri A, Haupt R. Liver disease as risk factor for cystic fibrosis-related diabetes development. Acta Paediatr. 2007;96(5):736–9.

36. Pals FH, Verkade HJ, Gulmans VAM, et al. Cirrhosis associated with decreased survival and a 10-year lower median age at death of cystic fibrosis patients in the Netherlands. J Cyst Fibros. 2019;18(3):385–9.

37. Bodewes FA, van der Doef HP, Houwen RH, Verkade HJ. Increase of serum γ-glutamyltransferase associated with development of cirrhotic cystic fibrosis liver disease. J Pediatr Gastroenterol Nutr. 2015;61(1):113–8.

38. Leung DH, Narkewicz MR. Cystic fibrosis-related cirrhosis. J Cyst Fibros. 2017;16(Suppl 2):S50–61.

39. Kondo T, Maruyama H, Sekimoto T, et al. Reversed portal flow: clinical influence on the long-term outcomes in cirrhosis. World J Gastroenterol. 2015;21(29):8894–902.

40. Ling SC, Ye W, Leung DH, et al. Liver ultrasound patterns in children with cystic fibrosis correlate with noninvasive tests of liver disease. J Pediatr Gastroenterol Nutr. 2019;69(3):351–7.

41. Durieu I, Pellet O, Simonot L, Durupt S, Bellon G, Durand DV, Minh VA. Sclerosing cholangitis in adults with cystic fibrosis: a magnetic resonance cholangiographic prospective study. J Hepatol. 1999;30(6):1052–6.

42. Lemaitre C, Dominique S, Billoud E, et al. Relevance of 3D cholangiography and transient elastography to assess cystic fibrosis-associated liver disease. Can Respir J. 2016;2016:4592702.

43. Lewindon PJ, Shepherd RW, Walsh MJ, et al. Importance of hepatic fibrosis in cystic fibrosis and the predictive value of liver biopsy. Hepatology. 2011;53(1):193–201.

44. Leung DH, Khan M, Minard CG, Guffey D, Ramm LE, Clouston AD, Miller G, Lewindon PJ, Shepherd RW, Ramm GA. Aspartate aminotransferase to platelet ratio and fibrosis-4 as biomarkers in biopsy validated pediatric cystic fibrosis liver disease. Hepatology. 2015;62:1576–83.

45. Stonebraker JR, Ooi CY, Pace RG, Corvol H, Knowles MR, Durie PR, Ling SC. Features of severe liver disease with portal hypertension in patients with cystic fibrosis. Clin Gastroenterol Hepatol. 2016;14(8):1207–15.

46. Friedrich-Rust M, Schlueter N, Smaczny C, Eickmeier O, Rosewich M, Feifel K, Herrmann E, Poynard T, Gleiber W, Lais C, Zielen S, Wagner TO, Zeuzem S, Bojunga J. Non-invasive measurement of liver and pancreas fibrosis in patients with cystic fibrosis. J Cyst Fibros. 2013;12(5):431–9.

47. Gominon AL, Frison E, Hiriart JB, Vergniol J, Clouzeau H, Enaud R, Bui S, Fayon M, de Ledinghen V, Lamireau T. Assessment of liver disease progression in cystic fibrosis using transient elastography. J Pediatr Gastroenterol Nutr. 2018;66(3):455–60.

48. Calvopina DA, Chatfield MD, Weis A, et al. MicroRNA sequencing identifies a serum microRNA panel, which combined with aspartate aminotransferase to platelet ratio index can detect and monitor liver disease in pediatric cystic fibrosis. Hepatology. 2018;68(6):2301–16.

49. Colombo C, Battezzati PM, Podda M, Bettinardi N, Giunta A. Ursodeoxycholic acid for liver disease associated with cystic fibrosis: a double-blind multicenter trial. The Italian Group for the Study of Ursodeoxycholic Acid in Cystic Fibrosis. Hepatology. 1996;23(6):1484–90.

50. Colombo C, Castellani MR, Balistreri WF, et al. Scintigraphic documentation of an improvement in hepatobiliary excretory function after treatment with ursodeoxycholic acid in patients with cystic fibrosis and associated liver disease. Hepatology. 1992;15(4):677–84.
51. Lindblad A, Glaumann H, Strandvik B. A two-year prospective study of the effect of ursodeoxycholic acid on urinary bile acid excretion and liver morphology in cystic fibrosis-associated liver disease. Hepatology. 1998;27(1):166–74.
52. Van der Feen C, van der Doef HPJ, van der Ent CK, Houwen RHJ. Ursodeoxycholic acid treatment is associated with improvement of liver stiffness in cystic fibrosis patients. J Cyst Fibros. 2016;15(6):834–8.
53. Cheng K, Ashby D, Smyth R. Ursodeoxycholic acid for cystic fibrosis-related liver disease. Cochrane Database Syst Rev. 2017;9:CD000222.
54. Turck D, Braegger CP, Colombo C, et al. ESPEN-ESPGHAN-ECFS guidelines on nutrition care for infants, children, and adults with cystic fibrosis. Clin Nutr. 2016;35(3):557–77.
55. Pozler O, Krajina A, Vanicek H, et al. Transjugular intrahepatic portosystemic shunt in five children with cystic fibrosis: long-term results. Hepato-Gastroenterology. 2003;50(52):1111–4.
56. Ledder O, Haller W, Couper RTL, Lewindon P, Oliver M. Cystic fibrosis: an update for clinicians. Part 2: Hepatobiliary and pancreatic manifestations. J Gastroenterol Hepatol. 2014;29:1954–62.
57. Debray D, Lykavieris P, Gauthier F, Dousset B, Sardet A, Munck A, Laselve H, Bernard O. Outcome of cystic fibrosis-associated liver cirrhosis: management of portal hypertension. J Hepatol. 1999;31(1):77–83.
58. Lupi A, Barbiero G, Battistel M, Ferrarese A, Loy M, Feltracco P, Stramare R, Burra P, Senzolo M. Transjugular intrahepatic portosystemic shunt in non-cirrhotic portal hypertension related to cystic fibrosis in a lung transplant patient. J Cyst Fibros. 2020;
59. Linnane B, Oliver MR, Robinson PJ. Does splenectomy in cystic fibrosis related liver disease improve lung function and nutritional status? A case series. Arch Dis Child. 2006;91(9):771–3.
60. Louis D, Duc ML, Reix P, Chazalette JP, Durieu I, Feigelson J, Bellon G. Partial splenectomy for portal hypertension in cystic fibrosis related liver disease. Pediatr Pulmonol. 2007;42(12):1173–80.
61. Morrell MR, Kiel SC, Pilewski JM. Organ transplantation for cystic fibrosis. Semin Respir Crit Care Med. 2019;40(6):842–56.
62. Freeman AJ, Sellers ZM, Mazariegos G, et al. A multidisciplinary approach to pretransplant and posttransplant management of cystic fibrosis-associated liver disease. Liver Transpl. 2019;25(4):640–57.
63. Colombo C, Costantini D, Rocchi A, et al. Effects of liver transplantation on the nutritional status of patients with cystic fibrosis. Transpl Int. 2005;18(2):246–55.
64. Nash KL, Collier JD, French J, et al. Cystic fibrosis liver disease: to transplant or not to transplant? Am J Transplant. 2008;8(1):162–9.
65. Molmenti EP, Squires RH, Nagata D, et al. Liver transplantation for cholestasis associated with cystic fibrosis in the pediatric population. Pediatr Transplant. 2003;7(2):93–7.
66. Nash EF, Volling C, Gutierrez CA, Tullis E, et al. Outcomes of patients with cystic fibrosis undergoing lung transplantation with and without cystic fibrosis-associated liver cirrhosis. Clin Transpl. 2012;26:34–41.
67. Dowman JK, Watson D, Loganathan S, et al. Long-term impact of liver transplantation on respiratory function and nutritional status in children and adults with cystic fibrosis. Am J Transplant. 2012;12(4):954–64.
68. Black SM, Woodley FW, Tumin D, Mumtaz K, Whitson BA, Tobias JD, Hayes D Jr. Cystic fibrosis associated with worse survival after liver transplantation. Dig Dis Sci. 2016;61(4):1178–85.
69. Desai CS, Gruessner A, Habib S, Gruessner R, Khan KM. Survival of cystic fibrosis patients undergoing liver and liver-lung transplantations. Transplant Proc. 2013;45(1):290–2.
70. Usatin DJ, Perito ER, Posselt AM, Rosenthal P. Under utilization of pancreas transplants in cystic fibrosis recipients in the United Network Organ Sharing (UNOS) data 1987-2014. Am J Transplant. 2016;16(5):1620–5.

71. Colombo C. Mutation-targeted personalised medicine for cystic fibrosis. Lancet Respir Med. 2014;2(11):863–5.
72. Burgel PR, Munck A, Durieu I, Chiron R, Mely L, Prevotat A, Murris-Espin M, Porzio M, Abely M, Reix P, Marguet C, Macey J, Sermet-Gaudelus I, Corvol H, Bui S, Lemonnier L, Dehillotte C, Da Silva J, Paillasseur JL, Hubert D, French Cystic Fibrosis Reference Network Study Group. Real-life safety and effectiveness of lumacaftor-ivacaftor in patients with cystic fibrosis. Am J Respir Crit Care Med. 2020;201(2):188–97.
73. Debray D, Narkewicz MR, Bodewes FAJA, Colombo C, Housset C, de Jonge HR, Jonker JW, Kelly DA, Ling SC, Poynard T, Sogni P, Trauner M, Witters P, Baumann U, Wilschanski M, Verkade HJ. Cystic fibrosis-related liver disease: research challenges and future perspectives. J Pediatr Gastroenterol Nutr. 2017;65(4):443–8.
74. Witters P, Libbrecht L, Roskams T, Boeck KD, Dupont L, Proesmans M, Vermeulen F, Strandvik B, Lindblad A, Stéphenne X, Sokal E, Gosseye S, Heye S, Maleux G, Aerts R, Monbaliu D, Pirenne J, Hoffman I, Nevens F, Cassiman D. Noncirrhotic presinusoidal portal hypertension is common in cystic fibrosis-associated liver disease. Hepatology. 2011;53(3):1064–5.
75. Wu H, Vu M, Dhingra S, Ackah R, Goss JA, Rana A, Quintanilla N, Patel K, Leung DH. Obliterative portal venopathy without cirrhosis is prevalent in pediatric cystic fibrosis liver disease with portal hypertension. Clin Gastroenterol Hepatol. 2019;17(10):2134–6.
76. Scott-Jupp R, Lama M, Tanner MS. Prevalence of liver disease in cystic fibrosis. Arch Dis Child. 1991;66(6):698–701.

Low Phospholipid-Associated Cholelithiasis (LPAC)

7

Annarosa Floreani and Christophe Corpechot

7.1 Introduction

Low phospholipid-associated cholelithiasis (LPAC), synonym gallbladder disease 1, OMIN #600803, has been described firstly in 2001 as "intrahepatic and gallbladder cholesterol-cholelithiasis" due to a mutation of the ABCB4 gene which codes for protein MDR3 [1, 2]. It was later defined as a clinical syndrome characterized by at least two of the following criteria: (1) Age below 40 years at the onset of symptoms; (2) Recurrence of pain after cholecystectomy; (3) Intrahepatic echogenic foci or microlithiasis [3] (Fig. 7.1). There was also noticed a history of gallstones in first-degree relatives [2].

This is a rare condition, but it must be suspected in all cases of juvenile cholelithiasis. In fact, initially it had been considered responsible for less than 5% of symptomatic cases of gallstones [2, 4]. More recently it has been shown that LPAC affects up to 25% of women under 30 years of age with symptomatic cholelithiasis [5].

A. Floreani (✉)
Scientific Consultant, Scientific Institute for Research, Hospitalization and Healthcare (IRCCS) Negrar, Verona, Italy

Senior Scholar University of Padova, Padova, Italy
e-mail: annarosa.floreani@unipd.it

C. Corpechot
Reference Center for Inflammatory Biliary Diseases and Autoimmune Hepatitis, Hepatology Department, Saint-Antoine Hospital, Paris, France

Assistance Publique–Hôpitaux de Paris (APHP), Paris, France

INSERM UMR_S938, Saint-Antoine Research Center, Sorbonne University, Paris, France

© Springer Nature Switzerland AG 2021
A. Floreani (ed.), *Diseases of the Liver and Biliary Tree*,
https://doi.org/10.1007/978-3-030-65908-0_7

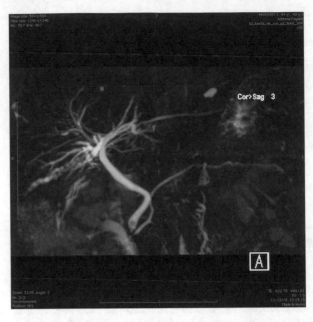

Fig. 7.1 T2w Magnetic Resonance Cholangiography: multiple calculi within dilatations of intra-hepatic biliary ducts in the right lobe and a pre-papillary common bile duct stone

7.2 Genetics

LPAC syndrome is associated with mutation of the *ABCB4* gene located on chromosome 7, locus 21 (7q21) which codes for protein MDR3 [1, 3]. MDR3 is a phospholipid floppase responsible for transport of phospholipids into bile. As consequence of the altered gene product a reduced concentration of phospholipids is present into bile, thus a decreased amount of phosphatidylcholine is excreted in the bile canaliculi. In the absence of phosphatidylcholine there is an impaired solubilization of cholesterol through the micelles which become unstable. As consequence, the cholesterol precipitates and forms calculi.

Indeed, the reduced concentration of phosphatidylcholine is responsible for the development of a wide range of cholangiopathies, from infancy to the adulthood (Table 7.1). The typical hallmarks of this disorder in infancy include high levels of gamma-glutamyl-transferase (GGT) and the typical markers of cholestasis [6–8]. It is noteworthy that hepatocellular carcinoma and intrahepatic cholangiocarcinoma have been documented in patients with *ABCB4*/MDR3 mutations. [9].

In a study including 156 patients with LPAC, a genetic variant of *ABCB4* gene was only found in 50% of cases; clinical features were similar in the groups with and without these variants, suggesting that unexplored regions of the gene or different genes could be involved [10]. Mutations are mostly heterozygous frameshift, nonsense or missense, but homozygous missense mutations have also been reported.

Table 7.1 Disease spectrum of MDR3 mutations

Childhood
• Neonatal cholestasis
• Progressive Familial Intrahepatic Cholestasis 3 (PFIC3)
Adulthood
• Low phospholipid-associated cholelithiasis (LPAC)
• Intrahepatic cholestasis of pregnancy (ICP)
• Drug-induced cholestasis
• Progressive Familial Intrahepatic Cholestasis 3 (PFIC3)

Indeed, a heterozygous *ABCB4* mutation has been detected in a woman who developed choledocholithiasis in adolescence, followed by cholestasis of pregnancy, and finally biliary cirrhosis at the age of 47 [11]. LPAC has also been described in two siblings with combined features with progressive familial intrahepatic cholestasis (PFIC) 3 [12]. However, the association between LPAC and biliary cirrhosis is rare, and patients presenting with the LPAC phenotype are not at particular risk of developing biliary cirrhosis later in adulthood.

Several hypotheses have been suggested to explain the lack of mutations in ABCB4 gene in patients with LPAC [13]: (1) Mutation in unexplored region of a gene (introns); (2) Mutation on a gene promoter; (3) Mutation in a regulatory region; (4) Mutation of another gene or another biliary carrier (*ABCB11* or *BSEP*, *ABCC2*, *ABCG5/ABCG8*, etc.); (5) Synonymous mutation influencing production or regulation of the gene.

7.3   Clinical Characteristics

LPAC syndrome affects generally young adults, with a female/male ratio of 3:1 [10]. In the large French cohort of 156 patients, the mean age at the onset of symptoms was 38.7 years for men and 29.1 years for women [10]. The onset in childhood and adolescence is quite uncommon [14]. The biliary stones present in LPAC syndrome are yellow and saturated with cholesterol in consequence of the elevated cholesterol/phospholipid ratio in the bile. By comparison, gallstone disease is frequent as high as 10% in the general population, with a prevalence rate >50% at 50 years of age in both men and women (Table 7.2, ref. 15). Gallstone disease is frequently associated to metabolic syndrome, and the rate of gallstone disease increases with advancing age, and in 20% of cases there are symptoms of disease or complications [15].

The clinical hallmark of LPAC syndrome is biliary pain leading to cholecystectomy in 90% of cases [3], due to residual intrahepatic lithiasis, Oddi dysfunction, or residual lithiasis in the common bile duct. After cholecystectomy there is also a recurrence of acute cholangitis, or pancreatitis, due to intrahepatic lithiasis or lithiasis migration [3]. Indeed, intrahepatic lithiasis can predispose to recurrent cholangitis and eventually to secondary biliary cirrhosis as a consequence of the aggression

Table 7.2 Clinical characteristics of LPAC syndrome in comparison with classical gall-stone disease

	LPAC syndrome	Classical gallstone disease
Age at onset of symptoms	Before 30 years	After 45 years
Associate conditions	Conditions linked to *ABCB4* mutations	Metabolic syndrome
Female/male ratio	3:1	1.5:1
Family history	Symptomatic intrahepatic lithiasis in first-degree relatives	Gallstones frequent in relatives
Imaging	Gallstones and intrahepatic lithiasis	Gallstones
Intrahepatic cholestasis of pregnancy (female patients)	50% of cases	Rare
Complications (pancreatitis, cholangitis, migration of calculi)	Frequent	Rare
Recurrence of pain after cholecystectomy	Frequent	Very rare

of hydrophobic bile acids [3, 10, 16]. The differential diagnosis includes congenital abnormalities of the biliary tree, i.e. Caroli disease, primary and secondary sclerosing cholangitis, and cholangiocarcinoma.

About 50% of women with LPAC syndrome who became pregnant do experience intrahepatic cholestasis of pregnancy (ICP) [10]. This condition is characterized by cholestasis, itching, and altered liver function tests mostly in the third trimester of pregnancy [17]. Another possible association is the drug-induced cholestasis following administration of amoxicillin, clavulanic acid, and risperidone [18]. Moreover, patients with a MDR3 mutation have a threefold increased risk of cholestatic drug-induced liver damage from oral contraceptives, psychotropic drugs, proton-pump inhibitors, and some antibiotics [18]. The phenotype of PFIC3 rarely associated with LPAC is caused by several biallelic variations (≥70% missense) [19].

7.4 Diagnosis

Ultrasound examination may detect gallstones and intrahepatic stones that appear as heterogeneous and echoic foci centred on the intrahepatic ducts, or as "comet-tail artefact" [20]. Magnetic resonance cholangiopancreatography (MRCP) shows the presence of intrahepatic stones and eventually, mild or moderate dilations. Such dilations may be present in one or two segments, or may be diffuse.

To confirm the diagnosis, ABCB4 genotyping is recommended in the index case and in the first-degree relatives.

7.5   Treatment

Standard therapy consists in ursodeoxycholic acid (UDCA) administration (13–15 mg/kg/day) which is beneficial for symptoms of disease. UDCA has several mechanisms of action including (1) protection of injured cholangiocytes against toxic effect of bile acids; (2) stimulation of impaired biliary secretion; (3) stimulation of detoxification of hydrophobic bile acids; (4) inhibition of apoptosis of hepatocytes [21]. Actually, no further agent is recommended in the management of LPAC. Nevertheless, on the experimental point of view two new medications might be used in the future for this condition. Interestingly, 24-ursodeoxycholic acid (*nor*-UDCA), a derivative of UDCA has been found highly effective in the mouse model of knockout mice (*Abcb4*$^{-/-}$) that closely reproduce the human cholangiopathies, such as PFIC3 and primary sclerosing cholangitis (PSC); in such animal model it has been shown to have superior anti-inflammatory, anti-fibrotic, and anti-proliferative effects compared to UDCA [22]. Recently, *nor*-UDCA has been successfully tested clinically in patients with PSC [23], thus it might have a potential indication also for patients with LPAC. Moreover, an engineered fibroblast growth factor 19 (FGF19), variant NGM282 has been assayed in murine model deficient in Mdr2 [24]. This agent produced remarkable effects on liver enzymes, liver histology, and bile acid homeostasis. Up to now, the engineered NGM282 has been tested in a phase 3 clinical trial for primary biliary cholangitis [25] but has a potential background to be translated also to patients with LPAC.

Cholecystectomy is indicated in case of symptomatic gallstones. However, bile stone recurs in many cases after cholecystectomy, thus endoscopic retrograde cholangiopancreatography (ERCP) should be performed. Moreover, rarely major liver surgery should be performed. The surgical approach for intrahepatic calculi should be individualized. Due to the expected need for long-term access to the intrahepatic biliary ducts, procedures such as hepatic-cutaneous jejunostomy with subcutaneous access loop have been proposed [26]. In case of complications, i.e. hepatic atrophy, abscesses, large intrahepatic stones, and malignancy, surgical resection may be appropriate. Patients with end-stage liver disease may be candidates for liver transplantation.

References

1. Rosmorduc O, Poupon R, Hermelin B. MDR3 gene defect in adults with symptomatic intrahepatic and gallbladder cholesterol cholelithiasis. Gastroenterology. 2001;120:1459–67.
2. Rosmorduc O, Hermelin B, Boelle P-Y, Parc R, Taboury J, Poupon R. *ABCB4* gene-mutation-associated cholelithiasis in adults. Gastroenterology. 2003;125:452–9.
3. Rosmorduc O, Poupon R. Low phospholipid associated cholelithiasis: association with mutation in the MDR3/*ABCB4* gene. Orphan J Rare Dis. 2007;3:29.
4. Erlinger S. Low phospholipid-associated cholestasis and cholelithiasis. Clin Res Hepatol Gastroenterol. 2012;36(Suppl 1):S36–40.
5. Condat B, Zanditenas D, Barbu V, Hauuy M-P, Parfait B, Elò Naggar A, et al. Prevalence of low phospholipid-associated cholelithiasis in young female patients. Dig Liver Dis. 2013;45:915–9.

 6. Gonzales E, Davit-Spraul A, Baussan C, Buffet C, Maurice M, Jacquemin E. Liver diseases related to MDR3 (*ABCB4*) gene deficiency. Front Biosci. 2009;14:4242–56.
 7. Davit-Spraul A, Gonzales E, Baussean C, Jacquemin E. The spectrum of liver disease related to *ABCB4* gene mutations: pathophysiology and clinical aspects. Semin Liver Dis. 2010;30:134–46.
 8. Colombo C, Vajro P, De Giorgio D, Coviello DA, Costantino L, Torniello L, et al. Clinical features and genotype-phenotype correlations in children with progressive familial intrahepatic cholestasis type 3 related to *ABCB4* mutations. J Pediatr Gastroenterol Nutr. 2011;52:73–83.
 9. Wendum D, Barbu V, Rosmorduc O, Arrivè L, Flejou J-F, Poupon R. Aspects of liver pathology in adult patients with MDR3/*ABCB4* gene mutations. Virchows Arch. 2012;460:281–98.
10. Poupon R, Rosmorduc O, Boelle PY, et al. Genotype-phenotype relationship in the low phospholipid associated cholelithiasis syndrome: a study of 156 consecutive patients. Hepatology. 2013;58:1105–10.
11. Lucena JF, Herrero JI, Quiroga J, et al. A multidrug resistance 3 gene mutation causing cholelithiasis, cholestasis of pregnancy, and adulthood biliary cirrhosis. Gastroenterology. 2003;124:1037–42.
12. Poupon R, Barbu V, Chamonard P, Wendum D, Rosmorduc O, Housset C. Combined features of low phospholipid-associated cholelithiasis and progressive familial intrahepatic cholestasis 3. Liver Int. 2009;30:327–31.
13. Goubault P, Brunel T, Rode A, Bancel B, Mohkam K, Mabrut J-Y. Low phospholipid associated cholelithiasis (LPAC) syndrome: a synthetic review. J Visc Surg. 2019;156:319–28.
14. Bitar A, Grunow J, Steele M, Sferra TJ. Early presentation of low phospholipid-associated cholelithiasis syndrome. Clin Pediatr. 2014;53:194–7.
15. Lammert F, Gurasamy K, Ko CW, Miquel J-F, Mendez-Sanchez N, Portincasa P, et al. Gallstones. Nat Rev Dis Prim. 2016;2:1–17.
16. Denk GU, Bikker H, Deprez RHLD, Terpstra V, Van Der Loos C, Beuers U, et al. ABCB4 deficiency: a family saga of early cholelithiasis, sclerosing cholangitis and cirrhosis and a novel mutation in the ABCB4 gene. Hepatol Res. 2010;40:937–41.
17. Floreani A, Gervasi MT. New insights on intrahepatic cholestasis of pregnancy. Clin Liver Dis. 2016;20:177–89.
18. Lang C, Meier Y, Stieger B, Beuers U, Lang T, Kerb R, et al. Mutations and polymorphisms in the bile salt export pump and the multidrug resistance protein 3 associated with drug-induced liver injury. Pharmacogenet Genomics. 2007;17:47–60.
19. Delaunay J-L, Durand-Schneider A-M, Dossier C, Falguires T, Gautherot J, Davit-Spraul A, et al. A functional classification of *ABCB4* variations causing progressive familial intrahepatic cholestasis type 3. Hepatology. 2016;63:1620–31.
20. Poupon R, Arrivè L, Rosmorduc O. The cholangiographic features of severe forms of ABCB4/MDR3 deficiency-associated cholangiopathy in adults. Gastroenterol Clin Biol. 2010;34:380–7.
21. Paumgartner G, Beuers U. Mechanisms of action and therapeutic efficacy of ursodeoxycholic acid in cholestatic liver disease. Clin Liver Dis. 2004;8:68–81.
22. Fichert P, Wagner M, Marschall HU, Fuchbichler A, Zollner G, Tsybrovsky O, et al. *24-nor*Ursodeoxycholic acid in the treatment of sclerosing cholangitis in Mdr2 (Abcb4) knockout mice. Gastroenterology. 2006;130:465–81.
23. Fickert P, Hirschfield GM, Denk G, Marschall H-U, Altorjay I, Farkkila M, et al. *nor*Ursodeoxycholic acid improves cholestasis in primary sclerosing cholangitis. J Hepatol. 2017;67:549–58.
24. Zhou M, Learned RM, Rossi SJ, De Paoli AM, Tian H, Ling L. Engineered fibroblast grow factor 19 reduces liver injury and resolves sclerosing cholangitis in Mdr2-deficient mice. Hepatology. 2016;63:914–29.
25. Mayo M, Wigg AJ, Legget BA, Arnold H, Thompson AJ, Weltman M, et al. NGM282 for treatment of patients with primary biliary cholangitis: a multicentre, randomized, double-blind, placebo-controlled trial. Hepatol Commun. 2018;2:1037–50.
26. Kassem M, Sorour MA, Ghazal A-H, El-Haddad HM, El-Riwini MT, El-Bahrawy HA. Management of intrahepatic stones: the role of subcutaneous hepaticojejunal access loop. A prospective cohort study. Int J Surg 2014;12:886–92.

Part III

Autoimmune Cholangiopathies

Primary Biliary Cholangitis

8

Annarosa Floreani

8.1 Introduction

Primary biliary cholangitis (PBC), formerly known as primary biliary cirrhosis, is a chronic cholestatic liver disease firstly described by Addison and Gull in 1851 [1]. It is a chronic progressive liver disease characterized by chronic cholestasis, which can lead to cirrhosis, liver failure, and death. PBC involves predominantly females with a female/male (*F/M*) ratio of 9:1 [2]. This *F/M* ratio has been described in several series of patients, unless, more recently, it has been observed more incident cases of males with PBC (Table 8.1, [3–12]). Unless the majority of the recent studies have been performed with administrative data, the *F/M* ratio tends to be lower than previously reported. Patients are typically diagnosed in their 50s, but the disease can affect patients as young as 20, as well as very old patients. Epidemiological studies across North America, Europe, Asia, and Australia showed an estimated incidence of 0.9–5.8 per 100,000 per year. The prevalence is variable between 2 and 58 patients per million people; there are wide geographical differences, however (Table 8.2, [6, 12–15]).

PBC is considered an autoimmune disease. In favor of this hypothesis, there are the following evidences: (a) a nearly specific association with antimitochondrial antibodies (AMA), which are present in 95% of cases; (b) the strong association with other autoimmune diseases, such as Sjogren's syndrome, Hashimoto thyroiditis, rheumatoid arthritis, etc. The cons to the autoimmune theory are: (a) the lack of response to immunosuppressive treatment; (b) the geographical clustering suggesting either environmental factors or infectious diseases; (c) a genetic predisposition

A. Floreani (✉)
Scientific Consultant, Scientific Institute for Research, Hospitalization and Healthcare (IRCCS) Negrar, Verona, Italy

Senior Scholar University of Padova, Padova, Italy
e-mail: annarosa.floreani@unipd.it

© Springer Nature Switzerland AG 2021
A. Floreani (ed.), *Diseases of the Liver and Biliary Tree*,
https://doi.org/10.1007/978-3-030-65908-0_8

Table 8.1 F:M ratio in PBC cohorts after 2000

Author	Year	Country	No. of patients	F:M	Methodology
Prince [3]	2001	UK	770	8:1	Case finding
Sood [4]	2004	Australia	249	9:1	Case finding
Sakauchi [5]	2005	Japan	9761	9:1	Case finding
Myers [6]	2009	Canada	137	5:1	Administrative data
Floreani [7]	2011	Italy	327	17:1	Prospective cohort
Lleo [8]	2011	Italy (Lombardy)	2970	2.3:1	Administrative data
Lleo [8]	2011	Denmark	722	4.2:1	Administrative data
Kanth [7]	2017	USA	71	19:1	Case finding
Lu [8]	2018	USA	3408	3.9:1	Data records
Marschall [9]	2019	Sweden	5350	4:1	Administrative data
Marzioni [11]	2019	Italy	412	4.5:1	Data records

Table 8.2 Prevalence and incidence of PBC in study populations reported after 2000

Author	Country	Period	Prevalence per million	Incidence per million	Method
Myers [6]	Canada	1996–2002	100–227	30.3	Population-based
Marschall [12]	Sweden	1987–2014	50–346	26	Case finding
Baldursdottir [13]	Iceland	1991–2010	3.83	0.24–0.34	Case finding
Pla [14]	Spain	1990–2002	195	17.2	Case finding
Delgado [15]	Israel	1990–2010	225	10–20	Case finding

[16]. Although the etiology remains unknown, the pathogenesis consists of a complex immune mediate process resulting from a genetic susceptibility and a number of trigger factors, which are unknown. Indeed, PBC can be triggered by an immune-mediated response to an autoantigen, which leads to a progressive destruction of bile ducts, chronic cholestasis, and eventually progressive fibrosis with cirrhosis and portal hypertension. Due to the lack of tolerance, bile epithelial cells become antigen-presenting cells for the immunologic attack by CD4+ and CD8+ lymphocytes. Intracellular adhesion molecules are strongly expressed on cholangiocytes and also salivary and lacrimal gland epithelial cells, suggesting a common pathogenic mechanism. Moreover, a dysregulation of apoptosis can lead to loss of tolerance and to the development of autoimmune reaction: (a) throughout the enhancement of inflammatory response; (b) triggering autoimmunity due to an abnormal presentation of autoantigens by the apoptotic fragments; (c) interfering with the recruitment of lymphocytes.

A number of xenobiotics, microbial antigens, and a variety of chemical products (i.e., hair dye, nail polish) have been hypothesized as exogenous proteins acting through the mechanisms of molecular mimicry to trigger the immune-mediated damage on biliary epithelial cells [17]. Among those: *Escherichia coli*, *Novosphingobium aromaticivorans*, *Borrelia burgdoferi*, *Mycobacterium gordonae*, *Pseudomonas aeruginosa*, which have been shown a shared sequence homology, with a cross reactivity by autoantibodies against the pyruvate dehydrogenase complex-E2 (the most important epitope of AMA). Moreover, another pathogenic mechanism exploring the cholangiocyte damage has been explored, that is, a defect in the "biliary umbrella" under physiological conditions is responsible for the exchange of Cl^- and HCO_3^- and maintains an intact glycocalyx [18]. Indeed, the "biliary umbrella" acts as a protection against the toxic hydrophobic bile acid monomers that are present in human bile. In PBC, a reduced expression of the anion exchanger 2 (AE2), which is responsible for Cl^-/HCO_3^- exchange, has been observed, leading to a toxic composition of bile. This, in turn, causes an enhanced vulnerability of cholangiocytes and periportal hepatocytes toward the attack of hydrophobic bile acids.

8.2 Diagnosis

PBC should be suspected in patients with biochemical signs of cholestasis, particularly with abnormal serum alkaline phosphatase (ALP), even in absence of specific symptoms, namely, pruritus or fatigue. Pruritus typically affects patients with PBC in a rate ranging between 40 and 80% with an increased perception toward the afternoon and night. Women in fertile age report itching before menstruation. In fact, estrogen receptors are located on keratinocytes and may influence changes in skin hydration and collagen composition as well; moreover, estrogens may influence pH changes leading to the activation of the proteinase-activated receptor-2, a well-known itch mediator [19]. Fatigue is a nasty symptom, only partially understood. Several factors can be responsible for fatigue, including: autonomic dysfunction, peripheral muscle dysfunction, central cerebral abnormalities, progesterone metabolites, and increase in different cytokines and adipokines (IL6, IL18, leptin, r-HT) [20]. Fatigue may be assayed by specific questionnaires: fatigue impact scale, PBC-40, and fatigue severity score. A patient with PBC may present at physical examination signs of cholestasis: skin lipid deposits (xanthomata and periorbital xanthelasmas), cracked skin, and hyperpigmentation. At least 60% of patients can also present an associated extrahepatic condition with typical signs: dry eyes, CREST syndrome, clubbing of the fingers, and Raynaud phenomenon. Very few cases can present initially with symptoms of end-stage liver disease, particularly with conditions related to portal hypertension.

8.2.1 Biochemistry

Serological tests of cholestasis include increase in ALP and gamma-glutamyl transpeptidase, and later in the course of the disease, conjugated hyperbilirubinemia. Elevation of IgM is also important for autoimmune cholangiopathies: as in primary sclerosing cholangitis, an increase in serum IgM can be observed in more than 50% of cases. Serum transaminases are usually only slightly elevated, except in the variant of the overlap syndrome with autoimmune hepatitis, in which serum transaminases are often upper than five times the normal range. Serum cholesterol is often increased due to cholestasis; the lipid profile in PBC is characterized by hypercholesterolemia with normal LDL and HDL cholesterol, whereas the "atherosclerotic profile" (high LDL and low HDL cholesterol) may be associated in patients with PBC and metabolic syndrome.

The hallmark of the disease is the positivity of AMA, which can be detected by immunofluorescence (IF) or ELISA, and is present in 95% of patients with PBC. AMA can be associated to other nonorgan-specific autoantibodies, in particular, antinuclear antibodies (ANA), which can be found in 30–50% of cases in PBC. However, two subtypes of ANA, namely anti-sp-100 and anti-gp-210, are considered specific for PBC. Anti-sp-100 is the main antigenic target of multiple nuclear dot (MND) reactivity. Anti-gp-210 is a glycoprotein integrated in the nuclear pore complex of nuclear membrane. In patients with a clinical suspicion of PBC, but negative for AMA, is of fundamental importance to test both sp-100 and gp-210 antibodies. Another specific pattern of ANA in IF is the anti-centromere pattern, which is associated to a portal hypertension phenotype.

8.2.2 Liver Biopsy

Liver biopsy is not essential for the diagnosis of PBC [21]. However, it is recommended when there is a clinical suspicion of PBC, but PBC-specific antibodies are absent, or in case of overlap syndrome with autoimmune hepatitis, or in case of association with nonalcoholic steatohepatitis (NASH). The histopathologic features of PBC include four histological stages according to Scheuer's [22] and Ludwig's classification [23]. Stage I is characterized by a lymphocytic cholangitis showing a disruption of biliary epithelium surrounding the bile ducts with florid periductular inflammation. Stage II is characterized by bile duct loss and ductular reaction with a dense inflammatory infiltrate forming granulomata, and eventually interface hepatitis. Stage III is characterized by fibrous septa and more prominent bile duct loss. Finally, stage IV is characterized by the presence of cirrhosis with broad fibrous septa surrounding the parenchyma. A more recent staging system proposed by Nakanuma [24] includes grading score for inflammation, fibrosis, and bile duct loss.

8.2.3 Imaging

Ultrasound in PBC has a role in advanced stages, specifically in the case of cirrhosis for screening of hepatocellular carcinoma (HCC) as in all types of liver disease. Nuclear magnetic resonance (NMR) may, in rare cases, be useful for the differential diagnosis with other types of cholestasis (cholangiocarcinoma, primary and secondary sclerosing cholangitis).

8.2.4 Natural History

PBC may remain asymptomatic for many years, all the while the disease may silently progress toward end-stage liver disease and liver failure. Over the past 30 years, the disease has been changed from a symptomatic disease characterized by symptoms of portal hypertension to a mild disease with a long, natural history and an out-patient follow-up. In the past '80s, case finding was based on the positivity for AMA, even in the absence of altered liver function tests, often in rheumatology setting. The probability that patients with isolated positivity for AMA can present at baseline or during follow-up a histological-proven PBC is very high, ranging between 16 and 83% (Table 8.3, [25–29]). Due to these findings, an annual follow-up of patients with isolated AMA positivity is mandatory, as suggested by EASL guidelines [21]. Moreover, if a patient with isolated AMA, even in absence of raised liver function tests, presents symptoms of cholestasis or an associated autoimmune condition, a liver biopsy is indicated for confirmation of liver damage.

The clinical presentation of PBC has changed over the years. Whereas, most patients presented with an advanced histological stage in earlier decades, nowadays, most patients present during an asymptomatic stage. The Global PBC cohort, including 4805 patients diagnosed between 1970 and 2014 from 17 centers across Europe and North America, has been recently evaluated [30]. The mean age at diagnosis increased by 2–3 years per decade from 46.9±10.1 years in the 1970s to 57.0±12.1 years from 2010 onward. The proportion of patients presenting with mild biochemical disease increased from 41.3% in the 1970s to 72.2% in the 1990s and remained relatively stable thereafter. The overall cumulative incidence of major events (ascites, variceal bleeding, and/or encephalopathy) was 9.1% after 10 years of follow-up but decreased over time to 5.8% after the year 2000 [31].

HCC may be a complication of patients with advanced PBC. The major risk factors correlated with the development of HCC are: male gender, lack of response to UDCA treatment, and the presence of cirrhosis.

8.2.5 Treatment

UDCA in a dose of 13–15 mg/kg/day is the first-line treatment of PBC. Its mechanism of action is not completely understood, but it is widely accepted that affects cholestasis on different levels. UDCA is believed to protect hepatocytes from toxic

Table 8.3 AMA +ve subjects with normal liver function tests

Author	N	Median follow-up (years)	Development of PBC
Dahlqvist [25]	66	7	1 (16.6%)
Mitchison [26]	29	8.7	5 (31.3%)
Metcalf [27]	24	17.8	22 (83%)
Sun [28]	67	–	55 (82.1%)
Berdichevski [29]	6	–	4 (67%)

Table 8.4 Definitions of biochemical response to ursodeoxycholic acid in patients with primary biliary cholangitis

Criteria	Definition
Barcelona [32]	ALP decline of >40% after 1 year of UDCA
Paris I [33]	ALP <3×ULN, AST <2×ULN, and bilirubin <1 mg/dL after 1 year of UDCA
Rotterdam [34]	Normalization of bilirubin and albumin concentrations after treatment with UDCA when one or both parameters were abnormal before treatment or normal bilirubin or albumin concentrations after treatment when both were abnormal at entry, after 1 year of UDCA
Paris II [35]	ALP and AST <1.5×ULN and normal total bilirubin after 1 year of UDCA
Toronto [36]	ALP <1.67 ULN at 2 years of UDCA
Ehime [37]	GGT decline by >70% of baseline or normal level after at least 6 months of UDCA
Mayo [38]	ALP level <2 times ULN at 2 years of UDCA

Alkaline phosphatase (ALP), aspartate transaminase (AST), gamma-glutamyl transpeptidase (GGT), ursodeoxycholic acid (UDCA), upper limit of normal (ULN)

bile acids by increasing the hydrophilicity of the circulating endogenous bile acid pool. It stimulates ductular and hepatocellular bile acid secretion by modulation of gene transcription and posttranscriptional events, leading to a regulation of the transport protein bile salt export pump (BSEP) and multidrug resistance-associated protein 2 (MRP2). Moreover, UDCA has an apoptotic effect and an immune modulatory effect as well. Several controlled trials showed a significant reduction of bilirubin, ALP, and transaminases in patients treated with UDCA, but despite overall promising results, RCTs failed to show a therapeutic benefit on transplant-free survival. An observational study on 192 UDCA-treated patients who achieve a reduction of ALP of at least 40% have a better transplant-free survival compared to the survival of so-called "nonresponders" to UDCA [32]. In the following years, a number of different criteria have been evaluated in order to discriminate responsive patients from nonresponders (Table 8.4, [32–38]). The use of UDCA improves transplant-free survival, regardless of disease stage and the observed biochemical response [39]. However, approximately one-third of patients have an inadequate biochemical response to UDCA. For these patients, there is the need for second-line treatment to reduce the risk of mortality and liver transplant.

8.2.5.1 Second-Line Treatment

Obeticholic acid (OCA) is the only registered agent for second-line treatment in patients nonresponders to UDCA after 1-year treatment (with ALP >1.5 upper the normal range) or intolerant to UDCA. OCA is a synthetic derivative of chenodeoxycholic acid, agonist of farnesoid X receptor (FXR), and has several mechanisms of action: (a) regulation of bile acid transport; (b) anti-inflammatory properties; (c) antifibrotic mechanisms [40]. Due to the induction of bile acid signaling pathway via fibroblast growth factor-19 (FGF-19), OCA has a more potent hepatoprotective effects than UDCA. OCA obtained the FDA approval in 1916 on the basis of an international multicenter phase III RCT of 216 patients [41]. The primary end point was an ALP level of less than 1.67 times the upper limit of the normal range, with a reduction of at least 15% from baseline, and a normal total bilirubin level. The primary end point was reached in 46–50% of patients treated with OCA after 12 months of treatment. Thereafter, all patients were switched to receive OCA in an extension phase. One hundred ninety-three patients were treated during the open-label extension [42]. In this 3-year interim analysis, OCA was well tolerated, and the performance of OCA was stable during this period. Survival benefit of add-on OCA has not yet to be confirmed. Pruritus is the major side effect of the drug and can be treated with the reduction of dosage and/or with temporary discontinuation of the drug. OCA is contraindicated in patients with serum bilirubin above two times the normal. In case of Child-Pugh B or C, patients should be started on 5 mg once weekly rather than daily, as advised in other PBC patients.

8.2.5.2 Fibrates

Fibrates are hypolipidemic agents with anticholestatic, anti-inflammatory, and anti-fibrotic effects. Fibrates are agonists of the peroxisome proliferator-activated receptors (PPARs), which belong to the superfamily of nuclear receptors. PPAR is known to exist in three isoforms: α, β/δ, and γ. These isoforms are encoded by distinct genes and have different patterns of distribution. Fenofibrate is the PPAR-α agonist, which stimulates the transcription and protein expression of multidrug resistance protein 3 (MDR3) and increases the biliary excretion of phosphatidylcholine. Bezafibrate is a nonselective PPAR agonist, targeting the three isoforms in equivalent concentrations. A number of clinical trials have assessed the potential efficacy of fibrates in PBC patients, in particular, in combination with UDCA [43]. Most studies have been limited by small sample size, yet the results are encouraging. However, the strongest evidence in favor of efficacy of fibrates originates from the placebo-controlled trial with BEZURSO [44]. This trial, enrolling 100 patients with PBC with incomplete response to UDCA, assessed the role of add-on 400 mg/day bezafibrate vs. placebo. In total, 67% of bezafibrate-treated patients achieved normalization of ALP, and 30% reached the primary end point after 2-year treatment (normalization of bilirubin, ALP, transaminases, and albumin). Interestingly, there was a marked reduction in pruritus, and this beneficial effect on this symptom was also observed in a Spanish cohort with 48 patients treated with bezafibrate over a median period of 38 months. Caution in the use of fibrates is represented by renal impairment and an eventual liver toxicity; in fact, in small number of patients both transaminases and creatinine flares have been reported.

8.2.5.3 Budesonide

Budesonide is a potent glucocorticoid with a 90% first-pass effect through the liver, and potential systemic side effects lower than classical steroids. Budesonide was the first second-line therapy for PBC, unless with conflicting results. After the first placebo-controlled trial conducted in 39 patients with early PBC, which reported a marginal beneficial effect of budesonide accompanied by worsening osteoporosis

[45], other reports failed to show a real effect in amelioration in biochemistry and symptoms of the disease. Moreover, the most important caveat for the use of budesonide was the cirrhotic stage, where a potential risk for portal thrombosis exists. Finally, a 3-year multicenter trial was terminated early because of slow recruitment and an insufficient power to detect a significant histological difference between treatment groups, although normalization occurred in 35% of the treated arm [46].

8.2.5.4 Other Strategies

A selective PPARδ-agonist (seladelpar) was tested in a 12-week double-blind, randomized, placebo-controlled, phase 2 trial [47]. Seventy patients with inadequate response or intolerance to UDCA were randomly assigned to placebo, seladelpar 50 mg/day, or seladelpar 200 mg/day. The primary outcome was the percentage change from baseline in ALP over 12 weeks. During recruitment, three patients treated with seladelpar developed fully reversible asymptomatic grade 3 alanine transferase increase, thus, the study was terminated early. Other strategies include: a dual PPAR α/δ-agonist (elafibranor), a fibroblast growth factor (FGF) 19-mimetics, a selective inhibitor of NOX1 and NOX4 enzymes (GKT831); the respective trials are still ongoing. Moreover, potential biological therapies are currently being studied extensively.

Liver transplantation is a therapeutic option when pharmacological interventions fail to adequately delay disease progression, in case of end-stage liver disease, and even in case of intractable pruritus.

8.2.6 Risk Stratification

PBC, even when treated, remains a progressive disease carrying the risk of progression toward end-stage liver disease and death. The EASL guidelines recommend evaluation of risk stratification according to high risk, moderate, and indeterminate [21]. The tools for stratification include:

1. Age and Gender: It has been established that the likelihood of response to UDCA therapy is less than 50% for a subject younger than 30 years, and more than 90% for those aged more than 70 years, and it is significantly higher in females compared to males [48]. The risk of male gender has not been confirmed thereafter but seems to have a higher risk for HCC development.
2. Liver Biochemistry: Bilirubin and ALP levels are the two strongest predictors of PBC prognosis [49]. They have been validated in two large cohorts, that is, Global-PBC and UK-PBC. The Globe score (www.globalpbc.com) was introduced in 2015 and was constructed using a derivation cohort of 2488 and a validation cohort of 1634 UDCA-treated patients. The UK-PBC risk score (www.uk-pbc.com) was developed in the same year in a nationwide cohort of 1916 English patients and validated in a cohort of 1249 UDCA-treated PBC patients. Both scores are biochemical variables on a continuous scale, resulting in more conservation of predictive information, that is, liver transplantation or death.

Importantly, they take into account biochemical response to UDCA after 1-year treatment. However, they seem to better predict the risk of progression in large cohorts than in a single patient.

3. Treatment Time Lag: More recently, a UDCA response score has been developed and validated in two historical cohorts of PBC patients: the UK-PBC and the Italian cohort of PBC patients [50]. Data show that an early interval (time lag) from PBC diagnosis and starting of UDCA treatment is positively correlated with the patient's outcome.

4. Liver Histology: Among histological parameters, ductular reaction has been shown to correlate with fibrosis extent, progression risk, and UDCA response. However, due to invasiveness of the procedure and the restricted indications for liver biopsy, this parameter has been evaluated in a limited number of liver samples.

5. Noninvasive Methods: Liver stiffness measurements by elastography have been shown to predict poor outcome. However, although elastography is not precise, it may provide useful information in the course of follow-up.

References

1. Addison T, Gull W. On a certain affection of the skin, vitilogoidea—a plana, b tuberosa. Guys Hosp Rep. 1851;7:265–76.
2. Carey EJ, Ali AH, Lindor KD. Primary biliary cirrhosis. Lancet. 2015;386:1565–75.
3. Prince MI, Chetwynd A, Diggle P, Jarner M, Metcalf JV, James OF. The geographical distribution of primary biliary cirrhosis in a well-defined cohort. Hepatology. 2001;34:1083–8.
4. Sood S, Gow PJ, Christie JM, Angus PW. Epidemiology of primary biliary cirrhosis in Victoria, Australia: high prevalence in migrant populations. Gastroenterology. 2004;127:470–5.
5. Sadauchi F, Mori M, Zeniya M, Toda G. A cross-sectional study of primary biliary cirrhosis in Japan: utilization of clinical data when patients applied to receive public financial aid. J Epidemiol. 2005;15:24–8.
6. Myers RP, Shaheen AAM, Fong A, Burak KW, Wan A, Swain MG, et al. Epidemiology and natural history of primary biliary cirrhosis in a Canadian health region: a population-based study. Hepatology. 2009;50:1884–92.
7. Floreani A, Caroli D, Variola A, Rosa Rizzotto E, Antoniazzi S, Chiaramonte M, et al. A 35-year follow-up in a large cohort of patients with primary biliary cirrhosis seen at a single centre. Liver Int. 2011;31:361–8.
8. Lleo A, Jepsen P, Morenghi E, Carbone M, Morone L, Battezzati PM, et al. Evolving trends in female to male incidence and male mortality of primary biliary cholangitis. Sci Rep. 2016;6:1–8.
9. Kanth R, Shresta R, Rai I, VanWormer JJ, Roy PK. Incidence of primary biliary cholangitis in a rural Midwestern population. Clin Med Res. 2017;15:13–8.
10. Lu M, Zhou Y, Halter IV, Romanelli RJ, VanWormer JJ, Rodriguez CV, et al. Increasing prevalence of primary biliary cholangitis and reduced mortality with treatment. Clin Gastroenterol Hepatol. 2018;16:1342–50.
11. Marzioni M, Bassanelli C, Ripellino C, Urbinati D, Alvaro D. Epidemiology of primary biliary cholangitis in Italy: evidence from a real-world data base. Dig Liver Dis. 2019;51:724–9.
12. Marschall HU, Henriksson I, Lindberg S, Soderdahl F, Thuresson M, Wahlin S, Ludvigsson JF. Incidence, prevalence, and outcome of primary biliary cholangitis in a nationwide Swedish population-based cohort. Sci Rep. 2019;9:1–8.

13. Baldursdottir TR, Bergmann OM, Jonasson JG, Ludviksson BR, Axelsson TA, Bjornsson E. The epidemiology and natural history of primary biliary cirrhosis: a nationwide population-based study. Eur J Gastroenterol Hepatol. 2012;24:824–30.
14. Pla X, Vergara M, Gil M, Dalman B, Cisterò B, Bella RM, Real J. Incidence, prevalence and clinical course of primary biliary cirrhosis in a Spanish community. Eur J Gastroenterol Hepatol. 2007;19:859–64.
15. Delgado J-S, Vodonos A, Delgado B, Jotkowitz A, Rosenthal A, Fich A, Novak V. Primary biliary cirrhosis in Southern Israel: a 20-year follow-up study. Eur J Intern Med. 2012;23:e193–8.
16. Webb GI, Siminovitch KA, Hirschfield GM. The immunogenetics of primary biliary cirrhosis: a comprehensive review. J Autoimmun. 2015;64:42–52.
17. Invernizzi P, Battezzati PM, Crosignani A, Perego F, Poli F, Morabito A, et al. Peculiar HLA polymorphisms in Italian patients with primary biliary cirrhosis. J Hepatol. 2003;38:401–6.
18. Beuers U, Hohenester S, de Buy Wenniger LJ, Kremer AE, Jansen PL, Elferink RP. The biliary $HCO(3)(-)$ umbrella: a unifying hypothesis on pathogenetic and therapeutic aspects of fibrosing cholangiopathies. Hepatology. 2010;52:1489–96.
19. Rimoin LP, Kwatra SG, Yosipovitch G. Female-specific pruritus from childhood to postmenopause: clinical features, hormonal factors, and treatment considerations. Dermatol Ther. 2013;26:157–67.
20. Jopson L, Dyson J, Jones DE. Understanding and treating fatigue in primary biliary cirrhosis and primary sclerosing cholangitis. Clin Liver Dis. 2016;20:131–42.
21. European Association for the Study of the Liver. EASL clinical practice guidelines: the diagnosis and management of patients with primary biliary cholangitis. J Hepatol. 2017;67:145–72.
22. Scheuer PJ. Primary biliary cirrhosis. Proc R Soc Med. 1967;60:1257–60.
23. Ludwig J, Dickson ER, McDonald GS. Staging of chronic non-suppurative cholangitis (syndrome of primary biliary cirrhosis). Virchows Arch. 1978;379:103–12.
24. Nakanuma Y, Tsuneyama K, Gershwin ME, et al. Pathology and immunopathology of primary biliary cirrhosis with emphasis on bile duct lesions: recent progress. Semin Liver Dis. 1995;15:313–28.
25. Dahlqvist G, Gaouar F, Carrat F, Meurisse S, Chazouilleres O, Poupon R, et al. Large-scale characterization study of patients with antimitochondrial antibodies but non-established primary biliary cholangitis. Hepatology. 2017;65:152–63.
26. Mitchison HC, Bassendine MF, Hendrick A, et al. Positive antimitochondrial antibody but normal alkaline phosphatase: is this primary biliary cirrhosis? Hepatology. 1986;6:1279–84.
27. Melcalf JV, Mitchison HC, Palmer JM, Jones DE, Bassendine MF, James OF. Natural history of early primary biliary cirrhosis. Lancet. 1996;348:1399–402.
28. Sun C, Xiao X, Yan L, Sheng L, Wang Q, Jiang P, et al. Histologically proven AMA-positive primary biliary cholangitis but normal serum alkaline phosphatase: is alkaline phosphatase truly a surrogate marker? J Autoimmun. 2019;99:33–8.
29. Berdichevski T, Cohen-Ezra O, Pappo O, Ben-Ari Z. Positive antimitochondrial antibody but normal serum alkaline phosphatase levels: could it be primary biliary cholangitis? Hepatol Res. 2017;47:742–6.
30. Murillo Perez CF, Goet JC, Lammers WJ, Gulamhusein A, van Buuren HR, Ponsioen CY, et al. Milder disease stage in patients with primary biliary cholangitis over a 44-year period: a changing natural history. Hepatology. 2018;67:1920–30.
31. Harms MH, Lammers WJ, Thornburn D, Corpechot C, Invernizzi P, Janssen HLA, et al. Major hepatic complications in ursodeoxycholic acid-treated patients with primary biliary cholangitis: risk factors and time trends in incidence and outcome. Am J Gastroenterol. 2018;113:254–64.
32. Pares A, Caballeria L, Rodes J. Excellent long-term survival in patients with primary biliary cirrhosis and biochemical response to ursodeoxycholic acid. Gastroenterology. 2006;130:715–20.
33. Corpechot C, Abenavoli L, Rabahi N, et al. Biochemical response to ursodeoxycholic acid and long-term prognosis in primary biliary cirrhosis. Hepatology. 2008;48:871–7.

34. Kuiper EMM, Hansen BE, de Vries RA, den Ouden-Muller JW, van Ditzhuijsen TJ, et al. Improved diagnosis of patients with primary biliary cirrhosis that have a biochemical response to ursodeoxycholic acid. Gastroenterology. 2009;136:1281–7.
35. Corpechot C, Chazouilleres O, Poupon R. Early primary biliary cirrhosis: biochemical response to treatment and prediction of long-term outcome. J Hepatol. 2011;55:1361–7.
36. Kumagi T, Guindi M, Fischer SE, Arenovich T, Abdalian R, Coltesen C, et al. Baseline ductopenia and treatment response predict long-term histological progression in primary biliary cirrhosis. Am J Gastroenterol. 2010;105:2186–94.
37. Azemoto N, Kumagi T, Abe M, Konishi I, Matsuura B, Yoichi H, Onji M. Biochemical response to ursodeoxycholic acid predicts long-term outcome in Japanese patients with primary biliary cirrhosis. Hepatol Res. 2011;41:310–7.
38. Angulo P, Lindor KD, Therneau TM, et al. Utilization of the Mayo risk score in patients with primary biliary cirrhosis receiving ursodeoxycholic acid. Liver. 1999;19:115–21.
39. Harms MH, van Buuren HR, Corpechot C, Thornburn D, Janssen HLA, Lindor KD, et al. Ursodeoxycholic acid treatment and liver transplantation-free survival in patients with primary biliary cholangitis. J Hepatol. 2019;7:357–65.
40. Pellicciari R, Fiorucci S, Camaioni E, et al. 6 alpha-ethyl-chenodeoxycholic acid (6-ECDCA), a potent and selective FXR agonist endowed with anticholestatic activity. J Med Chem. 2002;45:3569–72.
41. Nevens F, Andreone P, Mazzella G, Strasser SI, Bowlus C, Invernizzi P, et al. A placebo-controlled trial of obeticholic acid in primary biliary cholangitis. N Engl J Med. 2016;375:631–43.
42. Trauner M, Nevens F, Shifmann ML, Drenth JPH, Bowlus CL, Vargas V. Long-term efficacy and safety of obeticholic acid for patients with primary biliary cholangitis: a 3-year results of an international open-label extension study. Lancet Gastroenterol Hepatol. 2019;4:445–53.
43. Floreani A, Mangini C. Primary biliary cholangitis: old and novel therapy. Eur J Int Med. 2018;47:1–5.
44. Corpechot C, Chazouilleres O, Rousseau A, Le Gruyer A, Habersetzer F, Mathurin P, et al. A placebo-controlled trial of bezafibrate in primary biliary cholangitis. N Engl J Med. 2018;378:2171–81.
45. Leuchner M, Maier KP, Schlichting J, Strahl S, Hermann G, Dahm HH, et al. Oral budesonide and ursodeoxycholic acid for treatment of primary biliary cirrhosis: results of a prospective double-blind trial. Gastroenterology. 1999;117:918–25.
46. Hirschfield GM, Kupcinskas L, Ott P, Beuers U, Bergquist AM, Farkkila M, et al. Results of a randomized controlled trial of budesonide add-on therapy in patients with primary biliary cholangitis and an incomplete response to ursodeoxycholic acid. J Hepatol. 2018;68:S38 (Abs).
47. Jones D, Boudes PF, Swain MG, Bowlus CL, Galambos MR, Bacon BR, et al. Seladelpar (MBX-8025), a selective PPAR-delta agonist, in patients with primary biliary cholangitis with an inadequate response tauroursodeoxycholic acid: a double-blind, randomized, placebo-controlled, phase 2, proof-of-concept study. Lancet Gastroenterol Hepatol. 2017;2:716–26.
48. Carbone M, Mells GF, Pells G, Dawwas MF, Newton JL, Heneghan MA, et al. Sex and age are determinants of the clinical phenotype of primary biliary cirrhosis and response to ursodeoxycholic acid. Gastroenterology. 2013;144:560–9.
49. Lammers WJ, van Buuren HR, Hirschfield GM, Janssen HL, Invernizzi P, Mason AL, et al. Levels of alkaline phosphatase and bilirubin are surrogate end points of outcomes of patients with primary biliary cirrhosis: an international follow-up study. Gastroenterology. 2014;147:1338–49.
50. Carbone M, Nardi A, Flack S, Carpino G, Varvaropulou N, Gavrila C, et al. Pretreatment prediction of response to ursodeoxycholic acid in primary biliary cholangitis: development and validation of the UDCA response score. Lancet Gastroenterol Hepatol. 2018;3:62634.

Primary Sclerosing Cholangitis

9

Laura Cristoferi, Alessio Gerussi, Marco Carbone, and Pietro Invernizzi

9.1 Definition and Epidemiology

Primary sclerosing cholangitis (PSC) is a chronic, cholestatic liver disease characterized by multifocal biliary strictures, usually affecting the intrahepatic and extrahepatic biliary tree [1]. The term "primary" implies that the diagnosis could be suspected after having excluded other known causes of secondary sclerosing cholangitis.

With a prevalence of less than 50 per 100,000, PSC is considered a rare disease. Population-based studies in PSC are scarce; prevalence is estimated up to 16.2 per 100,000, with a geographical gradient from Northern Europe and USA to Southern Europe and Asia, where a 10-to-100-fold lower prevalence has been shown [1–3]. Studies from Northern Europe suggest that both incidence and prevalence are increasing [3, 4]. The reason of the increment may reflect an actual increase in disease occurrence, but also better detection related to higher awareness or availability of better diagnostic techniques, such as endoscopic retrograde cholangiography (ERCP) and magnetic resonance cholangiography (MRCP) [5].

L. Cristoferi (✉)
Division of Gastroenterology, Center for Autoimmune Liver Diseases, Department of Medicine and Surgery, University of Milano-Bicocca, Monza, Italy

European Reference Network on Hepatological Diseases (ERN RARE-LIVER), San Gerardo Hospital, Monza, Italy

Bicocca Bioinformatics Biostatistics and Bioimaging Centre-B4, School of Medicine and Surgery, University of Milano-Bicocca, Monza, Italy
e-mail: l.cristoferi@campus.unimib.it

A. Gerussi · M. Carbone · P. Invernizzi
Division of Gastroenterology, Center for Autoimmune Liver Diseases, Department of Medicine and Surgery, University of Milano-Bicocca, Monza, Italy

European Reference Network on Hepatological Diseases (ERN RARE-LIVER), San Gerardo Hospital, Monza, Italy

© Springer Nature Switzerland AG 2021
A. Floreani (ed.), *Diseases of the Liver and Biliary Tree*,
https://doi.org/10.1007/978-3-030-65908-0_9

Age at diagnosis in PSC ranges from childhood to the sixth to seventh decade, with an average age at diagnosis from 30 to 40 years old [1].

PSC has a strong association with inflammatory bowel disease (IBD) that varies significantly across countries. It goes from 60% to 80% observed in Northern Europe and United States patients to 34–37% reported for Asian patients [6, 7]. PSC is usually diagnosed after IBD, but it may also precede it or being diagnosed after liver transplantation (LT) for PSC [8, 9]. Conversely, PSC affects approximately 8% of patients with IBD and often runs a subclinical course in female patients and Crohn's disease (CD). However, despite the subclinical course of some patients, PSC should always be excluded in IBD patients, given the increased risk for colorectal and biliary malignancies.

9.2   Pathogenesis

The pathogenesis of PSC is still poorly understood. Current available evidence supports the theory of a multifactorial etiology, with the combination of a predisposing genetic background and environmental factors.

Several pieces of evidence support the role of genetic predisposition in PSC pathogenesis. Siblings of patients with PSC and IBD have an enhanced risk of developing PSC (11-fold and 8-fold, respectively). A genome-wide association studies (GWAS) of large cohorts of PSC patients has shown an association with human leukocytes antigen (HLA) that is more than 1000 times stronger than any other genetic association, which supports the notion of PSC as immune-mediated condition [10]. HLA and minor genetic associations detected in the GWAS analyses support a pathogenetic role for T cells [10–12].

Along with genetic factors, the association between PSC and IBD may shed light on some pathogenetic aspects. Three hypotheses, which might coexist, may explain the link between enteric inflammation seen in IBD and the development of PSC. First, an altered composition of gut microbiota ("intestinal dysbiosis") may produce potentially toxic immunostimulatory byproducts. Second, an increased permeability of intestinal mucosa ("leaky gut" hypothesis) due to inflammation could allow translocation of microbial toxins and bacteria to the hepatobiliary system. Third, gut bacteria or byproducts may trigger immune activation against biliary cells and consequent biliary injury [13].

Multiple studies have demonstrated that patients with PSC present reduced microbiota diversity, associated to prevalence of selected species, which are different from patients with IBD alone and healthy controls (HC). Significant abundance of *Veillonella, Enterococcus,* and *Streptococcus* has been found in different reports [14]. It is still unclear whether these organisms have pathogenic activity or represent a biomarker of severity of the disease [15].

Intestinal permeability has been found increased in both ulcerative colitis (UC) and CD. To date, no studies directly analyzed the increased permeability in PSC with and without IBD. An indirect way to test intestinal permeability is to assess for translocation of bacteria or microbial byproducts (i.e., lipopolysaccharide) across the gut barrier in portal circulation. After transplanting the microbiota of PSC-UC and UC patients and HC into germ-free mice, Nakamoto et al. reported that mice with PSC-UC microbiota had increased serum levels of endotoxin; intestinal bacteria were found in mesenteric lymph nodes [16].

The link between immune-mediated hepatobiliary injury and gut-derived factors has been suggested in animal models by showing that intestinal bacterial overgrowth and fecal administration of bacterial byproducts can lead to hepatobiliary inflammation resembling PSC [17, 18].

9.3   Clinical Presentation

Reaching a diagnosis of PSC is challenging since the clinical presentation mimics that of secondary sclerosing cholangitis (Fig. 9.1). The typical PSC patient is a 30–40-years old male with a concomitant diagnosis of IBD and elevated cholestatic liver enzymes. Considering the shared genetic autoimmune disposition, 25% of patients are diagnosed with extrahepatic autoimmune diseases, such as autoimmune thyroid disease, celiac disease, Type 1 diabetes, and rheumatoid arthritis. When IBD is associated (more frequently UC, 80%), the clinical phenotype of intestinal disease is different from classical IBD. In PSC, IBD is typically mild or asymptomatic, and it interests all the colonic mucosa with inflammation mainly localized to the right side, backwash ileitis, and rectal sparing. Unfortunately, although less frequent, severe colitis requiring biological treatment or colectomy is not uncommon in PSC patients.

Approximately 40–50% of patients with PSC are asymptomatic and come to medical attention for persistently abnormal serum liver enzymes. When symptoms occur, fatigue is the most common. Among the other symptoms, fever, pruritus, and chronic right upper quadrant discomfort are most commonly described. Abdominal

Fig. 9.1 Differential diagnosis of secondary sclerosing cholangitis that can mimic primary sclerosing cholangitis (PSC) [1] Might be a consequence of PSC

- Choledocholithiasis [1]
- Cholangiocarcinoma [1]
- Recurrent pyogenic cholangitis [1]
- IgG4-related cholangitis
- AIDS-related cholangiopathy
- Sarcoidosis
- Chronic biliary parasites infestation
- Recurrent pyogenic cholangitis
- Congenital causes (choledochal cysts, Caroli's syndrome, biliary atresia)
- Cystic fibrosis
- Eosinophilic cholangitis
- Mast cell cholangiopathy
- Histiocytosis X
- Ischaemic cholangitis
- Portal hypertensive biliopathy
- Sclerosing cholangitis in critically ill patients
- Surgical trauma

distention with ascites, hepatic encephalopathy, and jaundice may be present in patients evolved to end-stage liver disease.

PSC patients are prone to develop cholelithiasis and may report episodes of biliary colic or cholecystitis. Cholangitis occurs frequently but symptoms may be atypical, and standard definitions for cholangitis are not applicable; some patients report episodes of fever and chills, typically self-limiting within 24 h. In some patients, cholangitis could be recurrent, and they may benefit from empiric antibiotic treatment. No evidence supports rotating antibiotic strategy, which in turn might select multidrug resistant bugs. Recurrent bacterial cholangitis could constitute an indication for liver transplantation even in patients without end-stage liver disease, despite it is not associated with a worse prognosis for patients awaiting liver transplant.

When bacterial cholangitis is suspected, MRCP should be performed to identify any biliary strictures. Up to 45% of PSC patients are diagnosed with dominant stricture (DS) that represent a clinically significant stenosis within the extrahepatic biliary tree. A DS in PSC is defined with cholangiography as a stricture less than 1.5 mm diameter in the common bile duct, or less than 1 mm in the left or right main hepatic ducts within 2 cm of the hilum at ERCP [19]. Since ERCP is not used anymore for diagnostic aims in PSC, this definition is not directly applicable to MRCP findings because of the lack of spatial resolution and hydrostatic pressure present in ERCP. Thus, the evaluation of diameter is not applied strictly, but the decision for intervention is based on clinical significance of the stricture and its consequences on liver enzymes and symptoms.

9.3.1   Small-Duct PSC

Individuals with biochemical markers and histologic features suggestive of PSC with normal cholangiography can be classified as small-duct PSC [20]. It is still debatable whether this represents an earlier stage of the disease rather than a separate variant. A recent study suggested that approximately 25% of patients with small-duct PSC progress to large-duct PSC over an average of 8 years [21]. Several studies on small-duct PSC suggest a better prognosis for patients with this variant as compared to classic PSC patients. Cholangiocarcinoma does not seem to occur in patients with small-duct disease in the absence of progression to large-duct PSC. In small-duct PSC without IBD, a heightened suspicion of other biliary diseases (e.g., primary biliary cholangitis (PBC)) or secondary sclerosing cholangitis (e.g., related to genetic cholestasis resulting from ABCB4 mutations) is warranted [22].

9.3.2   PSC-AIH Syndrome

The prevalence of AIH in patients with PSC is 10% and patients are frequently younger [1]. Hence, further testing for AIH is appropriate among patients with PSC with higher-than-expected levels of aminotransferase. An elevation of transaminase and immunoglobulin G may be attributable to an associated AIH but may also be part of biliary disease. A possible association with AIH should be suspected in case of elevation of transaminase at least five times upper limits of normal (ULN), IgG at least 2×ULN, and typical or compatible histological findings. Liver histology is mandatory for the diagnosis of concomitant AIH.

On the same line, it appears also reasonable to recommend MRC among young patients with autoimmune hepatitis who have elevated serum alkaline phosphatase (ALP). In these patients, the response to immunosuppressive treatment is usually not complete respect to patients with AIH without PSC.

9.3.3 IgG4-Related Sclerosing Cholangitis

The biliary manifestation of IgG4-related disease (IgG4-RD), IgG4-related cholangitis (IRC) might also mimic PSC [23, 24]. IgG4-RD is a systemic fibroinflammatory disease with tumor-like swelling of involved organs, a lymphoplasmacytic infiltrate rich in IgG4+ plasma cells, variable degrees of storiform fibrosis, obliterative phlebitis, and often elevated serum IgG4 concentration [25]. The distinction between IRC and PSC with elevated IgG4 is important, as the cholangiographic changes of IRC may resolve completely upon corticosteroid treatment, and IRC is not a premalignant condition. Although both diseases classically affect men, PSC often occurs in a younger age group than IRC [26]. The prevalence of IBD is much lower in IRC (5%) than in PSC (70%) [27]. An approach for the diagnosis of IRC is the HISTORt criteria, which includes features on histology, imaging, serology, other organ involvement, and response to treatment with corticosteroids, and was initially utilized for the diagnosis of autoimmune pancreatitis and has been extended to include additional IgG4-related biliary diseases [28]. Serum IgG4 measurement has insufficient accuracy, and cutoff values have not been identified: slight elevations up to 5 g/L or 4×ULN occur in patients with PSC not fulfilling IRC criteria. Additional evaluation of IgG4/IgG1-ratio (>0.24 indicates IRC) or blood IgG4/IgG RNA ratio using real-time PCR (elevated in IRC) has been reported to improve delineation of IgG4 disease and could enhance the diagnostic algorithm [29, 30].

9.4   Diagnosis

The diagnosis of PSC is radiological and made upon the exclusion of known causes of secondary sclerosing cholangitis (Fig. 9.1). The diagnostic gold standard is now considered MRCP, with acceptable sensitivity and specificity (86% and 94%, respectively). Compared with ERCP for initial screening, MRCP is less invasive, presents fewer complications (i.e., post-ERCP pancreatitis), and is more cost-effective [31, 32]. The diagnosis of PSC is generally made in the setting of chronic cholestasis, in particular, elevations of serum ALP levels along with cholangiographic evidence of multifocal strictures, which may involve the intrahepatic (<25%) or extrahepatic duct (<5%), or both (50–80%) (Fig. 9.2). Diffuse involvement of the hepatobiliary system may be seen, including structuring of the

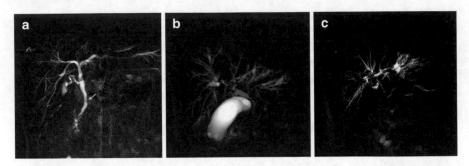

Fig. 9.2 Three-dimensional-gated T2 magnetic resonance cholangiopancreatography (MRCP) showing typical features of large-duct primary sclerosing cholangitis with irregular narrowing of bile ducts, stenoses, and focal dilatation of bile ducts. In (**a**) is shown choledochal irregular narrowing, while in (**b, c**) is most evident the alteration of intrahepatic bile ducts

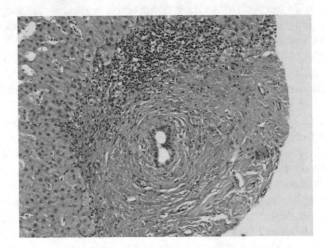

Fig. 9.3 Reproduced with permission from Nicola Zucchini, San Gerardo Hospital, Monza. Portal tracts with bile ducts surrounded by periductal onion-skin concentric fibrosis with a mild portal inflammatory cell infiltrate (hematoxylin and eosin stain [H&E])

gallbladder, cystic duct, and pancreatic duct. Although MRCP is recommended as the initial imaging modality for the diagnosis of PSC, ERCP may be necessary in patients with a nondiagnostic MRCP or for those who require therapeutic intervention for bile duct strictures.

Liver biopsy is rarely required to establish the diagnosis and is not considered necessary [33]. A liver biopsy, if performed, will show changes consistent with PSC, but the characteristic "onion skin" fibrosis is infrequent (Fig. 9.3). Given the absence of pathognomonic characteristics, liver biopsy is often interpreted as "compatible" with PSC.

The biochemical hallmark of PSC is chronic cholestasis, characterized by an elevation of serum levels of ALP and gamma-glutamyl transferase (GGT). ALP and GGT may vary throughout the course of disease and may also be normal.

Serum alanine aminotransferase (ALT) and aspartate aminotransferase (AST) levels may also be elevated to 2–3× ULN. Serum bilirubin and albumin levels are usually normal at the time of diagnosis but may become increasingly abnormal in patients with advanced disease, malignancy, or superimposed choledocholithiasis. Hypergammaglobulinemia is not a common finding, although IgM levels are found to be increased in 50% of patients [34]. Detectable autoantibodies are found in as many as 97% of patients with PSC, but none of them is disease specific. In particular, anti-smooth muscle antibodies (ASMA) and antinuclear antibodies (ANA), which can be seen in up to 75% of patients. Perinuclear antineutrophil cytoplasmic antibody (p-ANCA) and anti-p40 autoantibody can also be detected in 30–80% of patients with PSC and UC.

Full colonoscopy with biopsy is recommended at diagnosis of PSC in all patients without known IBD in order to diagnose subclinical colitis [35].

9.5 Prognosis

Patients with PSC have a four-fold increased risk of mortality compared to the general population. In almost half of the patients with PSC, liver transplantation (LT) is needed after 10–15 years from symptoms' onset [36, 37]. However, a Dutch population-based study showed a median survival from diagnosis to liver transplantation or PSC-related death of 21.3 years [3]. This difference might be due to referral bias that may confound studies on natural history of PSC, with more serious ill patients more often referred to tertiary centers.

Despite the overall poor prognosis, a proportion of patients may never need transplant. The most frequent causes of PSC-related death are cholangiocarcinoma (CCA) (32%), liver failure (15%), transplant-related complications (9%), and colorectal cancer (8%); it turns out that the major impact on life expectancy in PSC is derived by the increased risk of malignancies [3].

9.5.1 Cholangiocarcinoma

Cholangiocarcinoma (CCA) is the most common PSC-related cause of death. It usually occurs in 1–2% of patients per year, and it is frequently detected within the first 3 years after the initial diagnosis. Median age at diagnosis is 47 years [3, 38]. To date, international guidelines do not recommend specific surveillance strategies for CCA. However, in a recent study, a significantly higher 5-year overall survival (68% versus 20%) has been showed in patients who had undergone surveillance for biliary tract cancers [39].

Early stage CCA is asymptomatic and hinders the distinction between CCA and PSC alone [40]. Clinical presentation of CCA depends on its localization. In fact, perihilar and extrahepatic CCA often present with jaundice and ALP elevation, while intrahepatic CCA typically present with mass lesion and deterioration of liver function tests, but no jaundice. Since disease progression may share the same symptoms of CCA (i.e., weight loss, abdominal pain, jaundice, and increase of cholestatic markers), high levels of suspicion are needed. When CCA is suspected, diagnosis relies on a combination of tumor marker CA 19.9, combined contrast MRI/MRC, biliary brush cytology, including cytogenetic testing and histology.

Utility of serum CA 19.9 alone is limited, as it lacks both sensitivity and specificity, since it is negative in 7% of cases and may be increased in cholangitis or other malignancies. Combined magnetic resonance imaging (MRI) and MRCP show instead the highest sensitivity and specificity (89% and 75%, respectively) and are preferred for the detection of small lesions [40, 41]. Computed tomography or MRI alone lack diagnostic accuracy in early CCA due to the difficult distinction between benign and inflammatory lesions from malignant ones.

In case of clinical or radiological suspicion of CCA, invasive imaging techniques, including ERCP, endoscopic extra or intraductal ultrasound, and cholangioscopy, are necessary to obtain cytological and histological samples required for definitive diagnosis of dysplasia or CCA. Routine brush cytology detects CCA with low sensitivity (40%) and is highly dependent on operator's and pathologist's experience and to the location of the lesion. To improve the brushing sensitivity, repeated brushing or fluorescence in situ hybridization (FISH) may be considered. Cholangioscopy allows direct biliary visualization and targeted biopsy of the dominant stricture; yet, its accuracy is still under evaluation (33%) [42]. As regards the surveillance strategy, some experts propose annual MRI/MRCP or ultrasound in combination with CA19-9, followed up by ERCP, with biliary brush cytology and FISH in cases of clinical or radiological suspicion of CCA [22].

Surgery is the only potentially curative treatment and is the standard approach for resectable CCA. For patients with unresectable CCA, the available systemic therapies are of limited effectiveness.

The advances of the research on CCA pathogenetic pathways are prompting to identify new promising therapeutic targets (i.e., isocitrate dehydrogenase (IDH)-1 mutations and fibroblast growth factor receptor (FGFR)-2 fusions).

9.5.2 Gallbladder Neoplasia

PSC involvement of the gallbladder and cystic duct and concurrent abnormalities, such as gallstone disease, are seen in approximately 41% of patients with PSC [43]. This population is also at an increased risk of developing gallbladder neoplasia with a frequency reported to 2.5–3.5%. The American guidelines recommend annual ultrasound and cholecystectomy if gallbladder polyps lesions are detected, regardless of the size [44].

9.5.3 Colorectal Cancer

The risk of colorectal dysplasia and cancer is significantly higher (approximately four- to five-fold) among patients with PSC-IBD compared with those with IBD alone [45]. The risk is much higher in patients with PSC and UC. PSC-IBD patients tend to be diagnosed with colorectal cancer (CRC) or dysplasia on average 20 years earlier than patients without PSC [3] with a cumulative incidence after 20 and 30 years of 6 and 13%, respectively. These data support the surveillance strategy of colonoscopy annually or biannually in patients with IBD and every 5 years in patients without IBD. Dye-based chromoendoscopy is increasingly recommended to facilitate detection of flat lesions with dysplasia [46, 47]. CRC and dysplasia in PSC patients are most often located in the right colon, which are associated with a worse prognosis when compared with left-sided colon cancer [48].

9.5.4 Hepatocellular Cancer

Hepatocellular carcinoma (HCC) occurs in patients with PSC-related cirrhosis. However, incidence rate of HCC appears to be slightly lower compared to patients with cirrhosis secondary to other etiologies. Standard surveillance is recommended in this population of patients with liver ultrasound every 6 months.

9.6 Risk Stratification

The highly variable natural history of PSC, with possible intercurrent clinical events (e.g., cholangitis, biliary lithiasis) that could be dissociated from the severity of underlying liver disease with consequent fluctuant clinical symptoms and serum cholestasis marker, makes the prognostic assessment of these patients challenging. Indeed, reliable and solid prognostic tools able to estimate prognosis at individual level are still not available in PSC.

9.6.1 Prognostic Models

Several models have been built for risk stratification purpose. The most widely used is Mayo risk score (MRS) [49]. However, the weight of variables reflecting end-stage liver disease (e.g., bilirubin, albumin, AST, and variceal bleeding) and its relatively short horizon (4 years) limits its use in early stages.

In 2018, a novel prognostic model, the Amsterdam-Oxford model (AOM), was developed [50]. It considered up to 15-year survival probability and included seven prognostic variables: PSC subtype (large- vs. small-duct), age at PSC diagnosis, ALP, AST, total bilirubin, albumin, and platelets. A large multicenter study in patients with PSC further validated the AOM for discriminative performance and good prediction both at PSC diagnosis and follow-up [51].

In 2019, the UK-PSC prognostic model was developed using a large cohort of 1001 patients from the entire United Kingdom, including patients both from transplant and nontransplant hospital, reducing selection bias [52]. They identified some variables associated to short-term (2 years) and long-term (10 years) disease survival. By using this dichotomous approach for risk stratification, they improved C-statistic from 0.78 to 0.81 for short-term prediction and to 0.85 for long-term prediction.

9.6.2   Serum Biomarkers: ALP and Enhanced Liver Fibrosis (ELF)

Similarly to PBC, ALP has been incorporated in all prognostic models in PSC, and drug development trials on PSC have used ALP levels variation as a primary endpoint [53–55]. However, the high variability in the disease course represents a caveat to consider ALP a more accurate marker of long-term prognosis rather than short-term outcome [52]. A recent study by Trivedi et al. analyzed data from a phase 2 trial evaluating safety and efficacy of simtuzumab in large-duct PSC patients; large variations in intraindividual and interindividual serum levels of ALP were found without significant associations between serum ALP levels and disease progression over a 2-year period [56].

In 2015, the enhanced liver fibrosis (ELF) score in PSC was developed [57]. It consists in the analysis of serum levels proteins normally released during collagen deposition: hyaluronic acid, tissue inhibitor of metalloproteinases-1, and propeptide of type III procollagen. This score was showed to be a potent and independent prognostic marker for prediction of transplant-free survival in PSC [57]. Furthermore, in the same study conducted by Trivedi et al. mentioned above, variations in ELF score were smaller, and scores determined at multiple time points associated with fibrosis progression and development of cirrhosis. Unfortunately, its use is not currently widespread due to its poor availability, mainly related to cost issues [56].

9.6.3   Imaging-Based Risk Assessment

The limitations of available risk stratification tools and the progress in medical radiology have fostered the development of noninvasive tools to assess disease progression and fibrosis. The most widely performed noninvasive radiological examination to study biliary tree is MRCP. However, despite its high sensitivity and specificity for diagnostic purpose, its use as a prognostic tool is limited by the qualitative evaluation of images and the interobserver variability [58].

Another promising noninvasive liver diagnostic imaging tool is vibration-controlled transient elastography (VCTE). In a French monocentric study [59], baseline liver stiffness measurements (LSM) as well as its changes over time have been associated with clinical outcomes. However, the role of dominant and cholestasis in influencing LSM in PSC has yet to be ascertained and further studies are needed. Recently, Cazzagon et al. have demonstrated that the combined use of radiological score based on MRCP and VCTE identifies three subgroups of patients with low, medium, or high risk of developing adverse outcomes [60].

9.7   Treatment

To date, no established medical therapy able to halt disease progression has been registered for PSC. Liver transplantation is the unique curative option, but PSC may recur in the liver transplant.

9.7.1   Medical Management

9.7.1.1 Symptom Management

The most manageable symptom is pruritus. In case of rapid worsening of the symptom, dominant strictures should be sought and actively managed. First-line medical therapy includes bile acid sequestrant cholestyramine, which is often poorly tolerated. In case of persistence or intolerance, second-line therapies include rifampicin and naltrexone. The FITCH trial has recently proved the beneficial effect of bezafibrate on cholestasis pruritus [61]. Pruritus in advanced disease is often refractory to medical management and might be an indication for liver transplantation when quality of life is severely compromised. At present, no specific therapies for fatigue exist.

9.7.1.2 UDCA

UDCA has been extensively studied as potential drug for PSC. However, while reducing ALP and other liver enzymes, the evidence is not sufficient to claim that UDCA halts disease progression [62]. Nonetheless, UDCA remains widely used, typically at doses around 15–20 mg/kg daily [3, 15, 19]. Whether the use of moderate dose UDCA is efficacious in the prevention of CRC in those with PSC-IBD or biliary neoplasia is still to be ascertained [63]. A large multicenter-randomized controlled trial comparing high dose of UDCA (28–30 mg/kg) vs. placebo showed higher serious adverse events in the treatment group than the placebo group [64]; thus, international guidelines advise against the use of high doses in PSC [19, 44].

9.7.1.3 Immunosuppressive Therapy

PSC does not respond to traditional immunosuppressive approaches [22]. Previous trials with immunosuppressive drugs, such as prednisolone, budesonide, azathioprine, tacrolimus, methotrexate, mycophenolate mofetil, colchicine, penicillamine, and anti-tumor necrosis factor antibodies, were limited by small numbers [65–73].

When IgG4-related disease is suspected, a short-term trial of corticosteroid therapy might be indicated. However, in the absence of a prompt clinical or biochemical response, treatment should not be prolonged.

Similarly, patients with suspected overlap with AIH features should be treated following treatment algorithms for classic AIH [74, 75].

9.7.1.4 Antibiotics

The rationale behind administration of antibiotics is to change the composition of gut bacteria. Available data in PSC come from three randomized controlled trials and two uncontrolled studies, including metronidazole, minocycline, vancomycin, or rifaximin [76–79]. Despite the limited evidence, vancomycin, metronidazole (in association with UDCA), and minocycline can improve cholestatic markers in PSC. Nevertheless, in case the improvement on liver enzymes was validated, it would be still unclear whether these drugs affect long-term outcome.

9.7.1.5 New Potential Drugs

Based on new insights in the pathogenesis of PSC, there has been a growing interest in clinical trial in PSC. Several drugs are being investigated along the three major pathogenetic theories: modulation of bile acids, immunomodulants, and change of the microbiome. Table 9.1 summarizes the novel molecules and their targets in PSC.

9.7.2 Endoscopic Management

Endoscopic intervention with ERC should be performed in case of clinical and radiological suspicion of dominant strictures, with or without cholangitis, and of CCA.

In case of clinically significant strictures, endoscopic treatment is beneficial on symptoms with limited evidence as regards prognosis. The best interventional approach is still debated, and the choice between balloon dilation, with or without short-term stenting, remains operator-dependent.

Prophylactic antibiotics, anti-inflammatory drugs (i.e., diclofenac or indometacin), and prophylactic pancreatic stent should be considered based on the higher risk of cholangitis and pancreatitis post-ERC in PSC patients.

In case of CCA suspicion, repeated brush cytology with FISH study and cholangioscopy (when available) may increase the diagnostic accuracy.

9.7.3 Liver Transplantation

Considering the lack of durable pharmacologic and endoscopic therapy, LT remains the sole curative option in patients with end-stage liver disease.

PSC is an established indication for LT in patients with end-stage liver disease, pruritus refractory to therapy, or recurrent bacterial cholangitis [80, 81]. In Northern Europe, LT is evaluated also in case of biliary dysplasia. Furthermore, some reports suggest in favor of LT for hilar CCA that could be considered in conjunction with neoadjuvant chemotherapy and radiation, but further studies are needed to extend the indication [82, 83].

In specific clinical circumstances, patients with PSC may be offered additional MELD points to improve their priority for receiving a donor organ for liver transplantation. MELD exception points can be approved by the United Network for Organ Sharing Regional Review Board for the following indications:

1. Recurrent episodes of cholangitis, with >2 episodes of bacteremia or >1 episode of sepsis

Table 9.1 Novel therapies in primary sclerosing cholangitis

Modulation of bile acids		
*nor*UDCA	Homologue of UDCA	NCT03872921
		Phase 3
OCA	FXR agonist	NCT02177136
		Phase 2
Cilofexor	Nonsteroidal FXR agonist	NCT03890120
		Phase 3
NGM282	FGF-19 analogue	NCT02704364
		Phase 2
All-trans retinoic acid (ATRA)	FXR/NR1H4 agonist	NCT03359174
		Phase 2
Bezafibrate	PPARα agonist	NCT 04309773
		Phase 3
Seladelpar	PPARδ agonist	NCT04024813
		Phase 2
Modulation of immunoregulation		
Cenicriviroc	C-C motif chemokine receptor (CCR) types 2 and 5 antagonist	NCT02653625
		Phase 2
Vedolizumab	α4β7 integrin blocker	NCT03035058
		Phase 3
Vidofludimus	DHODH and JAK/STAT and NFkB pathways inhibitor	NCT03722576
		Phase 2
Modulation of gut microbiome		
Vancomycin	Modulation of gut microbiome	NCT03710122
		Phase 3
Metronidazole or vancomycin		NCT01085760
		Phase 1
Minocycline	Modulation of gut microbiome	NCT00630942
		Phase 1
Fecal microbiome transplantation (FMT)	Modulation of gut microbiome	NCT02424175
		Phase 1–2
Antifibrotic therapies		
Simtuzumab	LOXL-2 inhibitor	NCT01672853
		Phase 2
Other treatments		
Sulfasalazine	Unclear	NCT03561584
		Phase 2
Mitomycin C	Inhibitor of the synthesis of cellular DNA, RNA, and proteins	NCT01688024

2. Cholangiocarcinoma <3 cm in diameter, without evidence of metastasis, undergoing treatment through an institutional review board-approved clinical trial
3. Intractable pruritus

In one of four patients, PSC recurs after LT and to date, no special immunosuppressant regimens disease-specific are recommended.

Most patients tolerate recurrent disease without significant morbidity or mortality, but progressive disease can occur in as many as one-third of patients with recurrent PSC.

References

1. Hirschfield GM, Karlsen TH, Lindor KD, Adams DH. Primary sclerosing cholangitis. Lancet. 2013;382(9904):1587–99.
2. Boonstra K, Beuers U, Ponsioen CY. Epidemiology of primary sclerosing cholangitis and primary biliary cirrhosis: a systematic review. J Hepatol. 2012;56(5):1181–8.
3. Boonstra K, Weersma RK, van Erpecum KJ, Rauws EA, Spanier BWM, Poen AC, et al. Population-based epidemiology, malignancy risk, and outcome of primary sclerosing cholangitis. Hepatology. 2013;58(6):2045–55.
4. Molodecky NA, Kareemi H, Parab R, Barkema HW, Quan H, Myers RP, et al. Incidence of primary sclerosing cholangitis: a systematic review and meta-analysis. Hepatology. 2011;53(5):1590–9.
5. Bakhshi Z, Hilscher MB, Gores GJ, Harmsen WS, Viehman JK, LaRusso NF, et al. An update on primary sclerosing cholangitis epidemiology, outcomes and quantification of alkaline phosphatase variability in a population-based cohort. J Gastroenterol. 2020;55(5):523–32.
6. Boonstra K, Van Erpecum KJ, Van Nieuwkerk KMJ, Drenth JPH, Poen AC, Witteman BJM, et al. Primary sclerosing cholangitis is associated with a distinct phenotype of inflammatory bowel disease. Inflamm Bowel Dis. 2012;18(12):2270–6.
7. Tanaka A, Tazuma S, Okazaki K, Tsubouchi H, Inui K, Takikawa H. Nationwide survey for primary sclerosing cholangitis and IgG4-related sclerosing cholangitis in Japan. J Hepatobiliary Pancreat Sci. 2014;21(1):43–50.
8. Wörns MA, Lohse AW, Neurath MF, Croxford A, Otto G, Kreft A, et al. Five cases of de novo inflammatory bowel disease after orthotopic liver transplantation. Am J Gastroenterol. 2006;101(8):1931–7.
9. Joo M, Abreu-E-Lima P, Farraye F, Smith T, Swaroop P, Gardner L, et al. Pathologic features of ulcerative colitis in patients with primary sclerosing cholangitis: a case-control study. Am J Surg Pathol. 2009;33(6):854–62.
10. Karlsen T, Franke A, Melum E, Kaser A, et al. Genome-wide association analysis in primary sclerosing cholangitis. Gastroenterology. 2010;138:1102–11.
11. Liu J, Hov J, Folseraas T, et al. Dense genotyping of immune-related disease regions identifies nine new risk loci for primary sclerosing cholangitis. Nat Genet. 2013;45:670–5.
12. Ellinghaus D, Jostins L, Spain SL, Cortes A, Bethune J, Han B, et al. Analysis of five chronic inflammatory diseases identifies 27 new associations and highlights disease-specific patterns at shared loci. Nat Genet. 2016;48(5):510–8.
13. Dean G, Hanauer S, Levitsky J. The role of the intestine in the pathogenesis of primary sclerosing cholangitis: evidence and therapeutic implications. Hepatology. 2020;72(3):1127–38.
14. Steck N, Hoffmann M, Sava IG, Kim SC, Hahne H, Tonkonogy SL, et al. *Enterococcus faecalis* metalloprotease compromises epithelial barrier and contributes to intestinal inflammation. Gastroenterology. 2011;141:959.
15. Sabino J, Vieira-Silva S, Machiels K, Joossens M, Falony G, Ballet V, et al. Primary sclerosing cholangitis is characterised by intestinal dysbiosis independent from IBD. Gut. 2016;65(10):1681–9.
16. Nakamoto N, Sasaki N, Aoki R, Miyamoto K, Suda W, Teratani T, et al. Gut pathobionts underlie intestinal barrier dysfunction and liver T helper 17 cell immune response in primary sclerosing cholangitis. Nat Microbiol. 2019;4(3):492–503.
17. Hobson CH, Butt TJ, Ferry DM, Hunter J, Chadwick VS, Broom MF. Enterohepatic circulation of bacterial chemotactic peptide in rats with experimental colitis. Gastroenterology. 1988;94(4):1006–13.

18. Lichtman SN, Keku J, Schwab JH, Sartor RB. Hepatic injury associated with small bowel bacterial overgrowth in rats is prevented by metronidazole and tetracycline. Gastroenterology. 1991;100(2):513–9.

19. European Association for the Study of the Liver. EASL clinical practice guidelines: management of cholestatic liver diseases. J Hepatol. 2009;51(2):237–67.

20. Björnsson E, Olsson R, Bergquist A, Lindgren S, Braden B, Chapman RW, et al. The natural history of small-duct primary sclerosing cholangitis. Gastroenterology. 2008;134(4):975–80.

21. Angulo P, Maor-Kendler Y, Lindor KD. Small-duct primary sclerosing cholangitis: a long-term follow-up study. Hepatology. 2002;35(6):1494–500.

22. Karlsen TH, Folseraas T, Thorburn D, Vesterhus M. Primary sclerosing cholangitis—a comprehensive review. J Hepatol. 2017;67:1298–323.

23. Hamano H, Kawa S, Horiuchi A, Unno H, Furuya N, Akamatsu T, et al. High serum IgG4 concentrations in patients with sclerosing pancreatitis. N Engl J Med. 2001;344(10):732–8.

24. Löhr JM, Beuers U, Vujasinovic M, Alvaro D, Frøkjær JB, Buttgereit F, et al. European guideline on IgG4-related digestive disease—UEG and SGF evidence-based recommendations. United Eur Gastroenterol J. 2020;8(6):637–66.

25. Stone J, Zen Y, Deshpande V. IgG4-related disease. N Engl J Med. 2012;366:539–51.

26. Alderlieste YA, van den Elzen BDJ, Rauws EAJ, Beuers U. Immunoglobulin G4-associated cholangitis: one variant of immunoglobulin G4-related systemic disease. Digestion. 2009;79(4):220–8.

27. Ravi K, Chari ST, Vege SS, Sandborn WJ, Smyrk TC, Loftus EV. Inflammatory bowel disease in the setting of autoimmune pancreatitis. Inflamm Bowel Dis. 2009;15(9):1326–30.

28. Chari ST, Smyrk TC, Levy MJ, Topazian MD, Takahashi N, Zhang L, et al. Diagnosis of autoimmune pancreatitis: the Mayo Clinic experience. Clin Gastroenterol Hepatol. 2006;4(8):1010–6.

29. Boonstra K, Culver EL, de Buy Wenniger LM, van Heerde MJ, van Erpecum KJ, Poen AC, et al. Serum immunoglobulin G4 and immunoglobulin G1 for distinguishing immunoglobulin G4-associated cholangitis from primary sclerosing cholangitis. Hepatology. 2014;59(5):1954–63.

30. Doorenspleet ME, Hubers LM, Culver EL, Maillette de Buy Wenniger LJ, Klarenbeek PL, Chapman RW, et al. Immunoglobulin G4+ B-cell receptor clones distinguish immunoglobulin G4-related disease from primary sclerosing cholangitis and biliary/pancreatic malignancies. Hepatology. 2016;64(2):501–7.

31. Talwalkar JA, Angulo P, Johnson CD, Petersen BT, Lindor KD. Cost-minimization analysis of MRC versus ERCP for the diagnosis of primary sclerosing cholangitis. Hepatology. 2004;40(1):39–45.

32. Dave M, Elmunzer BJ, Dwamena BA, Higgins PDR. Primary sclerosing cholangitis: meta-analysis of diagnostic performance of MR cholangiopancreatography. Radiology. 2010;256(2):387–96.

33. Burak K, Angulo P, et al. Is there a role for liver biopsy in primary sclerosing cholangitis? Am J Gastroenterol. 2013;98(5):1155–8.

34. Newsome PN, Cramb R, Davison SM, Dillon JF, Foulerton M, Godfrey EM, et al. Guidelines on the management of abnormal liver blood tests. Gut. 2018;67:6–19.

35. Albert J, Arvanitakis M, Chazouilleres O, Dumonceau J-M, Färkkilä M, Fickert P, et al. Role of endoscopy in primary sclerosing cholangitis: European Society of Gastrointestinal Endoscopy (ESGE) and European Association for the Study of the Liver (EASL) clinical guideline. J Hepatol. 2017;66(6):1265–81.

36. Broomé U, Olsson R, Lööf L, Bodemar G, Hultcrantz R, Danielsson Å, et al. Natural history and prognostic factors in 305 Swedish patients with primary sclerosing cholangitis. Gut. 1996;38(4):610–5.

37. Tischendorf JJW, Hecker H, Krüger M, Manns MP, Meier PN. Characterization, outcome, and prognosis in 273 patients with primary sclerosing cholangitis: a single center study. Am J Gastroenterol. 2007;102(1):107–14.

38. Bergquist A, Ekbom A, Olsson R, et al. Hepatic and extrahepatic malignancies in primary sclerosing cholangitis. J Hepatol. 2002;36(3):321–7.
39. Ali AH, Tabibian JH, Nasser-Ghodsi N, Lennon RJ, DeLeon T, Borad MJ, et al. Surveillance for hepatobiliary cancers in patients with primary sclerosing cholangitis. Hepatology. 2018;67(6):2338–51.
40. Charatcharoenwitthaya P, Enders FB, Halling KC, Lindor KD. Utility of serum tumor markers, imaging, and biliary cytology for detecting cholangiocarcinoma in primary sclerosing cholangitis. Hepatology. 2008;48(4):1106–17.
41. Razumilava N, Gores GJ, Lindor KD. Cancer surveillance in patients with primary sclerosing cholangitis. Hepatology. 2011;54:1842–52.
42. Arnelo U, Von Seth E, Bergquist A. Prospective evaluation of the clinical utility of single-operator peroral cholangioscopy in patients with primary sclerosing cholangitis. Endoscopy. 2015;47(8):696–702.
43. Mendes F, Lindor KD. Primary sclerosing cholangitis: overview and update. Nat Rev Gastroenterol Hepatol. 2010;7:611–9.
44. Lindor KD, Kowdley KV, Harrison ME, American College of Gastroenterology. ACG clinical guideline: primary sclerosing cholangitis. Am J Gastroenterol. 2015;110(5):646–59.
45. Soetikno RM, Lin OS, Heidenreich PA, Young HS, Blackstone MO. Increased risk of colorectal neoplasia in patients with primary sclerosing cholangitis and ulcerative colitis: a meta-analysis. Gastrointest Endosc. 2002;56(1):48–54.
46. Kamiński MF, Hassan C, Bisschops R, Pohl J, Pellisé M, Dekker E, et al. Advanced imaging for detection and differentiation of colorectal neoplasia: European Society of Gastrointestinal Endoscopy (ESGE) guideline. Endoscopy. 2014;46:435–49.
47. Chapman R, Fevery J, Kalloo A, Nagorney DM, Boberg KM, Shneider B, et al. Diagnosis and management of primary sclerosing cholangitis. Hepatology. 2010;51:660–78.
48. Yahagi M, Okabayashi K, Hasegawa H, Tsuruta M, Kitagawa Y. The worse prognosis of right-sided compared with left-sided colon cancers: a systematic review and meta-analysis. J Gastrointest Surg. 2015;20(3):648–55.
49. Kim WR, Therneau TM, Wiesner RH, Poterucha JJ, Benson JT, Malinchoc M, et al. A revised natural history model for primary sclerosing cholangitis. Mayo Clin Proc. 2000;75(7):688–94.
50. De Vries EM, Wang J, Williamson KD, Leeflang MM, Boonstra K, Weersma RK, et al. A novel prognostic model for transplant-free survival in primary sclerosing cholangitis. Gut. 2018;67(10):1864–9.
51. Goet JC, Floreani A, Verhelst X, Cazzagon N, Perini L, Lammers WJ, et al. Validation, clinical utility and limitations of the Amsterdam-Oxford model for primary sclerosing cholangitis. J Hepatol. 2019;71(5):992–9.
52. Goode EC, Clark AB, Mells GF, Srivastava B, Spiess K, Gelson WTH, et al. Factors associated with outcomes of patients with primary sclerosing cholangitis and development and validation of a risk scoring system. Hepatology. 2019;69(5):2120–35.
53. Rupp C, Rössler A, Halibasic E, Sauer P, Weiss KH, Friedrich K, et al. Reduction in alkaline phosphatase is associated with longer survival in primary sclerosing cholangitis, independent of dominant stenosis. Aliment Pharmacol Ther. 2014;40(11–12):1292–301.
54. Lindström L, Hultcrantz R, Boberg KM, Friis-Liby I, Bergquist A. Association between reduced levels of alkaline phosphatase and survival times of patients with primary sclerosing cholangitis. Clin Gastroenterol Hepatol. 2013;11(7):841–6.
55. de Vries EMG, Wang J, Leeflang MMG, Boonstra K, Weersma RK, Beuers UH, et al. Alkaline phosphatase at diagnosis of primary sclerosing cholangitis and 1 year later: evaluation of prognostic value. Liver Int. 2016;36(12):1867–75.
56. Trivedi PJ, Muir AJ, Levy C, Bowlus CL, Manns M, Lu X, et al. Inter- and intra-individual variation and limited prognostic utility of serum alkaline phosphatase in a trial of patients with primary sclerosing cholangitis. Clin Gastroenterol Hepatol. 2020;22:S1542–3565(20)30994–0.
57. Vesterhus M, Hov JR, Holm A, Schrumpf E, Nygård S, Godang K, et al. Enhanced liver fibrosis score predicts transplant-free survival in primary sclerosing cholangitis. Hepatology. 2015;62(1):188–97.

58. Zenouzi R, Liwinski T, Yamamura J, Weiler-Normann C, Sebode M, Keller S, et al. Follow-up magnetic resonance imaging/3D-magnetic resonance cholangiopancreatography in patients with primary sclerosing cholangitis: challenging for experts to interpret. Aliment Pharmacol Ther. 2018;48(2):169–78.
59. Corpechot C, Gaouar F, El Naggar A, Kemgang A, Wendum D, Poupon R, et al. Baseline values and changes in liver stiffness measured by transient elastography are associated with severity of fibrosis and outcomes of patients with primary sclerosing cholangitis. Gastroenterology. 2014;146(4):970–979.e6.
60. Cazzagon N, Lemoinne S, El Mouhadi S, Trivedi PJ, Gaouar F, Kemgang A, et al. The complementary value of magnetic resonance imaging and vibration-controlled transient elastography for risk stratification in primary sclerosing cholangitis. Am J Gastroenterol. 2019;114(12):1878–85.
61. Bolier R, de Vries ES, Parés A, Helder J, Kemper EM, Zwinderman K, et al. Fibrates for the treatment of cholestatic itch (FITCH): study protocol for a randomized controlled trial. Trials. 2017;18(1):230.
62. Poropat G, Giljaca V, Stimac D, Gluud C. Bile acids for primary sclerosing cholangitis. Cochrane Database Syst Rev. 2011;2011(1):CD003626.
63. Wolf JM, Rybicki LA, Lashner BA. The impact of ursodeoxycholic acid on cancer, dysplasia and mortality in ulcerative colitis patients with primary sclerosing cholangitis. Aliment Pharmacol Ther. 2005;22(9):783–8.
64. Lindor KD, Kowdley KV, Luketic VAC, Harrison ME, McCashland T, Befeler AS, et al. High-dose ursodeoxycholic acid for the treatment of primary sclerosing cholangitis. Hepatology. 2009;50(3):808–14.
65. Boberg KM, Egeland T, Schrumpf E. Long-term effect of corticosteroid treatment in primary sclerosing cholangitis patients. Scand J Gastroenterol. 2003;38(9):991–5.
66. Angulo P, Jorgensen RA, Keach JC, Dickson ER, Smith C, Lindor KD. Oral budesonide in the treatment of patients with primary biliary cirrhosis with a suboptimal response to ursodeoxycholic acid. Hepatology. 2000;31(2):318–23.
67. Schramm C, Schirmacher P, Helmreich-Becker I, Gerken G, Zum Büschenfelde KHM, Lohse AW. Combined therapy with azathioprine, prednisolone, and ursodiol in patients with primary sclerosing cholangitis: a case series. Ann Intern Med. 1999;131(12):943–6.
68. Talwalkar JA, Gossard AA, Keach JC, Jorgensen RA, Petz JL, Lindor RNKD. Tacrolimus for the treatment of primary sclerosing cholangitis. Liver Int. 2007;27(4):451–3.
69. Knox TA, Kaplan MM. A double-blind controlled trial of oral-pulse methotrexate therapy in the treatment of primary sclerosing cholangitis. Gastroenterology. 1994;106(2):494–9.
70. Lankarani KB. Mycophenolate mofetil for the treatment of primary sclerosing cholangitis. Aliment Pharmacol Ther. 2005;21(10):1279–80.
71. Olsson R, Broomé U, Danielsson Å, Hägerstrand I, Järnerot G, Lööf L, et al. Colchicine treatment of primary sclerosing cholangitis. Gastroenterology. 1995;108(4):1199–203.
72. LaRusso NF, Wiesner RH, Ludwig J, MacCarty RL, Beaver SJ, Zinsmeister AR. Prospective trial of penicillamine in primary sclerosing cholangitis. Gastroenterology. 1988;95(4):1036–42.
73. Hommes DW, Erkelens W, Ponsioen C, Stokkers P, Rauws E, Van Der Spek M, et al. A double-blind, placebo-controlled, randomized study of infliximab in primary sclerosing cholangitis. J Clin Gastroenterol. 2008;42(5):522–6, [cited 2020 Aug 31].
74. Floreani A, Rizzotto ER, Ferrara F, Carderi I, Caroli D, Blasone L, et al. Clinical course and outcome of autoimmune hepatitis/primary sclerosing cholangitis overlap syndrome. Am J Gastroenterol. 2005;100(7):1516–22.
75. Gregorio GV, Portmann B, Karani J, Harrison P, Donaldson PT, Vergani D, et al. Autoimmune hepatitis/sclerosing cholangitis overlap syndrome in childhood: a 16-year prospective study. Hepatology. 2001;33(3):544–53.
76. Tabibian JH, Weeding E, Jorgensen RA, Petz JL, Keach JC, Talwalkar JA, et al. Randomised clinical trial: vancomycin or metronidazole in patients with primary sclerosing cholangitis—a pilot study. Aliment Pharmacol Ther. 2013;37(6):604–12.

77. Silveira M, Torok N, et al. Minocycline in the treatment of patients with primary sclerosing cholangitis: results of a pilot study. Am J Gastrol. 2009;104(1):83–8.
78. Tabibian JH, Gossard A, El-Youssef M, Eaton JE, Petz J, Jorgensen R, et al. Prospective clinical trial of rifaximin therapy for patients with primary sclerosing cholangitis. Am J Ther. 2017;24(1):e56–63.
79. Färkkilä M, Karvonen AL, Nurmi H, Nuutinen H, Taavitsainen M, Pikkarainen P, et al. Metronidazole and ursodeoxycholic acid for primary sclerosing cholangitis: a randomized placebo-controlled trial. Hepatology. 2004;40(6):1379–86.
80. Bjøro K, Brandsærter B, Foss A, Schrumpf E. Liver transplantation in primary sclerosing cholangitis, Seminars in liver disease, vol. 26. New York: Thieme Medical Publishers; 2006. p. 69–79.
81. Khungar V, Goldberg DS. Liver transplantation for cholestatic liver diseases in adults, Clinics in liver disease, vol. 20. Philadelphia: W.B. Saunders; 2016. p. 191–203.
82. Rea DJ, Heimbach JK, Rosen CB, Haddock MG, Alberts SR, Kremers WK, et al. Liver transplantation with neoadjuvant chemoradiation is more effective than resection for hilar cholangiocarcinoma. In: Annals of surgery. Philadelphia: Lippincott, Williams, and Wilkins; 2005. p. 451–61.
83. Darwish Murad S, Kim WR, Harnois DM, Douglas DD, Burton J, Kulik LM, et al. Efficacy of neoadjuvant chemoradiation, followed by liver transplantation, for perihilar cholangiocarcinoma at 12 US centers. Gastroenterology. 2012;143(1):88.

Immunoglobulin G4-Related Sclerosing Cholangitis

10

Atsushi Tanaka

10.1 Introduction

IgG4-related sclerosing cholangitis (IgG4-SC), also known as IgG4-associated cholangitis (IAC) or IgG4-related cholangitis (IRC), is a biliary tract manifestation of IgG4-related diseases (IgG4-RDs). IgG4-RDs are characterized by systemic, inflammatory, and sclerosing lesions with massive infiltrations by IgG4-positive lymphocytes involving multiple organs, including the eye, salivary and lacrimal glands, lungs, pancreas, retroperitoneum, kidneys, and vascular systems [1–5]. IgG4-SC is frequently accompanied by pancreatic involvement of IgG4-RDs, a condition termed as autoimmune pancreatitis (AIP) [6]. The clinical importance of IgG4-SC lies in its excellent response to corticosteroids, and thus, differential diagnosis from primary sclerosing cholangitis (PSC) and cholangiocarcinoma is crucial. In particular, a correct diagnosis of IgG4-SC resembling cholangiocarcinoma is extremely important to avoid a major, invasive, but unnecessary surgical intervention. Herein, the basic and clinical concept of IgG4-SC is comprehensively discussed. Clinical practice guidelines for IgG4-SC [7] or IgG4-related digestive disease [8] will help in further understanding this clinical condition.

10.2 History

Since the 1970s, cases of sclerosing cholangitis (SC) associated with chronic pancreatitis have sporadically appeared. In most reports, pancreatic and biliary involvements were diagnosed as chronic pancreatitis and PSC, respectively. Waldram et al. reported two SC cases associated with chronic pancreatitis, diabetes, and Sjögren

A. Tanaka (✉)
Department of Medicine, Teikyo University School of Medicine, Tokyo, Japan
e-mail: a-tanaka@med.teikyo-u.ac.jp

© Springer Nature Switzerland AG 2021
A. Floreani (ed.), *Diseases of the Liver and Biliary Tree*,
https://doi.org/10.1007/978-3-030-65908-0_10

syndrome in 1975 [9]. Sjögren et al. reported two PSC cases that responded to steroid therapy [10]. In 1991, Kawaguchi et al. reported lymphoplasmacytic sclerosing pancreatitis with cholangitis as a variant of PSC in Japan by studying surgical specimens [11]. Since 1996, a few cases of SC that met the diagnostic criteria of PSC, but presented a better clinical course than did the classic PSC, have been reported. These were reported as "atypical PSC" to discriminate them from the classic PSC [12]. The atypical PSC cases revealed characteristic findings, such as onset at older age, good response to steroid therapy and biliary drainage, no association with ulcerative colitis, and frequent association with characteristic chronic pancreatitis.

Furthermore, Hamano et al. conducted an epoch-making study in 2001, demonstrating significant elevation of serum IgG4 levels in patients with sclerosing pancreatitis [13]; Kamisawa et al. proposed this condition as a new clinicopathological entity in 2003 [14], newly coined as AIP, for which the clinical characteristics and treatment policies have been established [15, 16]. After establishment of the concept of AIP, "atypical PSC" cases described above have been reported as "SC with AIP" [17]. After establishment of the concept of IgG4-RD and reporting of isolated SC without AIP, these cases have been reported as IgG4-SC [18].

In 2008, Ghazale et al. analyzed a large database of patients with AIP at the Mayo Clinic and described the clinical profiles and responses to therapy of 53 patients with IAC [19]. Huggett et al. demonstrated in 2014 that AIP/IgG4-SC is associated with significant morbidity and mortality in a cohort of 115 patients, including 68 patients with IgG4-SC [20]. Xiao et al. reported the clinical characteristics and treatment responses of 39 patients with IAC in 2018 [21]. In Japan, my colleagues and I have regularly performed nationwide surveys of PSC and IgG4-SC since 2012 and described the clinical characteristics of 43 patients [22] and 527 patients with IgG4-SC [23]. Recently, we conducted another nationwide epidemiological survey, and the point prevalence was estimated by registration of 1026 patients with IgG4-SC [24].

10.3 Nomenclature

The nomenclature of the disease is somewhat confusing because of several nomenclatures. IgG4-SC, IAC [19, 21, 25], and IRC [8] are currently used in the literature for the biliary manifestation of IgG4-RDs.

The first appearance of this clinical entity in the title of the literature was in 2004, coined as IgG4-SC [18]. Thereafter, along with an increasing trend of studies, the term "IgG4-SC" has been mainly used by Japanese researchers who have contributed in identifying the disease concept of IgG4-RDs, AIP, and the biliary manifestation of IgG4-RDs; conversely, European researchers apparently prefer to use the term "IAC." During the International Symposium on IgG4-Related Disease, which was held in Boston in 2011, the researchers discussed the nomenclature and agreed that the term "related" rather than "associated" was preferred to express IgG4-RDs in specific organs, including the pancreas and bile ducts; they also emphasized the importance of including "sclerosing" in the nomenclature because it is important to link this condition with and distinguish it from PSC, even though "sclerosis" of the bile ducts is not always observed after successful treatment with corticosteroids [3]. As no international consensus in terms of alternative nomenclatures has been achieved, the term "IgG4-SC" has validity in the current scientific literature. Yet, a recent European guideline on IgG4-related digestive disease recommends the use of IRC because of the very reason that the term "sclerosing" may evoke PSC, a progressive disease without any effective treatment [8]. Undoubtedly, an identical term should be used in this biliary disorder, and another international consensus regarding the nomenclature is strongly warranted.

10.4 Etiology

Although a significant elevation in serum IgG4 levels is a hallmark of IgG4-SC and IgG4-RDs, the role of IgG4 remains unclear and enigmatic. IgG4 antibodies comprise the smallest fraction (<5%) of all IgG antibodies in the sera of healthy humans [26]. Patients with IgG4-SC and IgG4-RD exhibit a dramatic response to rituximab, an anti-CD20 antibody, indicating a pathogenic role of B-cell responses and Igs. Indeed, IgG4+ B-cell clones were identified in the blood and tissues of patients with IgG4-SC and disappeared upon corticosteroid treatment [27], suggesting the pathogenicity of IgG4 molecules, as observed in other autoimmune diseases, including pemphigus [28, 29] or idiopathic membranous glomerulonephritis [30]. Nevertheless, recent studies suggest an anti-inflammatory role of IgG4 in this disease. For instance, Shiokawa et al. demonstrated that subcutaneous injection of patient IgG, not control IgG, resulted in pancreatic injuries, which mimic AIP. Interestingly, while pancreatic injury was induced by injecting both IgG1 and IgG4, more destructive changes were induced by IgG1 than by IgG4. The potent pathogenic activity in patients with IgG1 was significantly inhibited by the injection of IgG4 [31]. IgG4-subtype autoantibodies remained undiscovered for a long time until the identification of anti-annexin A11 as an autoantigen, which was targeted by IgG4 as well as IgG1 autoantibodies [32]. Coincident with the findings of Shiokawa et al., IgG4 antibodies blocked the binding of IgG1 to annexin A11, supporting an anti-inflammatory role, not a pro-inflammatory role, of IgG4 in IgG4-RDs. In fact, IgG4 is biologically unable to activate Fc-gamma receptors on the effector cells owing to its low affinity and is, therefore, considered an anti-inflammatory Ig [26]. Moreover, IgG4 may be secondarily induced to reduce the extensive immune reaction in IgG4-RDs. In IgG4-RDs, Th2-cytokines, such as IL-4, IL-5, and IL-13, are significantly overexpressed, contributing to oligoclonal B-cell activation, plasma cell expansion, and extensive IgG4 production [33]. Taken together, IgG4 appears to be a two-sided antibody in the etiopathogenesis of IgG4-SC. IgG4 functions as a destructive and pathogenic molecule and at the same time may function as a protective antibody against a more harmful role of IgG1 when directed to the same epitopes [34].

10.5   Epidemiology and Demographics

Recently, our group conducted the first-ever epidemiological study to estimate the point prevalence of IgG4-SC in Japan [24]. In this study, we selected 1180 departments from health centers covering all over Japan and investigated the number of patients with IgG4-SC in 2018 in a questionnaire-based manner. The estimated number of patients and the point prevalence in Japan were 2742 (95% confidence interval [CI], 2683–2811) and 2.18 (95% CI, 2.13–2.23) per 100,000 population, respectively. The prevalence of IgG4-SC was 1.2 times higher than the point prevalence of PSC in Japan (1.80; 95% CI, 1.75–1.85), which was estimated using an identical method.

The demographics of patients with IgG4-SC in the USA [19], the UK [20], Japan [23], and China [21] are summarized in Table 10.1. IgG4-RDs are generally a male-dominant disease, and indeed, male sex was dominant in all case series of IgG4-SC. The age during presentation was similar among the three reports, indicating that patients in their 60s were at the highest risk of developing IgG4-SC. In Fig. 10.1, the age and sex distributions at presentation are shown for 1096 cases of IgG4-SC in Japan [24]. The patient age ranged from 21.7 to 92.8 years, and no patient developed IgG4-SC in childhood or adolescence, unlike PSC. The median age at diagnosis was 67.1 years. Male sex predominance is obvious at any age.

10.6   Diagnosis

To date, no single biomarker with high specificity and sensitivity has been found for the diagnosis of IgG4-SC. Elevation of serum IgG4 level, a hallmark of IgG4-RD in general, is not observed in all patients. Therefore, a combination of several clinical parameters, including blood biochemistry, imaging studies, histological studies, and presence of IgG4-RD in other organs, is needed; diagnostic criteria comprising these findings have been established and are currently used in clinical practice [19, 35].

Table 10.1 Comparison of the clinical features of immunoglobulin G4-related sclerosing cholangitis

Region	Year	N	Male sex (%)	Age at diagnosis (years)[a]	Most prevalent symptom at diagnosis (%)	Presence of AIP (%)
USA [19]	2008	53	85	62	Jaundice (77%)	92
UK [20]	2014	68	74	61	Jaundice (74%)	88
Japan [23]	2017	527	83	66	Jaundice (39%)	87
China [21]	2018	39	82	NA	Jaundice (67%)	90

Autoimmune pancreatitis (AIP), not available (NA)
[a]Average (USA), median (UK and Japan)

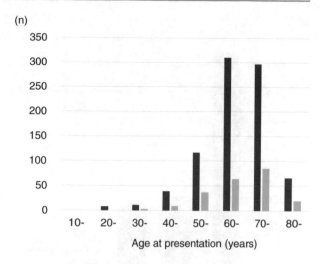

Fig. 10.1 Distributions of age at presentation in a Japanese cohort of 1096 patients with immunoglobulin G4-related sclerosing cholangitis [24]. Black and gray bars indicate the male and female patients, respectively

Symptoms at presentation. The most frequent symptom is jaundice due to obstruction of the extrahepatic bile ducts, especially at the distal portion of the bile ducts surrounded by the swollen pancreatic head, coinciding with a high frequency of AIP as comorbidities. In the cohort from the USA, the UK, and China, 77%, 74%, and 67% of patients with IgG4-SC had jaundice at presentation, respectively (Table 10.1) [19–21]. In the cohort from Japan, 428 out of 1096 patients (39%) developed jaundice at presentation, followed by pruritus (14%) and abdominal pain (13%), whereas 410 patients (37%) were diagnosed as having IgG4-SC without any symptoms (Fig. 10.2) [24]. The proportion of asymptomatic patients is higher in this cohort, owing to the higher chances of having blood tested for health checkups in Japan.

Blood chemistry and serology. Levels of cholestatic liver enzymes, serum alkaline phosphatase (ALP), and gamma-glutamyl transferase are elevated in most cases, as in other cholestatic liver diseases. Bilirubin levels are also elevated in patients with icterus. Although elevated levels of serum IgG4 are a hallmark of IgG4-SC, it is of note that 14% of patients exhibited serum IgG4 levels within normal levels at presentation (Fig. 10.3); therefore, the diagnosis of IgG4-SC cannot be denied even in a patient with normal IgG4 levels in the serum. Antinuclear antibodies were positive in only 39% of patients in the Japanese cohort. Although no disease-specific autoantibodies were reported in IgG4-SC, annexin A11 [32] and laminin 511-E8 [36] were recently identified as autoantigens in IgG4-RD and AIP, respectively. Anti-laminin 511-E8 antibody was detected in a patient with IgG4-SC with normal serum IgG4 levels and provided an important clue for diagnosis [37]. Further analyses with large-scale samples are strongly warranted to evaluate the diagnostic capability of these autoantibodies for IgG4-SC.

Imaging. It is extremely important to perform cholangiography, either endoscopic retrograde cholangiography (ERC) or magnetic resonance cholangiography, for the diagnosis of IgG4-SC. In characteristic cholangiograms of patients with IgG4-SC, diffuse or segmental narrowing of the intra and/or extrahepatic bile ducts

(n)

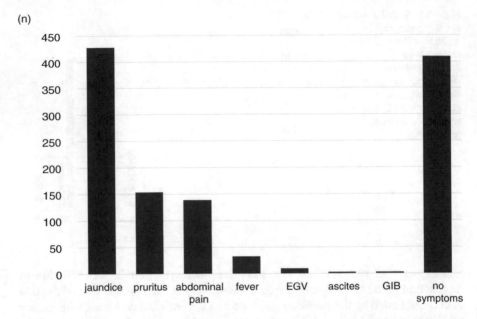

Fig. 10.2 Symptoms at presentation in a Japanese cohort of 1096 patients with immunoglobulin G4-related sclerosing cholangitis [24]. Esophagogastric varices (EGV), gastrointestinal bleeding (GIB)

Fig. 10.3 Proportion of serum immunoglobulin G4 levels at pretreatment in a Japanese cohort of 1096 patients with immunoglobulin G4-related sclerosing cholangitis [24]. Upper limit of normal (ULN)

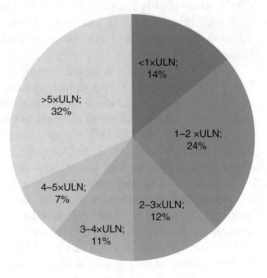

is observed, along with thickening of the bile duct wall; this helps distinguish IgG4-SC from PSC, pancreatic cancer, bile duct cancer, and hepatic hilar carcinoma.

Nakazawa et al. proposed a classification of cholangiograms in IgG4-SC (Fig. 10.4) [38]: intrapancreatic biliary strictures without any other stricture in the bile ducts (type 1), intrahepatic segmental (type 2a) and diffuse (type 2b) strictures in addition to intrapancreatic biliary strictures, both intrapancreatic and hilar lesions (type 3), and strictures in the hilar hepatic lesion (type 4). Type 1 is the most dominant, as observed in 64% of patients in the Japanese cohort [23], reflecting the frequent coexistence of AIP, as shown later; however, it could be very difficult to differentiate IgG4-SC from pancreatic cancer in cases without AIP. Types 2a, 2b, 3, and 4 were found in 5%, 8%, 11%, and 10% of patients, respectively. Types 3 and 4 mimic bile duct cancer or hepatic hilar carcinoma, and the differential diagnosis could be challenging.

Histology. When IgG4-SC is suspected on the basis of symptoms and blood chemistry, serology, and cholangiogram findings, specimens for histological examination should be obtained. The characteristic features of histology in IgG4-SC included (1) marked lymphoplasmacytic infiltration and fibrosis, (2) >10 IgG4-positive plasma cells per HPF, (3) storiform fibrosis, and (4) obliterative phlebitis [35]. A cutoff of >10 IgG4-positive cells per HPF was considered for biopsy-based diagnosis of IgG4-SC.

IgG4-SC is characterized by transmural-marked lymphoplasmacytic infiltration and fibrosis, which results in duct wall thickening. In contrast to PSC, in which the

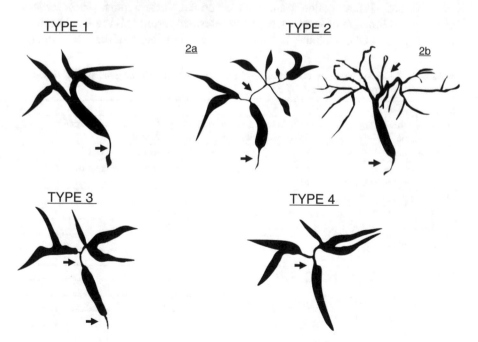

Fig. 10.4 Classification of cholangiographic findings of immunoglobulin G4-related sclerosing cholangitis [38]

emphasis of inflammation is the epithelium, no cell damage or inflammatory cell infiltration is observed in the epithelium [7]. Eosinophilic infiltration, storiform fibrosis, and/or obliterative phlebitis are commonly identified, and the latter two are particularly regarded as diagnostically important. Storiform fibrosis is an irregular swirling arrangement of collagen [39], and inflammatory cells are commonly observed. Obliterative phlebitis is an inflammatory lesion with inflammatory cells and fibrosis that obliterates the venous lumen [39].

Comorbidities. The presence of other organ involvement (OOI) in IgG4-RD greatly facilitates the diagnosis of IgG4-SC, and AIP was the most prevalent OOI, being present in 88–92% of patients (Table 10.1) [19–21, 24]. Other OOIs include dacryoadenitis and sialadenitis, retroperitoneal fibrosis, and involvement of the kidneys, lungs, and aorta. In the Japanese cohort, dacryoadenitis and sialadenitis and retroperitoneal fibrosis were observed in 22% and 12% of cases, respectively [24]. Regarding malignant diseases in the biliary tract, the development of cholangiocarcinoma was reported only in four cases (0.8%) in the Japanese cohort, indicating that the occurrence of cholangiocarcinoma is a rare event in patients with IgG4-SC.

Diagnostic criteria. As discussed, a combination of biomarkers and findings is required to diagnose IgG4-SC. In the USA and Europe, the histology, imaging, serology, OOI, and response to therapy criteria, which were originally designed for the diagnosis of AIP [40], have frequently been used for the diagnosis of IgG4-SC (or IAC) [19, 41, 42]. In 2012, the diagnostic criteria of IgG4-SC were established by the Japanese Biliary Association [35] (Table 10.2) to facilitate its appropriate diagnosis and differentiation from PSC or cholangiocarcinoma. These criteria involve a combination of imaging, serology (elevated serum IgG4 level), histological findings, and OOI. Definite diagnosis is made on the basis of the following: (1)

Table 10.2 Clinical diagnostic criteria of IgG4-related sclerosing cholangitis, as established by the Japanese Biliary Association in 2012[a]

Diagnostic items
(1) Biliary tract imaging reveals diffuse or segmental narrowing of the intrahepatic and/or extrahepatic bile ducts, associated with thickening of the bile duct wall
(2) Hematological examination presents elevated serum IgG4 levels (≥135 mg/dL)
(3) Coexistence of autoimmune pancreatitis, IgG4-related dacryoadenitis/sialadenitis, or IgG4-related retroperitoneal fibrosis
(4) Histopathological examination reveals:
(a) Marked lymphocytic and plasmacytic infiltration and fibrosis
(b) Infiltration of IgG4-positive plasma cells (>10 cells per HPF)
(c) Storiform fibrosis
(d) Obliterative phlebitis
Optional: effectiveness of steroid therapy
Diagnosis
Definite diagnosis: (1)+(3) or (1)+(2)+(4) (a+b or a+b+c or a+b+d)
Probable diagnosis: (1)+(2)+optional item
Possible diagnosis: (1)+(2)

Immunoglobulin (Ig)
[a]Adapted from Ohara et al. [35]

imaging findings and OOI; (2) imaging findings, observation of elevated IgG4 levels, and two typical histological findings: marked lymphocytic and plasmacytic infiltration and fibrosis and infiltration by IgG4-positive plasma cells; and (3) three typical histological findings: the two aforementioned and storiform fibrosis.

10.7   Differential Diagnosis

As mentioned previously, it is extremely important to differentiate IgG4-SC from PSC or pancreatobiliary malignancy, based on an excellent response of IgG4-SC to corticosteroids. Moreover, unnecessary major operations for pancreatobiliary cancer profoundly affecting the postoperative quality of life of patients can be avoided with a correct diagnosis of IgG4-SC. Nevertheless, it could be extremely challenging to do so, especially in distinguishing type 1 IgG4-SC from pancreatic cancer, type 2 from PSC and bile duct cancer, and types 3 and 4 from hepatic hilar cholangiocarcinoma.

PSC. While elevated IgG4 levels are found in 10–20% of patients with PSC [7], an ample elevation of serum IgG4 levels (e.g., $\geq 1.25 \times$ULN) may help in the differential diagnosis of IgG4-SC from PSC with excellent predictability [43]. The median IgG4/IgG1 ratio in IgG4-SC was significantly higher than that in PSC, indicating the utility of the IgG4/IgG1 ratio in clinical practice for differentiating IgG4-SC from PSC [44]. The IgG4/IgG RNA ratio determined by quantitative PCR may allow more accurate discrimination of IgG4-SC from PSC [42]. IgG1 and IgG2 [45] and unique patterns of glycosylation in IgG [46] may aid in the accurate diagnosis of IgG4-SC and PSC. Although experienced gastroenterologists are able to differentiate IgG4-SC from PSC by ERC findings with serum IgG4 levels in terms of imaging studies [47], an international panel suggested that ERC findings themselves did not provide sufficient reliability for correct diagnosis without additional clinical information [48]. The presence of comorbidities is very helpful for differentiation; OOI of IgG4-RD or inflammatory bowel diseases strongly support the diagnosis of IgG4-SC or PSC, respectively. Systemic examination is required for search, even though patients complain of no subjective symptoms. A scoring system employing age, OOI, and beaded appearance on ERC is proposed [49]. Administration of corticosteroids before confirmation of diagnosis ("steroid trials") may be a final option when diagnosis is extremely difficult, but is allowed only for a short-term, that is, 1–2 weeks [7].

Pancreatobiliary malignancies. While a number of reports showed cases of IgG4-SC that were misdiagnosed as cholangiocarcinoma before operation, others have demonstrated the reverse [50], possibly leading to a worse outcome. Elevated IgG4 levels are also found in 10–20% of patients with cholangiocarcinoma [7]. Although it was reported that the IgG4/IgG RNA ratio may also allow discrimination of IgG4-SC from biliary/pancreatic malignancies [42], further study by the same group denied this result later [51]. Imaging studies with intraductal ultrasonography (IDUS) or peroral cholangioscopy (POCS) are very helpful for differentiating IgG4-SC from cholangiocarcinoma [7]. IDUS findings of circular, symmetric wall thickness, a smooth inner and outer margin, and a homogeneous internal echo in the stricture as well as >0.8 mm of the bile duct wall in nonstricture regions strongly suggest IgG4-SC [52]. In POCS, findings of tortuous and dilated arteries in the bile ducts are suggestive of IgG4-SC and partially dilated arteries of cholangiocarcinoma [53].

Histological findings of biopsied samples obtained from the bile ducts or endoscopic ultrasound fine-needle aspiration from the pancreas are used for the final diagnosis of bile duct or pancreatic cancer when findings of malignancy are observed; however, a suspicion for carcinoma should be maintained even if not observed. The use of fluorescence in situ hybridization using transpapillary forceps biopsy specimens might be an option to differentiate cholangiocarcinoma from IgG4-SC [54]. Steroid trials should not be performed when a suspicion of pancreatobiliary cancer remains [7].

10.8 Management and Outcomes

It is well known that prednisolone (PSL) is efficient in treating IgG4-SC, as for other IgG4-RDs, although no randomized prospective trial of corticosteroids has been conducted for IgG4-SC. In the Japanese cohort, PSL was initiated in 462 patients (88%) following diagnosis [23]. In the US and UK cohorts, corticosteroid was administered in 57% and 85% of patients, respectively [19, 20]. The overall treatment responses in these retrospective observational study protocols were excellent. In the Japanese cohort, reduction in the ALP levels to <50% of the pretreatment levels or within the normal range was achieved in 395 patients (88% of documented cases), and alleviation of biliary strictures was noted on the imaging results of 376 patients (90% of documented cases). Endoscopic stents inserted for the treatment of obstructive jaundice should be removed within 2 weeks after corticosteroid administration [55]. Coincident with the excellent short-term efficacy of corticosteroids, the long-term outcome of IgG4-SC appears to be excellent. In Table 10.3, the

Table 10.3 Treatment and outcomes of patients with IgG4-SC

Region	Year	n	Follow-up period (months)	Corticosteroid treatment (%)	Progression to cirrhosis (%)	All-cause mortality (%)	LT	Mortality due to liver and bile duct diseases
USA [19]	2008	53	29.5[a]	30 (57%)	4 (7.5%)	7 (13%)	0	1 (1.9%)
UK [20]	2014	68	32.5	98 (85%)[b]	6 (5.2%)[a]	11 (9.6%)[a]	1	3 (2.6%)[a]
Japan [23]	2017	527	49.2	458 (88%)	N/A	26 (5%)	0	4 (0.8%)

Immunoglobulin G4-related sclerosing cholangitis (IgG4-SC), liver transplantation (LT)
[a] Mean follow-up period of patients treated with corticosteroids
[b] Proportion of 115 patients with autoimmune pancreatitis, including those without IgG4-SC

outcomes are summarized for the US, UK, and Japanese cohorts. During 4.1±3.1 years of follow-up in the Japanese cohort, 27 patients (5%) were reported to have died; however, only four patients died from liver or bile duct-related pathological conditions. No liver transplantation was performed in this cohort. Cirrhosis progression accounted for two deaths. The overall 5- and 10-year survival rates were 94.4% and 81.0%, respectively, and the 5- and 10-year survival rates from hepatobiliary disease-related deaths were 98.9% and 97.7%, respectively. Conversely, progression to cirrhosis was noted in 5.2% and 7.5% of patients in the UK and US cohorts, respectively. Mortality due to liver or bile duct complications was observed in only one case in the US cohort and in two cases liver failure and cholangiocarcinoma and one case that underwent liver transplantation in the UK cohort.

In contrast, relapse of IgG4-SC, that is, restenosis of the bile ducts, is commonly observed, particularly in patients for whom corticosteroid treatment is terminated. During the follow-up period, relapse of IgG4-SC was noted in 104 patients (19%) in the Japanese cohort. The cumulative rates of restenosis were 1.6%, 7.6%, and 16.5% at 1, 3, and 5 years after diagnosis, respectively. Nevertheless, the overall survival was similar between patients with and without restenosis. In the multivariate analysis, the presence of any symptoms at presentation and discontinuation of corticosteroid treatment were identified as factors independently associated with relapse [23]. A retrospective study at the Mayo Clinic demonstrated that rituximab maintenance therapy reduces the rate of relapse [56]. However, it is of note that a minority of patients with multiple organs affected, a more fibrotic phenotype, and multiple duct strictures may exhibit poor responses to corticosteroids [8, 57]. The efficacy of rituximab and other immunomodulatory agents, including thiopurines and mycophenolate mofetil, should be investigated in refractory cases in the near future.

10.9 Future Direction

IgG4-SC is a relatively new clinical entity, and a number of uncertainties still remain, including etiology, incidence and prevalence, risk factors, biomarkers for diagnosis (autoantibodies), natural history, and long-term outcomes. In particular, biomarkers with high specificity and sensitivity are required. Currently, the diagnosis of IgG4-SC is largely based on elevated serum IgG4 levels because imaging results could be challenging to interpret, and it could also be difficult to obtain adequate amounts of samples for histological examination. However, some patients with IgG4-SC have normal IgG4 levels. International and collaborative efforts are required to develop large-scale registries of patients with IgG4-SC and to validate the utility of novel biomarkers for the diagnosis of this disease.

References

1. Deshpande V, Zen Y, Chan JK, Yi EE, Sato Y, Yoshino T, Kloppel G, et al. Consensus statement on the pathology of IgG4-related disease. Mod Pathol. 2012;25:1181–92.

2. Khosroshahi A, Wallace ZS, Crowe JL, Akamizu T, Azumi A, Carruthers MN, Chari ST, et al. International consensus guidance statement on the management and treatment of IgG4-related disease. Arthritis Rheumatol. 2015;67:1688–99.

3. Stone JH, Khosroshahi A, Deshpande V, Chan JK, Heathcote JG, Aalberse R, Azumi A, et al. Recommendations for the nomenclature of IgG4-related disease and its individual organ system manifestations. Arthritis Rheum. 2012;64:3061–7.

4. Umehara H, Okazaki K, Masaki Y, Kawano M, Yamamoto M, Saeki T, Matsui S, et al. A novel clinical entity, IgG4-related disease (IgG4-RD): general concept and details. Mod Rheumatol. 2012;22:1–14.

5. Umehara H, Okazaki K, Masaki Y, Kawano M, Yamamoto M, Saeki T, Matsui S, et al. Comprehensive diagnostic criteria for IgG4-related disease (IgG4-RD). Mod Rheumatol. 2012;22:21–30.

6. Okazaki K, Uchida K, Ikeura T, Takaoka M. Current concept and diagnosis of IgG4-related disease in the hepato-bilio-pancreatic system. J Gastroenterol. 2013;48:303–14.

7. Kamisawa T, Nakazawa T, Tazuma S, Zen Y, Tanaka A, Ohara H, Muraki T, et al. Clinical practice guidelines for IgG4-related sclerosing cholangitis. J Hepatobiliary Pancreat Sci. 2019;26:9–42.

8. Löhr JM, Beuers U, Vujasinovic M, Alvaro D, Frøkjær JB, Buttgereit F, Capurso G, et al. European guideline on IgG4-related digestive disease—UEG and SGF evidence-based recommendations. United Eur Gastroenterol J. 2020;8:637–66.

9. Waldram R, Kopelman H, Tsantoulas D, Williams R. Chronic pancreatitis, sclerosing cholangitis, and sicca complex in two siblings. Lancet. 1975;1:550–2.

10. Sjögren I, Wengle B, Korsgren M. Primary sclerosing cholangitis associated with fibrosis of the submandibular glands and the pancreas. Acta Med Scand. 1979;205:139–41.

11. Kawaguchi K, Koike M, Tsuruta K, Okamoto A, Tabata I, Fujita N. Lymphoplasmacytic sclerosing pancreatitis with cholangitis: a variant of primary sclerosing cholangitis extensively involving pancreas. Hum Pathol. 1991;22:387–95.

12. Nakazawa T, Ohara H, Yamada T, Ando H, Sano H, Kajino S, Hashimoto T, et al. Atypical primary sclerosing cholangitis cases associated with unusual pancreatitis. Hepato-Gastroenterol. 2001;48:625–30.

13. Hamano H, Kawa S, Horiuchi A, Unno H, Furuya N, Akamatsu T, Fukushima M, et al. High serum IgG4 concentrations in patients with sclerosing pancreatitis. N Engl J Med. 2001;344:732–8.

14. Kamisawa T, Funata N, Hayashi Y, Eishi Y, Koike M, Tsuruta K, Okamoto A, et al. A new clinicopathological entity of IgG4-related autoimmune disease. J Gastroenterol. 2003;38:982–4.

15. Kamisawa T, Kim MH, Liao WC, Liu Q, Balakrishnan V, Okazaki K, Shimosegawa T, et al. Clinical characteristics of 327 Asian patients with autoimmune pancreatitis based on Asian diagnostic criteria. Pancreas. 2011;40:200–5.

16. Kamisawa T, Okamoto A, Wakabayashi T, Watanabe H, Sawabu N. Appropriate steroid therapy for autoimmune pancreatitis based on long-term outcome. Scand J Gastroenterol. 2008;43:609–13.

17. Nakazawa T, Ohara H, Sano H, Ando T, Aoki S, Kobayashi S, Okamoto T, et al. Clinical differences between primary sclerosing cholangitis and sclerosing cholangitis with autoimmune pancreatitis. Pancreas. 2005;30:20–5.

18. Zen Y, Harada K, Sasaki M, Sato Y, Tsuneyama K, Haratake J, Kurumaya H, et al. IgG4-related sclerosing cholangitis with and without hepatic inflammatory pseudotumor, and sclerosing pancreatitis-associated sclerosing cholangitis: do they belong to a spectrum of sclerosing pancreatitis? Am J Surg Pathol. 2004;28:1193–203.

19. Ghazale A, Chari ST, Zhang L, Smyrk TC, Takahashi N, Levy MJ, Topazian MD, et al. Immunoglobulin G4-associated cholangitis: clinical profile and response to therapy. Gastroenterology. 2008;134:706–15.

20. Huggett MT, Culver EL, Kumar M, Hurst JM, Rodriguez-Justo M, Chapman MH, Johnson GJ, et al. Type 1 autoimmune pancreatitis and IgG4-related sclerosing cholangitis is associated

with extrapancreatic organ failure, malignancy, and mortality in a prospective UK cohort. Am J Gastroenterol. 2014;109:1675–83.

21. Xiao J, Xu P, Li B, Hong T, Liu W, He X, Zheng C, et al. Analysis of clinical characteristics and treatment of immunoglobulin G4-associated cholangitis: a retrospective cohort study of 39 IAC patients. Medicine (Baltimore). 2018;97:e9767.

22. Tanaka A, Tazuma S, Okazaki K, Tsubouchi H, Inui K, Takikawa H. Nationwide survey for primary sclerosing cholangitis and IgG4-related sclerosing cholangitis in Japan. J Hepatobiliary Pancreat Sci. 2014;21:43–50.

23. Tanaka A, Tazuma S, Okazaki K, Nakazawa T, Inui K, Chiba T, Takikawa H. Clinical features, response to treatment, and outcomes of IgG4-related sclerosing cholangitis. Clin Gastroenterol Hepatol. 2017;15:920–6.e3.

24. Tanaka A, Mori M, Kubota K, Naitoh I, Nakazawa T, Takikawa H, Unno M, et al. Epidemiological features of immunoglobulin G4-related sclerosing cholangitis in Japan. J Hepatobiliary Pancreat Sci. 2020;27:598.

25. Roos E, Hubers LM, Coelen RJS, Doorenspleet ME, de Vries N, Verheij J, Beuers U, et al. IgG4-associated cholangitis in patients resected for presumed perihilar cholangiocarcinoma: a 30-year tertiary care experience. Am J Gastroenterol. 2018;113:765–72.

26. Bruhns P, Iannascoli B, England P, Mancardi DA, Fernandez N, Jorieux S, Daeron M. Specificity and affinity of human Fc-gamma receptors and their polymorphic variants for human IgG subclasses. Blood. 2009;113:3716–25.

27. Maillette de Buy Wenniger LJ, Doorenspleet ME, Klarenbeek PL, Verheij J, Baas F, Elferink RP, Tak PP, et al. Immunoglobulin G4+ clones identified by next-generation sequencing dominate the B-cell receptor repertoire in immunoglobulin G4-associated cholangitis. Hepatology. 2013;57:2390–8.

28. Parlowsky T, Welzel J, Amagai M, Zillikens D, Wygold T. Neonatal pemphigus vulgaris: IgG4 autoantibodies to desmoglein 3 induce skin blisters in newborns. J Am Acad Dermatol. 2003;48:623–5.

29. Rock B, Martins CR, Theofilopoulos AN, Balderas RS, Anhalt GJ, Labib RS, Futamura S, et al. The pathogenic effect of IgG4 autoantibodies in endemic pemphigus foliaceus (fogo selvagem). N Engl J Med. 1989;320:1463–9.

30. Beck LH Jr, Salant DJ. Membranous nephropathy: recent travels and new roads ahead. Kidney Int. 2010;77:765–70.

31. Shiokawa M, Kodama Y, Kuriyama K, Yoshimura K, Tomono T, Morita T, Kakiuchi N, et al. Pathogenicity of IgG in patients with IgG4-related disease. Gut. 2016;65:1322–32.

32. Hubers LM, Vos H, Schuurman AR, Erken R, Oude Elferink RP, Burgering B, van de Graaf SFJ, et al. Annexin A11 is targeted by IgG4 and IgG1 autoantibodies in IgG4-related disease. Gut. 2018;67:728–35.

33. Zen Y, Kawakami H, Kim JH. IgG4-related sclerosing cholangitis: all we need to know. J Gastroenterol. 2016;51:295–312.

34. Trampert DC, Hubers LM, van de Graaf SFJ, Beuers U. On the role of IgG4 in inflammatory conditions: lessons for IgG4-related disease. Biochim Biophys Acta Mol basis Dis. 2018;1864:1401–9.

35. Ohara H, Okazaki K, Tsubouchi H, Inui K, Kawa S, Kamisawa T, Tazuma S, et al. Clinical diagnostic criteria of IgG4-related sclerosing cholangitis 2012. J Hepatobiliary Pancreat Sci. 2012;19:536–42.

36. Shiokawa M, Kodama Y, Sekiguchi K, Kuwada T, Tomono T, Kuriyama K, Yamazaki H, et al. Laminin 511 is a target antigen in autoimmune pancreatitis. Sci Transl Med. 2018;10:eaaq0997.

37. Kato Y, Azuma K, Someda H, Shiokawa M, Chiba T. Case of IgG4-associated sclerosing cholangitis with normal serum IgG4 concentration, diagnosed by anti-laminin 511-E8 antibody: a novel autoantibody in patients with autoimmune pancreatitis. Gut. 2020;69(3):607–9.

38. Nakazawa T, Naitoh I, Hayashi K, Okumura F, Miyabe K, Yoshida M, Yamashita H, et al. Diagnostic criteria for IgG4-related sclerosing cholangitis based on cholangiographic classification. J Gastroenterol. 2012;47:79–87.

39. Zen Y. The pathology of IgG4-related disease in the bile duct and pancreas. Semin Liver Dis. 2016;36:242–56.
40. Chari ST, Smyrk TC, Levy MJ, Topazian MD, Takahashi N, Zhang L, Clain JE, et al. Diagnosis of autoimmune pancreatitis: the Mayo Clinic experience. Clin Gastroenterol Hepatol. 2006;4:1010–6; quiz 934.
41. Beuers U, Hubers LM, Doorenspleet M, Maillette de Buy Wenniger L, Klarenbeek PL, Boonstra K, Ponsioen C, et al. IgG4-associated cholangitis—a mimic of PSC. Dig Dis. 2015;33(Suppl 2):176–80.
42. Doorenspleet ME, Hubers LM, Culver EL, Maillette de Buy Wenniger LJ, Klarenbeek PL, Chapman RW, Baas F, et al. Immunoglobulin G4(+) B-cell receptor clones distinguish immunoglobulin G 4-related disease from primary sclerosing cholangitis and biliary/pancreatic malignancies. Hepatology. 2016;64:501–7.
43. Lian M, Li B, Xiao X, Yang Y, Jiang P, Yan L, Sun C, et al. Comparative clinical characteristics and natural history of three variants of sclerosing cholangitis: IgG4-related SC, PSC/AIH and PSC alone. Autoimmun Rev. 2017;16:875–82.
44. Boonstra K, Culver EL, de Buy Wenniger LM, van Heerde MJ, van Erpecum KJ, Poen AC, van Nieuwkerk KM, et al. Serum immunoglobulin G4 and immunoglobulin G1 for distinguishing immunoglobulin G4-associated cholangitis from primary sclerosing cholangitis. Hepatology. 2014;59:1954–63.
45. Vujasinovic M, Maier P, Maetzel H, Valente R, Pozzi-Mucelli R, Moro CF, Haas SL, et al. Immunoglobulin G subtypes-1 and 2 differentiate immunoglobulin G4-associated sclerosing cholangitis from primary sclerosing cholangitis. United Eur Gastroenterol J. 2020;8:584–93.
46. Culver EL, van de Bovenkamp FS, Derksen NIL, Koers J, Cargill T, Barnes E, de Neef LA, et al. Unique patterns of glycosylation in immunoglobulin subclass G4-related disease and primary sclerosing cholangitis. J Gastroenterol Hepatol. 2019;34:1878–86.
47. Takagi Y, Kubota K, Takayanagi T, Kurita Y, Ishii K, Hasegawa S, Iwasaki A, et al. Clinical features of isolated proximal-type immunoglobulin G4-related sclerosing cholangitis. Dig Endosc. 2019;31:422–30.
48. Kalaitzakis E, Levy M, Kamisawa T, Johnson GJ, Baron TH, Topazian MD, Takahashi N, et al. Endoscopic retrograde cholangiography does not reliably distinguish IgG4-associated cholangitis from primary sclerosing cholangitis or cholangiocarcinoma. Clin Gastroenterol Hepatol. 2011;9:800–3.e2.
49. Moon SH, Kim MH, Lee JK, Baek S, Woo YS, Cho DH, Oh D, et al. Development of a scoring system for differentiating IgG4-related sclerosing cholangitis from primary sclerosing cholangitis. J Gastroenterol. 2017;52:483–93.
50. Azeem N, Ajmera V, Hameed B, Mehta N. Hilar cholangiocarcinoma associated with immunoglobulin G4-positive plasma cells and elevated serum immunoglobulin G4 levels. Hepatol Commun. 2018;2:349–53.
51. de Vries E, Tielbeke F, Hubers L, Helder J, Mostafavi N, Verheij J, van Hooft J, et al. IgG4/IgG RNA ratio does not accurately discriminate IgG4-related disease from pancreatobiliary cancer. JHEP Rep. 2020;2:100116.
52. Nakazawa T, Naitoh I, Hayashi K. Usefulness of intraductal ultrasonography in the diagnosis of cholangiocarcinoma and IgG4-related sclerosing cholangitis. Clin Endosc. 2012;45:331–6.
53. Itoi T, Sofuni A, Itokawa F, Tsuchiya T, Kurihara T, Ishii K, Tsuji S, et al. Peroral cholangioscopic diagnosis of biliary-tract diseases by using narrow-band imaging (with videos). Gastrointest Endosc. 2007;66:730–6.
54. Kato A, Naitoh I, Miyabe K, Hayashi K, Kondo H, Yoshida M, Kato H, et al. Differential diagnosis of cholangiocarcinoma and IgG4-related sclerosing cholangitis by fluorescence in situ hybridization using transpapillary forceps biopsy specimens. J Hepatobiliary Pancreat Sci. 2018;25:188–94.
55. Miyazawa M, Takatori H, Kawaguchi K, Kitamura K, Arai K, Matsuda K, Urabe T, et al. Management of biliary stricture in patients with IgG4-related sclerosing cholangitis. PLoS One. 2020;15:e0232089.

56. Majumder S, Mohapatra S, Lennon RJ, Piovezani Ramos G, Postier N, Gleeson FC, Levy MJ, et al. Rituximab maintenance therapy reduces rate of relapse of pancreaticobiliary immuno-globulin G4-related disease. Clin Gastroenterol Hepatol. 2018;16:1947–53.
57. Liu W, Chen W, He X, Qu Q, Hong T, Li B. Poor response of initial steroid therapy for IgG4-related sclerosing cholangitis with multiple organs affected. Medicine (Baltimore). 2017;96:e6400.

Overlap Syndromes

11

Nora Cazzagon and Olivier Chazouillères

11.1 Introduction

Three well-defined rare autoimmune diseases, namely autoimmune hepatitis (AIH), primary biliary cholangitis (PBC), and primary sclerosing cholangitis (PSC) may affect the liver. AIH targets hepatocytes and is characterized by a predominant hepatocellular injury, whereas PBC and PSC target bile ducts and are characterized by predominant cholestatic features. These three diseases are generally differentiated easily on the basis of clinical, biochemical, serological, radiological, and histological findings (Table 11.1). However, patients may present at diagnosis or develop during follow-up, features of two diseases, typically PBC and AIH or PSC and AIH (Fig. 11.1). Overlapping features between PBC and PSC have been described only in a few case reports of variable quality and do not represent a real issue.

The term overlap syndrome is often used to describe these variant forms. Unfortunately, lack of universal agreement on what precisely constitutes an overlap syndrome has generated considerable confusion in the literature, and the clinical phenotypes of patients with the same overlap syndrome designation exhibit considerable heterogeneity [1]. As a result, "overlap syndrome" is one of the most abused descriptive term currently used in hepatology [2].

The three diseases share similar pathogenic themes of injury, including genetic predisposition relating to defect in immunological control of autoreactivity, as well

N. Cazzagon
Department of Surgery, Oncology and Gastroenterology, University of Padova, Padova, Italy

ERN RARE-LIVER Azienda Ospedale-Università di Padova, Padova, Italy

O. Chazouillères (✉)
Hôpitaux de Paris, Sorbonne University, INSERM, Reference Center for Inflammatory Biliary Diseases and Autoimmune Hepatitis & Saint-Antoine Research Center, Service d'Hépatologie, Saint-Antoine Hospital, Paris, France

ERN RARE-LIVER Saint-Antoine Hospital, APHP, Paris, France
e-mail: olivier.chazouilleres@aphp.fr

© Springer Nature Switzerland AG 2021
A. Floreani (ed.), *Diseases of the Liver and Biliary Tree*,
https://doi.org/10.1007/978-3-030-65908-0_11

Table 11.1 Features of autoimmune liver diseases

	AIH	PBC	PSC
Gender	Female > male (4:1)	Female > male (9:1)	Male > female (2:1)
Coexisting IBD	3–10% (PSC should be excluded)	Not characteristic	**Up to 80%**
ANA	70–80%	30–50% (some specific)	30–70%
ASMA	**70–80%**	May be present: <10%	0–80%
AMA	5–10%	**95%**	Coincidental
p-ANCA	Up to 90%	0–5%	25–95%
Immunoglobulins	IgG elevated	IgM elevated in most	IgG elevated (2/3) and IgM (45%) elevated
Cholangiography	Usually normal	Normal	**Multifocal stricturing** (not in small-duct PSC)
Interface hepatitis	**Characteristic**	Variably present	Variably present
Biliary changes	10%	**Inflammatory duct lesion**	**Onion-skin periductal fibrosis** (<30%)
Response to immunosuppression	Yes	Mild	Minimal

AIH autoimmune hepatitis, *AMA* antimitochondrial antibody, *ANA* antinuclear anti-body, *ASMA* anti-smooth-muscle antibody, *IBD* inflammatory bowel disease, *pANCA* perinuclear anti-neutrophil cytoplasmic antibody, *PBC* primary biliary cholangitis, *PSC* primary sclerosing cholangitis
Most characteristic features are indicated in bold

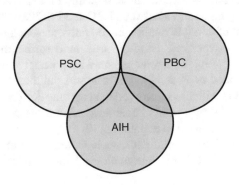

Fig. 11.1 Overlap syndromes of the classical autoimmune liver diseases. PBC-PSC overlap syndrome is an extremely rare (and even controversial) condition. Autoimmune hepatitis (AIH), primary biliary cholangitis (PBC), primary sclerosing cholangitis (PSC)

as environmental triggers, which precipitate a persistent breakdown in self-tolerance, and liver disease represents the result of a cell and antibody-mediated immunological attack against liver-specific targets.

The overlap syndrome pathogenesis is highly debated, and it remains unclear whether two distinct diseases coexist in one patient; whether these forms are an own entity or whether they represent a variant form of either disease (PBC, PSC, or

AIH). The latter seems to be the most appropriate since a predominant phenotype can be identified in most cases. For example, in PBC-AIH overlap, it has been proposed that overlap represents an "hepatitic" form of PBC in genetically susceptible individuals (HLA-B8, DR3- or DR4-positive) [3]. This would fit with the hypothesis that immune-mediated disease can develop ("secondary" AIH) in any susceptible host if, for some reason, the local milieu becomes pro-inflammatory. In this regard, the name overlap that strongly suggests the presence of two distinct diseases could be a misnomer. As a result, according to the EASL AIH and PBC guidelines, the preferred terminology to describe these conditions is now "variants forms," primarily variants forms of the cholestatic autoimmune liver disease with autoimmune features [4, 5]. By contrast, recent British and US PBC guidelines still use the term "overlap" [6, 7].

A key point is that no autoimmune liver disease has an absolute diagnostic test (the possible exception being PBC), and there is intrinsic scope for individuals to present with overlapping features of more than one of these conditions although, in most cases, it is possible to define one primary disorder ("dominant" disease). Overlapping presentations include: biochemical overlap (AST or ALT>5 ULN in patients with PSC or PBC; or ALP>3ULN in patients with AIH), serological overlap (positive ASMA in AMA-positive PBC; or positive AMA in AIH), histological overlap (interface hepatitis on liver biopsy with biliary lesions indicative of PBC or PSC), radiologic overlap (cholangiographic abnormalities associated with clinical features of AIH), and finally, varying combinations of the above. However, these overlapping presentations have various significance, the weaker being probably immunoserology. Indeed, autoantibody profile should never be used in isolation but rather interpreted in conjunction with biochemical, radiological, and histological features. Laboratory features lack sensitivity considering that cholestasis in itself can cause raised ALT levels in the absence of inflammation and that cirrhosis can lead to high IgG levels in the absence of histological hepatitis. By contrast, a good-quality cholangiogram and/or liver biopsy interpretation are the strongest means to diagnose overlap. Finally, it should be kept in mind that the diagnosis of AIH is, at least in part, a diagnosis of exclusion and that other causes of liver damage have to be ruled out, including intercurrent drug-induced liver injury and occasionally, hepatitis E.

The aim of this chapter is to describe the overlap syndrome (OS) between primary biliary cholangitis and autoimmune hepatitis (PBC-AIH) and primary sclerosing cholangitis and autoimmune hepatitis (PSC-AIH), especially focusing on the clinical presentation, the diagnostic criteria, including the histological features, the therapy and the natural history of OS, and finally, the association with extrahepatic autoimmune disorders.

It should be kept in mind that OS should not be overdiagnosed in order not to expose PBC or PSC patients unnecessarily to the risk of steroid side effects. On the other hand, tragic consequences of a missed opportunity of instituting immunosuppressive therapy in overlap patients have occasionally been reported [8]. The low prevalence of overlap syndromes has made it impracticable to perform randomized controlled trials. As a consequence, treatment of OS is largely empiric.

11.2 Clinical Features of Overlap Syndromes

It is generally assumed that PBC-AIH OS is present in around 8–10% of adult patients with PBC or AIH, even if these frequencies are quite variable in different studies depending of the diagnostic criteria applied and the size of the population included [9]. The reported prevalence figures of PSC-AIH OS vary greatly due to the lack of precise and strict diagnostic criteria. When the revised International Autoimmune Hepatitis Group (IAIHG) criteria were applied to a large series of PSC patients, the prevalence of PSC-AIH overlapping features ranged from 7 to 14% [9]. On the other hand, cholangiographic abnormalities typical of PSC are found in AIH patients at a various prevalence depending on the age of patients evaluated: 2–10% in adults (41% if ulcerative colitis (UC) is present) and up to 50% in children [10].

PBC-AIH OS may present simultaneously or consecutively and the former presentation is more frequent. The simultaneous occurrence of PBC and AIH is characterized by a hepatitic and cholestatic profile at the same time, an elevation of both serum immunoglobulin G (IgG) and immunoglobulin M (IgM), the positivity of autoantibodies characterizing the two diseases, and the presence of histological features of both PBC and AIH [11, 12]. The sequential development of PBC-AIH OS may present in two different modalities. In most cases, PBC is the first diagnosis, and AIH occurs 6 months–14 years after the initial diagnosis of PBC [13–16]. More rarely, patients with AIH may develop PBC within 1–20 years after the initial diagnosis of AIH [14–19]. The sequential development of overlap should be suspected when a hepatitic or a cholestatic flare appears during the course of the disease, or when an incomplete response to standard treatment is observed. In these cases, a diagnostic workup, including liver biopsy, to exclude or confirm the presence of OS is recommended [5, 9]. Unfortunately, the development of sequential overlap is unpredictable. Symptoms of PBC-AIH OS are usually fatigue and pruritus and the latter seems to be less frequent in these patients compared to patients with pure PBC [20, 21]. Other reported symptoms are malaise, abdominal pain, weight loss, and general symptoms of chronic liver diseases. As in pure PBC or AIH, age at diagnosis of PBC-AIH OS is variable, but some studies have suggested that patients with OS are younger at diagnosis than those with pure PBC [20, 22].

PSC-AIH OS has been described in both children and adults and is assumed to exist in a considerable part of mainly young patients with autoimmune liver disease. In adults, AIH and PSC may be concurrent or sequential in their occurrence, typically with AIH presenting first, as illustrated by a case series of AIH patients becoming cholestatic and resistant to immunosuppressive therapy [23]. AIH is more rarely diagnosed in patients with an original diagnosis of PSC. Symptoms of PSC-AIH OS, similarly to PBC-AIH OS, are highly nonspecific and include fatigue and pruritus but symptoms may be absent in a relevant percentage of patients. Age at diagnosis of PSC-AIH OS was suggested to be lower than in patients with PSC [24].

11.3   Diagnosis of Overlap Syndromes

The diagnosis of OS is based on the concomitant presence or sequential development of biochemical, serological, histologic, and, for PSC, cholangiographic features of the two diseases.

11.3.1 Diagnostic Criteria of PBC-AIH Overlap

The most widely applied criteria for PBC-AIH OS are the so-called Paris criteria, which were derived by the end of 1990s by identifying 12 patients with PBC-AIH OS among PBC patients by the presence of PBC and AIH, either simultaneously or consecutively [11]. For the diagnosis of each disease, the presence of at least two of the following three accepted criteria was required:

Criteria for PBC:
1. Serum alkaline phosphatase (AP) levels at least two times the upper limit of normal (ULN) values or serum gamma-glutamyl transpeptidase (GGT) levels at least five times the ULN values
2. A positive test for antimitochondrial antibodies (AMAs) and
3. A liver biopsy specimen showing florid bile duct lesions

Criteria for AIH:
1. Serum alanine transaminase (ALT) levels at least five times the ULN values
2. Serum immunoglobulin G (IgG) levels at least two times the ULN values or a positive test for anti-smooth muscle antibodies (ASMAs) and
3. A liver biopsy showing moderate or severe periportal or periseptal lymphocytic piecemeal necrosis [11]

Other studies published in the same period defined the presence of PBC-AIH OS by applying less strict histological and clinical criteria of both diseases [3] or even by employing, in AMA-positive patients, the original IAIHG score for diagnosing AIH [12]. Subsequently, studies applied the revised AIH score [25] or the simplified AIH score [26] to PBC patients to retrospectively identify patients treated with corticosteroids, but these scores were shown to be less performant compared to Paris criteria [27] since they were not originally developed to diagnose cholestatic variants of AIH. At present, Paris criteria are the most widely applied [13, 15, 20–22, 27–30], and most experts agree that these criteria provide a diagnostic template that can be consistently applied. The 2009 European Association of the Study of the Liver guidelines on the management of cholestatic liver diseases endorsed the Paris criteria for the diagnosis of PBC-AIH OS and specified that histologic evidence of moderate to severe lymphocytic piecemeal necrosis (interface hepatitis) was mandatory for the diagnosis of PBC-AIH OS [31]. Moreover, the same guidelines stated that PBC-AIH OS should always be suspected in PBC patients in case of poor response to UDCA because of potential therapeutic implications [31]. Nevertheless, there are still several areas of uncertainty, including the cutoffs for IgG/gamma-globulins and transaminases levels to indicate liver biopsy and the grade of hepatitis activity to indicate immunosuppression [5]. Indeed, the recent EASL guidelines on AIH recommend treatment for patients with AIH at lower cutoffs for transaminase or IgG levels and a histological mHAI score as low as 4 [4]. Indeed, Paris criteria may not identify patients with less severe forms of OS, which did not fulfill the biochemical criteria or serological criteria despite the presence of histologic features of both PBC and AIH. To overcome these limitations, a new scoring classification for PBC-AIH OS was recently proposed, but this score needs to be externally validated before its dissemination since is potentially associated with an overestimation of diagnosis of PBC-AIH OS [32].

11.3.2 Diagnostic Criteria of PSC-AIH OS

Despite the absence of precise and strict criteria, the diagnosis of PSC-AIH OS is made in a patient with overt cholangiographic or histological features of PSC, together with robust histological features of AIH concurrently or historically [1, 9] (Table 11.2). The diagnosis of large-duct PSC should always be established on the base of typical cholangiographic findings (alternating strictures and dilatations of intra and/or extrahepatic bile ducts), keeping in mind that an intrahepatic biliary tree, which simulates a sclerosing pattern, can be observed in any liver disease with extensive fibrosis. One study evaluated 79 patients with a confirmed diagnosis of AIH and found that 10% of patients had MRI findings consistent with a

Table 11.2 Proposed criteria for a diagnosis of overlap syndrome

Presence of at least two of the three accepted key criteria required for diagnosis of each disease:	
PBC	1. AP ≥ 2 ULN and/or GGT ≥ 5 ULN
	2. AMA ≥ 1/40 or PBC-specific ANA
	3. Florid bile duct lesions (liver biopsy)
PSC (causes of secondary SC excluded)	1. AP ≥ 2 ULN and/or GGT ≥ 5 ULN
	2. Typical cholangiographic abnormalities
	3. Periductal fibrosis (liver biopsy)
	NB: some cases of overlap with "small-duct" PSC
AIH	1. ALT ≥ 5 ULN
	2. IgG levels ≥ 2 ULN[a] or ASMA ≥ 1/80
	3. Moderate or severe periportal or periseptal lymphocytic piecemeal necrosis (liver biopsy) (mandatory)

PBC primary biliary cholangitis, *PSC* primary sclerosing cholangitis, *AIH* autoimmune hepatitis, *AP* alkaline phosphatase, *AMA* antimitochondrial antibody, *ANA* antinuclear anti-body, *GGT* gamma-glutamyl transferase, *ASMA* anti-smooth-muscle antibody
[a]20 g/L tends to be the usual proposed cutoff

cholangiopathy, suggesting the presence of PSC-AIH OS. These patients were characterized by lower age at diagnosis, higher baseline ALP, and higher bilirubin at the time of MRI and greater lobular activity at the time of liver biopsy [33]. On the other hand, a French study reported that one quarter of AIH patients had mild MRCP abnormalities of intrahepatic bile ducts in 24% of AIH patients, which were associated with the presence of advanced fibrosis, but finally a definite diagnosis of concurrent sclerosing cholangitis was made in only 1.7% of AIH [34].

Some cases of small-duct PSC (normal cholangiogram)-AIH OS have also been reported, but it can be argued that approximately 10% of patients with typical AIH, with or without ulcerative colitis, may have histological features of bile duct injury as extensively discussed below.

In children, the hepatitic feature can be very dominant and up to 50% of pediatric AIH (clinical and/or evidence of liver disease associated with circulating autoantibodies) have cholangiographic abnormalities suggestive of PSC, including some (25%) without any histological features of bile duct injury or biochemical cholestasis [10]. Inflammatory bowel disease (IBD) was present in 44% of these children compared to 20% of those with AIH alone. The term "autoimmune sclerosing cholangitis (AISC)" was introduced by Mieli-Vergani's group to describe this variant of AIH in pediatric patients [10]. Evolution from AIH to AISC has been documented, supporting the view that they could be part of the same pathogenic process. It has been proposed that at least some adult PSC cases may represent an advanced, at times "burnt out," stage of AISC, but whether childhood AISC and adult PSC belong to the same disease spectrum remains to be established. These findings suggest also the need of an investigation of the biliary tree at least with MRCP in all children with a diagnosis of AIH. At present, this variant seems unique for children, as a prospective study in adults with AIH was negative, and thus, in the absence of cholestatic indices, MRCP screening does not seem justified in adult-onset AIH [34]. However, in particular cases, such as in young adults with AIH and cholestatic features or inflammatory bowel disease and in AIH patients with remaining cholestasis despite adequate immunosuppression, MRCP for the detection of possible underlying or coexistent PSC is recommended [35].

11.3.3 Biochemical Features of Overlap Syndromes

Patients with PBC-AIH OS are typically characterized by hepatitic and cholestatic profile and an elevation of both immunoglobulin G and immunoglobulin M. In comparison with patients with pure PBC, patients with PBC-AIH OS showed, as expected, higher transaminases, higher gamma-globulins, and higher IgG. Otherwise, compared to patients with pure AIH, PBC-AIH OS patients show higher AP, both at baseline and also during remission, higher GGT, and IgM, but lower transaminases and bilirubin. Similarly, patients with PSC-AIH OS had higher serum globulins, transaminases, and IgG levels than PSC alone [24, 36].

11.3.4 Serology of Overlap Syndromes

Serum autoantibodies are frequently described in autoimmune liver disease, and their presence is used to subclassify disease.

PBC-AIH OS may present serological pattern of both PBC and AIH, however, the concomitant presence of autoantibodies of the two diseases is not sufficient for the diagnosis of OS and, moreover, is not predictive of the sequential development of OS in a patient with a previous diagnosis of PBC or AIH [37]. Type-I AIH is typically characterized by antinuclear antibodies (ANA) and/or ASMAs, while type-II AIH is characterized by anti-liver kidney microsomal type-I (anti-LKM-1) antibodies, which are mostly directed toward the human cytochrome P450IID6, or rarely anti-liver cytosol (anti-LC) antibodies. Anti-soluble liver pancreas antigen (SLA/LP) antibodies were originally thought to identify a third group of AIH, but more than 75% of anti-SLA/LP-positive patients are also ANA- and/or SMA-positive. PBC is characterized by anti-mitochondrial autoantibodies (AMA) positivity in up to 95% of patients. ANA positivity is also reported in 30–50% of patients, but, in PBC, some ANA are directed against specific antigens, namely gp210 and sp100. The presence of anti-gp210 and/or anti-sp100 antibodies in PBC patients is more often observed in AMA-negative patients, and their identification supports the diagnosis of PBC in patients with biochemical features of cholestasis. The serological pattern of reactivity of PBC-AIH OS has been largely reported and is characterized by AMA positivity in 60–100% of patients, SMA positivity in up to 75% of patients (lower in Eastern population), ANA positivity in 33–100% of cases with PBC-specific ANA (i.e., anti-gp210 and anti-sp100) positivity reported in up to 55% of ANA-positive cases [38]. Among ANA-positive OS, several immunofluorescence pattern of ANA in OS are possible: homogeneous in 28–33% of cases, speckled pattern in 33–43%, nuclear rim in 14–33%, and anti-centromere in 7–14% [11, 39]. Anti-SLA was reported in 7–33% of PBC-AIH OS, and since these antibodies had the highest specificity for AIH among AIH-related autoantibodies [40], some authors suggested that the presence of anti-SLA/LP antibodies could be helpful in the diagnosis of a "variant" syndrome of PBC with AIH features and that immunosuppressive treatment should be offered to these patients when a relevant inflammatory activity is suspected [3, 41]. The presence of anti-LKM-1 has been poorly reported in adult patients with OS and varies between 1 and 7% in different studies. Anti-double-strand DNA (anti-dsDNA) positivity was reported in 38–60% of patients with PBC-AIH OS diagnosed according to Paris criteria [38, 39, 42], and this frequency was significantly higher than in patients with pure PBC (3%) and pure AIH (26%) [39]. Interestingly, the concomitant positivity for anti-dsDNA and AMA seemed highly specific (98%) for the diagnosis of PBC-AIH OS, with a reported likelihood ratio for a positive and a negative test of 28 and 0.5, respectively [39]. Overlap of AMA-negative PBC with AIH has also been reported [11], but in these cases, the diagnosis of overlap is highly challenging because histological biliary injury may also be observed in "pure" AIH as a collateral damage in the context of a marked inflammation (see below). As a consequence, a diagnosis of overlap in these patients lacking "specific" PBC autoantibodies can be reasonably made only if marked biochemical cholestasis and/or granulomatous (not purely lymphocytic) cholangitis are present.

Atypical nonspecific antibodies directed against neutrophil cytoplasmic antigens (ANCA), distinct from those seen in microscopic polyangiitis or Wegener's granulomatosis, are detectable in up to 88% of patients with PSC, UC ($\approx$87%), and AIH (50–96%) [43]. Differently from systemic vasculitis, ANCA titers do not correlate with disease activity in autoimmune liver disease and in inflammatory bowel disease [44, 45]. In patients with PSC-AIH OS, the prevalence of ANCA reactivity appeared comparable to that observed in PSC patients, but the presence of non-organ-specific autoantibodies appeared higher in the former group [24]. ANA (8–77%) and ASMA (up to 83%) reactivity is also variably reported in PSC [46], and in patients with PSC-AIH OS, their prevalence appears similar to that observed in patients with AIH [36].

11.3.5 Liver Biopsy in Overlap Syndromes

Liver biopsy is considered a prerequisite for the diagnosis of AIH [4, 47], and it is mandatory in clinical practice when an OS is suspected [5, 9]. Histological features of PBC-AIH OS were extensively reported and include in most cases the concomitant presence of typical findings of both diseases (Fig. 11.2). The most frequent histological finding in AIH is the presence of lymphocytic interface hepatitis, which is characterized by the presence of lymphocytic, often lymphoplasmacytic,

Fig. 11.2 Histological features of PBC-AIH overlap syndrome. Lymphocytic cholangitis (star) and diffuse interface hepatitis (arrow) (HE-staining, original magnification ×100). (Courtesy of Pr Dominique Wendum)

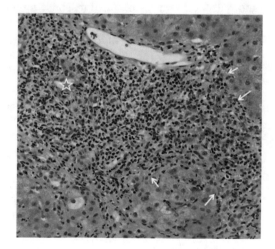

inflammatory infiltrates invading the limiting plate and extending from portal tracts into acinar tissue with hepatocyte injury [48, 49]. Interface hepatitis differs from biliary interface modifications (previously described as "biliary interface activity"), that is, the consequence of major cholestasis and associates ductular reaction, neutrophilic inflammation, and cholate stasis of periportal hepatocytes [50] (Fig. 11.2). Nevertheless, lymphocytic interface hepatitis is not pathognomonic of AIH since it can be also seen in approximately 25% of PBC and PSC patients [9], in drug-related liver injury, and also in viral hepatitis. PBC histological hallmarks are chronic nonsuppurative destructive cholangitis, which is characterized by lymphocytic infiltration of the biliary epithelium, biliary epithelial cells senescence, and bile duct loss, with areas of macrophage-rich fibrosis replacing bile ducts in portal tracts. However, interface hepatitis develops at some degree in untreated pure PBC and is associated with disease progression [51, 52]. In a study comparing 41 PBC patients with interface hepatitis and 43 AIH treatment-naïve patients, the degree of interface hepatitis did not differ between the two groups, but, in AIH, a higher score of lobular hepatitis with zonal or even bridging necrosis, focal hepatocellular necrosis, hepatitic rosette formation, and emperipolesis was observed compared to PBC [53]. Moreover, hepatocellular injuries associated with interface and lobular hepatitis in AIH seems not be identical to PBC and by analyzing immunophenotypes of infiltrating inflammatory cells and infiltrating plasma cells with respect to immunoglobulin classes [52–54]. On the other hand, pure AIH may be characterized in one quarter of patients by bile duct injury, variously characterized by nondestructive, destructive cholangitis, and even ductopenia [55]. Other groups reported much higher prevalence of biliary damage in AIH [56, 57].

The general opinion is that bile duct injury in AIH is reliably a collateral injury associated with an exuberant inflammatory process due to a possible promiscuous nature of the immune-mediated response targeting not only hepatocytes, but also cholangiocytes [55, 58], and the presence of bile duct injury and ductular reaction in AIH do not necessarily imply a change in therapeutic management in such cases [55, 59].

PSC is characterized by a progressive and chronic injury possibly occurring in small, medium, and large bile ducts with inflammatory and obliterative concentric periductal fibrosis, so-called onion skin fibrosis, leading to biliary strictures and eventually occlusion. Although periductal fibrosis is regarded as typical for PSC, its frequency and localization varies greatly in adult patients with PSC [60–62], moreover, certain heterogeneity in distribution of portal and septal fibrosis, ductular reaction, and portal lymphocyte infiltrations can be observed in the liver of patients with PSC [63]. Thus, it appears clear that in case of suspicion of PSC-AIH OS based on cholangiographic findings, a liver biopsy without typical histological finding of PSC does not exclude the diagnosis of OS. However, PSC-AIH OS is typically characterized by the concomitant presence of periductal fibrosis and diffuse interface hepatitis (Fig. 11.3).

In clinical practice, the good-quality liver biopsy interpretation is key, and a specialist review of liver biopsies has a major added value [64].

Fig. 11.3 Histological features of
PSC-AIH overlap syndrome.
Sclerosing cholangitis (star) and
lymphocytic interface hepatitis
(arrow) (HE-sstaining, original
magnification ×100). (Courtesy of Pr
Dominique Wendum)

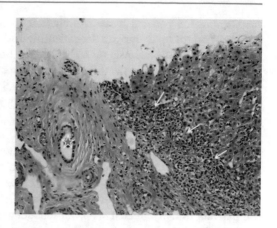

11.4 Course of Overlap Syndromes and Therapy

Patients with PBC-AIH OS seems to have a more severe disease compared to conventional PBC as illustrated by a higher frequency of extensive fibrosis at presentation, despite a younger age in some reports [22]. In PBC patients, ursodeoxycholic acid (UDCA) (15 mg/kg/day) leads to slowed progression of fibrosis and liver failure, in particular, in patients who demonstrate an adequate biochemical response to therapy [65, 66], which can be assessed according qualitative binary definitions (Barcelona [67], Paris I and II [65, 68], Toronto [69], and Rotterdam [66] criteria) or continuous scores (Globe score [70] and UK-PBC score [71]). Patients who respond to UDCA therapy have a significantly better transplant-free survival than nonresponders. On the other hand, PBC patients presenting with significant interface hepatitis at liver biopsy may show a rapid progression of fibrosis and, in this situation, the institution of immunosuppression has to be considered [12, 72, 73]. Moreover, patients who are nonresponders to UDCA, with persistent cholestatic enzyme elevation, showed a clear benefit after starting second-line therapy with obeticholic [74, 75] acid (OCA) or fibrates [76]. On the other hand, once the diagnosis of AIH is achieved, the institution of immunosuppressive therapy, based on the use of steroids (usually prednisone/prednisolone) monotherapy or in combination with azathioprine, is mandatory [4, 47]. The goal of therapy in AIH is the achievement of biochemical remission, defined as normalization of transaminases and IgG, and histological remission, defined as score of inflammatory activity below 4/18 according to the modified HAI grading [77].

Patients with overlapping features of PBC and AIH showed, in most of cases, a positive response to the immunosuppressive and UDCA combination therapy [3, 11–18, 20–22, 29, 38, 39, 73, 78–81], but the criteria of response for the single diseases have not yet been validated in PBC-AIH OS, and thus the evaluation of response in OS patients remains a challenge. Chazouillères et al. retrospectively reported about 17 patients with OS, identified according Paris criteria, and followed up for a mean interval time of 7.5 years. Among them, 11 patients were initially treated with UDCA alone and the remaining six with UDCA and immunosuppressive drugs (initially prednisone/prednisolone 0.5 mg/kg/day monotherapy, progressively tapered and subsequent addition of azathioprine or mycophenolate mofetil as corticosteroids-sparing agents). Only three patients treated with UDCA alone were responders (in terms of transaminases <2ULN and IgG<16 g/L), and a subsequent liver biopsy showed a decreased or stable inflammatory activity and no increase in fibrosis after a median time of 4.5 years was reported. The eight nonresponders to UDCA alone showed, in subsequent liver biopsy, an increase of activity in 38% of cases and of fibrosis in 89% of patients without cirrhosis at baseline. By contrast, all six patients initially treated with immunosuppressive and UDCA in combination were responders, and subsequent liver biopsies showed a decreased or stable activity in 67% and 17% of cases, respectively, and a stability of fibrosis in all noncirrhotic patients. Seven nonresponders to UDCA monotherapy were then treated with immunosuppressants, and after 4 years, liver biopsy available in three showed decrease or stable fibrosis. Finally, one nonresponder to UDCA monotherapy declined immunosuppression and follow-up biopsy showed an increase of fibrosis. The efficacy of immunosuppressive and UDCA combination therapy was confirmed in different studies, also including patients with sequential development of OS [3, 12, 16, 38]. Other data suggested that PBC-AIH OS patients less likely have a complete response to immunosuppressive agents compared to AIH alone, but, in these studies, UDCA therapy was not given in combination from the beginning but subsequently added during the follow-up [18, 82]. Only one study reported on 16 patients retrospectively identified with PBC-AIH OS a similar percentage of biochemical improvement after UDCA compared to patients with PBC alone, but histological fibrosis course was not assessed, and thus no firm conclusions can be drawn from this study [28].

The more recent results of a large retrospective multicenter study (88 patients defined according to Paris criteria) have underlined the predictive role of the interface hepatitis degree. In this study, 30 patients received UDCA alone and 58 patients a combination of UDCA and immunosuppression (prednisone +/−azathioprine) as first-line therapy, and in patients with moderate interface hepatitis, UDCA alone or combination therapy had similar efficacy (80%) in terms of biochemical response, whereas in patients with severe hepatitis, efficacy of UDCA alone was much lower (14% vs. 71%, respectively). Second-line immunosuppressive agents (cyclosporine, tacrolimus, and mycophenolate) led to biochemical remission in half of the patients who were nonresponders to initial immunosuppression and UDCA combination [38]. The combination therapy with UDCA and immunosuppressive was shown to be effective also in PBC-AIH OS with cirrhosis decompensation at baseline [30], whereas UDCA monotherapy was associated to a lower remission rate and a lower transplant-free survival [38]. Anecdotical use of several different agents in association with UDCA or as third-line therapy in nonresponders to standard combination therapy was reported in PBC-AIH OS patients, such as budesonide in combination with UDCA [83], cyclophosphamide and cyclosporine [3, 22, 38], tacrolimus, mycophenolate mofetil, and methotrexate [38, 84]. Recently, OCA has been approved as a second-line therapy for PBC patients with an inadequate response to UDCA monotherapy [74]. Impressive results of fibrates have also been reported in these patients [76]. It's important to differentiate patients with "classical" PBC and nonresponse to UDCA from those with overlap who are also nonresponsive to UDCA. Whether the pleiotropic effects of fibrates or farnesoid X receptor agonists like OCA have sufficient immunosuppressive capacities and could be beneficial for overlap syndromes is currently unknown, but bezafibrate in association to UDCA was reported to be effective in one patient with OS [72]. Relapse after immunosuppressive agents' withdrawal was variably reported in different studies and occurs generally in a high percentage of patients [12, 18, 22]. However, these patients usually respond well to reintroduction of immunosuppressive agents. Chazouillères reported that one-third of patients successfully stopped immunosuppressive agents after a median interval time of 2.7 years and maintained persistent normal transaminases and no progression of fibrosis at subsequent biopsy was reported [73]. This rate of successful withdrawal seems higher than in classical AIH. Corticosteroid therapy in OS is generally safe, even in rare patients with decompensated cirrhosis [30], and is usually not associated with an increased risk of bone disease compared to UDCA alone [29].

The natural course of PBC-AIH OS is aggressive if an adequate therapy is not established due to the persistence of inflammatory activity and the progression of fibrosis. On the other hand, patients with OS, responders to appropriate therapy, showed a comparable liver transplant-free survival to patients with PBC [84] and AIH [18]. However, some studies suggested that patients with PBC-AIH OS are characterized by a higher rate of cirrhosis decompensation events and adverse outcomes compared to patients with PBC [20, 84]. In particular, in patients with decompensated cirrhosis, prognosis was strongly related to the efficacy of the combination therapy with UDCA and immunosuppressive agents [17, 30, 81]. Finally, Hispanics with PBC-AIH OS were suggested to have a more aggressive disease course than non-Hispanics [21].

Similar to PBC-AIH OS, there are no double-blind, randomized controlled trials in PSC-AIH OS. It should be kept in mind that, although immunosuppressants benefit the hepatitic component of AIH, no survival benefit has been demonstrated with UDCA in PSC. In addition, unlike in PBC and AIH, biochemical improvement in PSC does not necessarily translate into better clinical outcome. Various results of therapy (usually prednisolone and azathioprine with or without UDCA) have been reported in patients with PSC-AIH overlap [23, 24, 85, 86]. It is difficult to draw any firm conclusions because of the small number of patients, the usually retrospective nature of the studies and the heterogeneity of the regimens. The combination of UDCA and immunosuppressive therapy may improve liver biochemistry, and this approach has been advocated by EASL guidelines [31], whereas the AASLD guidelines recommend the use of corticosteroids and other immunosuppressive agents, and the IAIHG position is to consider immunosuppressive treatment with or without UDCA [9]. Unsurprisingly, patients with PSC-AIH overlap have a poorer outcome when compared to those with (treated) AIH alone, with more patients failing immunosuppressive therapy [18, 87, 88]. In the pediatric AISC form treated with immunosuppressants, liver biopsies may show improvement in inflammation, but cholangiographic appearances may progress, and transplant-free survival at 10 years (65%) is lower than in AIH (100%) [10]. In the series with the most homogeneous regimen (UDCA, prednisolone and azathioprine), including seven young adults with a mean follow-up of 8 years, the Mayo risk score did not increase and transplant-free survival was much better (100%) than that of 34 classical PSC (43%) with the same follow-up and treated with UDCA [24]. However, in the long-term (>10 years), long-term progression toward cirrhosis seems to occur in the majority of patients.

Liver transplantation (LT) for end-stage liver disease in OS (both PBC-AIH and PSC-AIH OS) is associated with a shorter duration from diagnosis to LT, a higher probability of recurrence of at least one disease, and a shorter median time to recurrence compared to patients with a single-autoimmune liver disease [89]. Moreover, the use of mycophenolate mofetil as part of immunosuppression and the presence of OS were independent predictive factors of recurrence. However, no differences in graft loss and patients' survival between patients with OS and patients with single-autoimmune liver disease were reported. In patients transplanted for OS, the recurrence in the graft can be characterized by the recurrence of OS or of a single disease [89].

In conclusion, the combination therapy of UDCA and immunosuppressive agents appears to be effective in patients with PBC-AIH OS to achieve biochemical remission, to reduce hepatic inflammation, and to prevent fibrosis progression. To date, it is recommended in patients with severe interface hepatitis at initial biopsy. Differently, patients with mild or moderate interface hepatitis and no advanced fibrosis may benefit of UDCA monotherapy, and, in these patients, immunosuppressive agents may be added in case of persistent biochemical activity as suggested by EASL guidelines. Otherwise, there are no criteria to evaluate response to therapy in PBC-AIH OS, neither the optimal time to perform a second biopsy to assess histological remission, and thus eventually support the decision regarding immunosuppressive drug withdrawal. Normalization of transaminases, IgG, and AP in these patients seems a reasonable target, but whether biochemical remission is indicative of absence or minimal histological activity in patients with PBC-AIH OS is still unknown. Similarly, the data presented above support the use of UDCA in combination with an immunosuppressive regimen in most patients with PSC-AIH OS patients despite the lack of adequate studies. However, the key point is that, even more than in PBC-AIH overlaps, treatments in PSC-AIH overlaps should be individualized based on biochemical, serological, cholangiographic, and histological findings. In patients with severe interface hepatitis, use of immunosuppressants is mandatory. In other cases (moderate interface hepatitis), our policy is, at present, similar to that of PBC-AIH OS and to start with UDCA monotherapy and add immunosuppressants only in case of inadequate biochemical response after 3 months of UDCA.

11.5 Extrahepatic Autoimmune Diseases Associated to Overlap Syndromes

Different concurrent autoimmune diseases may occur in the same patient, and this association has been described both in patients with multisystemic autoimmune diseases (e.g., rheumatoid arthritis, systemic sclerosis, systemic lupus erythematosus (SLE)) and also in patients with organ-specific autoimmune diseases (e.g., Graves' disease, myasthenia gravis, polymyositis) [90]. As in PBC and in AIH alone, patients with PBC-AIH OS may also present with one or more associated extrahepatic autoimmune disease (EHAD). In the first series of PBC-AIH OS diagnosed using Paris criteria, EHAD, including Sjogren's syndrome, Raynaud's phenomenon, and arthropathies, occurred in one-third of patients [11]. EHAD were reported in 27–91% of patients with PBC-AIH OS, depending on criteria applied for OS diagnosis. In the largest series of PBC-AIH OS, defined using Paris criteria, 44% of 71 patients with OS had an associated EHAD [91], and this frequency was comparable to that reported in AIH (42%) [92] and PBC patients (32–61%) [93, 94]. Autoimmune thyroid diseases, namely Hashimoto's thyroiditis and Graves' disease, are reported in 9–36% of patients with PBC-AIH OS [21, 72, 91] compared to 18% of patients with pure AIH [92] and 12% of patients with pure PBC [95]. Sjogren's syndrome occurred in 3–18% of patients with PBC-AIH OS [11, 21, 72, 81, 91], compared to 3% of AIH patients [92] and 34% of PBC patients [94]. Raynaud's phenomenon was reported in 8–9% of patients with OS [11, 96], in 2% of patients with AIH [92], and in 18% of patients with PBC [94]. Autoimmune arthropathies, including rheumatoid arthritis, were reported in 4–17% of patients with OS [11, 91], in 5% of patients with AIH [92], and in up to 10% of patients with PBC [94, 97, 98]. SLE was reported in 4% of 71 patients with PBC-AIH OS, in 3% of patients with AIH, and in 2% of patients with PBC. Among autoimmune cutaneous diseases, psoriasis was reported in 4% of PBC-AIH OS patients [91], whereas it is rarely reported in AIH and PBC patients. Vitiligo was reported in 3% of patients with PBC-AIH OS, in 1–2% of patients with AIH [92, 99], and together with other cutaneous autoimmune diseases in 5% of patients with PBC [94]. Celiac disease was described in 4% of PBC-AIH OS and in 1.4% of AIH and PBC patients [92, 94]. Other reported single case of EHAD associated to PBC-AIH OS included autoimmune hemolytic anemia, antiphospholipid syndrome, multiple sclerosis, membranous glomerulonephritis, sarcoidosis, systemic sclerosis, and temporal arteritis [91].

The most relevant association in PSC with EHAD is the presence of IBD in 50–80% of patients, and mainly UC. Differently, IBD is infrequent in AIH and if present, an abnormal cholangiogram can be found in up to 41% of patients [87]. In PSC-AIH OS, the frequency of IBD is higher than that reported in AIH alone but comparable to that observed in PSC. The presence of IBD in PSC patients is associated with an increased risk of colorectal cancer development, and for this reason, patients with PSC and PSC-AIH OS need to undergo a colonoscopy at the time of diagnosis. Moreover, annual endoscopic surveillance is recommended in patients with confirmed IBD to detect the prevalence of dysplasia. In patients without concomitant IBD, colonoscopy should be repeated when intestinal symptoms occur for every 5 years in asymptomatic patients [100].

The reported association and the sequential development of different autoimmune hepatic and/or extrahepatic disease support the concept that clinical expression of autoimmune diseases may be affected by multiple factors contributing to the development of additional autoimmune manifestations. Indeed, it's commonly believed that autoimmune conditions develop after an environmental trigger responsible to derange the immune system equilibrium in a genetically predisposed host. These alterations of the immune system may lead to the development of one autoimmune disease in some patients or several different clinical manifestations affecting different organs in other patients. This concept has been referred as the mosaic of autoimmunity by Shoenfeld and colleagues and implies that the integration of genetic, environmental, and hormonal factors into the etiology of autoimmune responses may emerge as different overlapping conditions [90, 101, 102].

11.6   PBC-PSC Overlap Syndrome

PBC overlapping with PSC has been reported only in a few case reports of variable quality and do not represent a real issue. Indeed, in most of these cases, the diagnosis of PBC-PSC was controversial due to lack of clear manifestation of both diseases, including the absence of associated inflammatory bowel disease [103–108]. As a consequence, the overlap between PBC and PSC still remains a controversial issue in the field of autoimmune liver diseases due to the small number of reported cases and the lack of properly defined diagnostic criteria.

11.7   Conclusions

Liver overlap syndromes do exist but are rare. Whatever the name used (e.g., variant PBC or PSC with autoimmune hepatitis features or variant autoimmune hepatitis with PBC or PSC features), recognition of autoimmune OS is of interest not only from a classification standpoint, but also, and more importantly, because of therapeutic and surveillance implications. OS should be diagnosed conservatively by using as strict criteria as possible. Appraisal has to be performed longitudinally rather than at a single point in time. Treatment decisions should be tailored to the individual and not be static. In most cases, it is possible to define one primary (dominant) disorder. As a rule, the dominant clinical feature should be treated first and therapy should be individualized and adjusted according to the response. In difficult cases, referral to a specialist center with a high volume of caseload with autoimmune liver diseases is recommended.

International effort for collection of a large database and discovery of more specific molecular signatures with the ability to identify subgroups within the spectrum of autoimmune liver disease should be encouraged.

Key Messages
- Some patients present with features of both primary biliary cholangitis (PBC) or primary sclerosing cholangitis (PSC) and autoimmune hepatitis (AIH), either simultaneously or consecutively.
- The term overlap syndrome (OS) is used to describe these settings, but lack of universal agreement on what precisely constitutes an OS has generated considerable confusion.
- The low prevalence of OS (roughly 10% of PBC and 11% of PSC) has made it impracticable to perform randomized controlled trials.
- It remains unclear whether this syndrome forms a distinct entity or, more likely, a variant of PBC, PSC, or AIH.
- Moderate to severe interface hepatitis is a fundamental component, and histology is vital in evaluating patients with overlap presentation. Use of the International Autoimmune Hepatitis Group criteria for the diagnosis of OS is not recommended.
- For PBC-AIH OS, EASL has provided diagnostic criteria, and, in most cases, it is possible to define one primary disorder ("dominant" disease), usually PBC.
- For PSC-AIH OS, there are no defined criteria, thus the diagnosis is based on the concomitant presence of histological, biochemical, serological, and radiological features of the two diseases.
- Patients with PBC-AIH OS seem to have a more severe disease compared to conventional PBC. Differently, PSC-AIH OS does not seem to have a worst outcome (when the AIH component is treated adequately) than conventional PSC.
- Treatment of OS is empiric and includes ursodeoxycholic acid (UDCA) for the cholestatic component and immunosuppressive agents for the hepatitic component, either simultaneously or sequentially. Immunosuppressive treatment in addition to UDCA is recommended in patients with severe interface hepatitis and deserves consideration in those with moderate interface hepatitis.
- The dominant clinical feature should be treated first and therapy adjusted according to the response.

References

1. Trivedi PJ, Hirschfield GM. Review article: overlap syndromes and autoimmune liver disease. Aliment Pharmacol Ther. 2012;36(6):517–33.
2. Heathcote EJ. Overlap of autoimmune hepatitis and primary biliary cirrhosis: an evaluation of a modified scoring system. Am J Gastroenterol. 2002;97(5):1090–2.
3. Lohse AW, zum Büschenfelde KH, Franz B, Kanzler S, Gerken G, Dienes HP. Characterization of the overlap syndrome of primary biliary cirrhosis (PBC) and autoimmune hepatitis: evidence for it being a hepatitic form of PBC in genetically susceptible individuals. Hepatology. 1999;29(4):1078–84.
4. European Association for the Study of the Liver. EASL clinical practice guidelines: autoimmune hepatitis. J Hepatol. 2015;63(4):971–1004.

5. Hirschfield GM, Beuers U, Corpechot C, Invernizzi P, Jones D, Marzioni M, et al. EASL clinical practice guidelines: the diagnosis and management of patients with primary biliary cholangitis. J Hepatol. 2017;67(1):145–72.
6. Lindor KD, Bowlus CL, Boyer J, Levy C, Mayo M. Primary biliary cholangitis: 2018 practice guidance from the American Association for the Study of Liver Diseases. Hepatology. 2019;69(1):394–419.
7. Hirschfield GM, Dyson JK, Alexander GJM, Chapman MH, Collier J, Hübscher S, et al. The British Society of Gastroenterology/UK-PBC primary biliary cholangitis treatment and management guidelines. Gut. 2018;67(9):1568–94.
8. van Leeuwen DJ, Sood G, Ferrante D, Lazenby AJ, Sellers MJ. A 38-year-old African American woman with an unusually rapid progression of "primary biliary cirrhosis": a missed opportunity! Semin Liver Dis. 2002;22(4):395–406.
9. Boberg KM, Chapman RW, Hirschfield GM, Lohse AW, Manns MP, Schrumpf E, et al. Overlap syndromes: the International Autoimmune Hepatitis Group (IAIHG) position statement on a controversial issue. J Hepatol. 2011;54(2):374–85.
10. Gregorio GV, Portmann B, Karani J, Harrison P, Donaldson PT, Vergani D, et al. Autoimmune hepatitis/sclerosing cholangitis overlap syndrome in childhood: a 16-year prospective study. Hepatology. 2001;33(3):544–53.
11. Chazouillères O, Wendum D, Serfaty L, Montembault S, Rosmorduc O, Poupon R. Primary biliary cirrhosis-autoimmune hepatitis overlap syndrome: clinical features and response to therapy. Hepatology. 1998;28(2):296–301.
12. Czaja AJ. Frequency and nature of the variant syndromes of autoimmune liver disease. Hepatology. 1998;28(2):360–5.
13. Bonder A, Retana A, Winston DM, Leung J, Kaplan MM. Prevalence of primary biliary cirrhosis-autoimmune hepatitis overlap syndrome. Clin Gastroenterol Hepatol. 2011;9(7):609–12.
14. Lindgren S, Glaumann H, Almer S, Bergquist A, Björnsson E, Broomé U, et al. Transitions between variant forms of primary biliary cirrhosis during long-term follow-up. Eur J Intern Med. 2009;20(4):398–402.
15. Efe C, Ozaslan E, Heurgué-Berlot A, Kav T, Masi C, Purnak T, et al. Sequential presentation of primary biliary cirrhosis and autoimmune hepatitis. Eur J Gastroenterol Hepatol. 2014;26(5):532–7.
16. Poupon R, Chazouilleres O, Corpechot C, Chrétien Y. Development of autoimmune hepatitis in patients with typical primary biliary cirrhosis. Hepatology. 2006;44(1):85–90.
17. Yoshioka Y, Taniai M, Hashimoto E, Haruta I, Shiratori K. Clinical profile of primary biliary cirrhosis with features of autoimmune hepatitis: importance of corticosteroid therapy. Hepatol Res. 2014;44(9):947–55.
18. Al-Chalabi T, Portmann BC, Bernal W, McFarlane IG, Heneghan MA. Autoimmune hepatitis overlaps syndromes: an evaluation of treatment response, long-term outcome and survival. Aliment Pharmacol Ther. 2008;28(2):209–20.
19. Dinani AM, Fischer SE, Mosko J, Guindi M, Hirschfield GM. Patients with autoimmune hepatitis who have antimitochondrial antibodies need long-term follow-up to detect late development of primary biliary cirrhosis. Clin Gastroenterol Hepatol. 2012;10(6):682–4.
20. Yang F, Wang Q, Wang Z, Miao Q, Xiao X, Tang R, et al. The natural history and prognosis of primary biliary cirrhosis with clinical features of autoimmune hepatitis. Clin Rev Allergy Immunol. 2016;50(1):114–23.
21. Levy C, Naik J, Giordano C, Mandalia A, O'Brien C, Bhamidimarri KR, et al. Hispanics with primary biliary cirrhosis are more likely to have features of autoimmune hepatitis and reduced response to ursodeoxycholic acid than non-Hispanics. Clin Gastroenterol Hepatol. 2014;12(8):1398–405.
22. Heurgué A, Vitry F, Diebold M-D, Yaziji N, Bernard-Chabert B, Pennaforte J-L, et al. Overlap syndrome of primary biliary cirrhosis and autoimmune hepatitis: a retrospective study of 115 cases of autoimmune liver disease. Gastroenterol Clin Biol. 2007;31(1):17–25.

23. Abdo AA, Bain VG, Kichian K, Lee SS. Evolution of autoimmune hepatitis to primary sclerosing cholangitis: a sequential syndrome. Hepatology. 2002;36(6):1393–9.
24. Floreani A, Rizzotto ER, Ferrara F, Carderi I, Caroli D, Blasone L, et al. Clinical course and outcome of autoimmune hepatitis/primary sclerosing cholangitis overlap syndrome. Am J Gastroenterol. 2005;100(7):1516–22.
25. Alvarez F, Berg PA, Bianchi FB, Bianchi L, Burroughs AK, Cancado EL, et al. International Autoimmune Hepatitis Group Report: review of criteria for diagnosis of autoimmune hepatitis. J Hepatol. 1999;31(5):929–38.
26. Hennes EM, Zeniya M, AlbertJ C, Parés A, Dalekos GN, Krawitt EL, et al. Simplified criteria for the diagnosis of autoimmune hepatitis. Hepatology. 2008;48(1):169–76.
27. Kuiper EMM, Zondervan PE, van Buuren HR. Paris criteria are effective in diagnosis of primary biliary cirrhosis and autoimmune hepatitis overlap syndrome. Clin Gastroenterol Hepatol. 2010;8(6):530–4.
28. Joshi S, Cauch-Dudek K, Wanless IR, Lindor KD, Jorgensen R, Batts K, et al. Primary biliary cirrhosis with additional features of autoimmune hepatitis: response to therapy with ursodeoxycholic acid. Hepatology. 2002;35(2):409–13.
29. Yokokawa J, Saito H, Kanno Y, Honma F, Monoe K, Sakamoto N, et al. Overlap of primary biliary cirrhosis and autoimmune hepatitis: characteristics, therapy, and long term outcomes. J Gastroenterol Hepatol. 2010;25(2):376–82.
30. Fan X, Zhu Y, Men R, Wen M, Shen Y, Lu C, et al. Efficacy and safety of immunosuppressive therapy for PBC-AIH overlap syndrome accompanied by decompensated cirrhosis: a real-world study. Can J Gastroenterol Hepatol. 2018;2018:1965492.
31. European Association for the Study of the Liver. EASL clinical practice guidelines: management of cholestatic liver diseases. J Hepatol. 2009;51(2):237–67.
32. Zhang W, De D, Mohammed KA, Munigala S, Chen G, Lai J-P, et al. New scoring classification for primary biliary cholangitis-autoimmune hepatitis overlap syndrome. Hepatol Commun. 2018;2(3):245–53.
33. Abdalian R, Dhar P, Jhaveri K, Haider M, Guindi M, Heathcote EJ. Prevalence of sclerosing cholangitis in adults with autoimmune hepatitis: evaluating the role of routine magnetic resonance imaging. Hepatology. 2008;47(3):949–57.
34. Lewin M, Vilgrain V, Ozenne V, Lemoine M, Wendum D, Paradis V, et al. Prevalence of sclerosing cholangitis in adults with autoimmune hepatitis: a prospective magnetic resonance imaging and histological study. Hepatology. 2009;50(2):528–37.
35. Lindor KD, Kowdley KV, Harrison ME, American College of Gastroenterology. ACG clinical guideline: primary Sclerosing cholangitis. Am J Gastroenterol. 2015;110(5):646–59; quiz 660.
36. Hunter M, Loughrey MB, Gray M, Ellis P, McDougall N, Callender M. Evaluating distinctive features for early diagnosis of primary sclerosing cholangitis overlap syndrome in adults with autoimmune hepatitis. Ulster Med J. 2011;80(1):15–8.
37. O'Brien C, Joshi S, Feld JJ, Guindi M, Dienes HP, Heathcote EJ. Long-term follow-up of antimitochondrial antibody-positive autoimmune hepatitis. Hepatology. 2008;48(2):550–6.
38. Ozaslan E, Efe C, Heurgué-Berlot A, Kav T, Masi C, Purnak T, et al. Factors associated with response to therapy and outcome of patients with primary biliary cirrhosis with features of autoimmune hepatitis. Clin Gastroenterol Hepatol. 2014;12(5):863–9.
39. Muratori P, Granito A, Pappas G, Pendino GM, Quarneti C, Cicola R, et al. The serological profile of the autoimmune hepatitis/primary biliary cirrhosis overlap syndrome. Am J Gastroenterol. 2009;104(6):1420–5.
40. Vergani D, Alvarez F, Bianchi FB, Cançado ELR, Mackay IR, Manns MP, et al. Liver autoimmune serology: a consensus statement from the committee for autoimmune serology of the International Autoimmune Hepatitis Group. J Hepatol. 2004;41(4):677–83.
41. Schulz L, Sebode M, Weidemann SA, Lohse AW. Variant syndromes of primary biliary cholangitis. Best Pract Res Clin Gastroenterol. 2018;34–35:55–61.

42. Nguyen HH, Shaheen AA, Baeza N, Lytvyak E, Urbanski SJ, Mason AL, et al. Evaluation of classical and novel autoantibodies for the diagnosis of primary biliary cholangitis-autoimmune hepatitis overlap syndrome (PBC-AIH OS). PLoS One. 2018;13(3):e0193960.
43. Levy C, Lindor KD. Primary sclerosing cholangitis: epidemiology, natural history, and prognosis. Semin Liver Dis. 2006;26(1):22–30.
44. Bansi DS, Bauducci M, Bergqvist A, Boberg K, Broome U, Chapman R, et al. Detection of antineutrophil cytoplasmic antibodies in primary sclerosing cholangitis: a comparison of the alkaline phosphatase and immunofluorescent techniques. Eur J Gastroenterol Hepatol. 1997;9(6):575–80.
45. Terjung B, Söhne J, Lechtenberg B, Gottwein J, Muennich M, Herzog V, et al. p-ANCAs in autoimmune liver disorders recognise human beta-tubulin isotype 5 and cross-react with microbial protein FtsZ. Gut. 2010;59(6):808–16.
46. Hov J-R, Boberg K-M, Karlsen T-H. Autoantibodies in primary sclerosing cholangitis. World J Gastroenterol. 2008;14(24):3781–91.
47. Manns MP, Czaja AJ, Gorham JD, Krawitt EL, Mieli-Vergani G, Vergani D, et al. Diagnosis and management of autoimmune hepatitis. Hepatology. 2010;51(6):2193–213.
48. Bach N, Thung SN, Schaffner F. The histological features of chronic hepatitis C and autoimmune chronic hepatitis: a comparative analysis. Hepatology. 1992;15(4):572–7.
49. Czaja AJ, Carpenter HA. Sensitivity, specificity, and predictability of biopsy interpretations in chronic hepatitis. Gastroenterology. 1993;105(6):1824–32.
50. Li MK, Crawford JM. The pathology of cholestasis. Semin Liver Dis. 2004;24(1):21–42.
51. Nakanuma Y, Zen Y, Harada K, Sasaki M, Nonomura A, Uehara T, et al. Application of a new histological staging and grading system for primary biliary cirrhosis to liver biopsy specimens: interobserver agreement. Pathol Int. 2010;60(3):167–74.
52. Christensen E, Crowe J, Doniach D, Popper H, Ranek L, Rodés J, et al. Clinical pattern and course of disease in primary biliary cirrhosis based on an analysis of 236 patients. Gastroenterology. 1980;78(2):236–46.
53. Kobayashi M, Kakuda Y, Harada K, Sato Y, Sasaki M, Ikeda H, et al. Clinicopathological study of primary biliary cirrhosis with interface hepatitis compared to autoimmune hepatitis. World J Gastroenterol. 2014;20(13):3597–608.
54. Lee H, Stapp RT, Ormsby AH, Shah VV. The usefulness of IgG and IgM immunostaining of periportal inflammatory cells (plasma cells and lymphocytes) for the distinction of autoimmune hepatitis and primary biliary cirrhosis and their staining pattern in autoimmune hepatitis-primary biliary cirrhosis overlap syndrome. Am J Clin Pathol. 2010;133(3):430–7.
55. Czaja AJ, Carpenter HA. Autoimmune hepatitis with incidental histologic features of bile duct injury. Hepatology. 2001;34(4 Pt 1):659–65.
56. Verdonk RC, Lozano MF, van den Berg AP, Gouw ASH. Bile ductal injury and ductular reaction are frequent phenomena with different significance in autoimmune hepatitis. Liver Int. 2016;36(9):1362–9.
57. de Boer YS, van Nieuwkerk CMJ, Witte BI, Mulder CJJ, Bouma G, Bloemena E. Assessment of the histopathological key features in autoimmune hepatitis. Histopathology. 2015;66(3):351–62.
58. Czaja AJ. Cholestatic phenotypes of autoimmune hepatitis. Clin Gastroenterol Hepatol. 2014;12(9):1430–8.
59. Czaja AJ, Muratori P, Muratori L, Carpenter HA, Bianchi FB. Diagnostic and therapeutic implications of bile duct injury in autoimmune hepatitis. Liver Int. 2004;24(4):322–9.
60. Wiesner RH, LaRusso NF, Ludwig J, Dickson ER. Comparison of the clinicopathologic features of primary sclerosing cholangitis and primary biliary cirrhosis. Gastroenterology. 1985;88(1 Pt 1):108–14.
61. Harrison RF, Hubscher SG. The spectrum of bile duct lesions in end-stage primary sclerosing cholangitis. Histopathology. 1991;19(4):321–7.
62. Chapman RW, Arborgh BA, Rhodes JM, Summerfield JA, Dick R, Scheuer PJ, et al. Primary sclerosing cholangitis: a review of its clinical features, cholangiography, and hepatic histology. Gut. 1980;21(10):870–7.

63. Olsson R, Hagerstrand I, Broome U, Danielsson A, Jarnerot G, Loof L, et al. Sampling variability of percutaneous liver biopsy in primary sclerosing cholangitis. J Clin Pathol. 1995;48(10):933–5.
64. Paterson AL, Allison MED, Brais R, Davies SE. Any value in a specialist review of liver biopsies? Conclusions of a 4-year review. Histopathology. 2016;69(2):315–21.
65. Corpechot C, Abenavoli L, Rabahi N, Chrétien Y, Andréani T, Johanet C, et al. Biochemical response to ursodeoxycholic acid and long-term prognosis in primary biliary cirrhosis. Hepatology. 2008;48(3):871–7.
66. Kuiper EMM, Hansen BE, de Vries RA, den Ouden-Muller JW, van Ditzhuijsen TJM, Haagsma EB, et al. Improved prognosis of patients with primary biliary cirrhosis that have a biochemical response to ursodeoxycholic acid. Gastroenterology. 2009;136(4):1281–7.
67. Parés A, Caballería L, Rodés J. Excellent long-term survival in patients with primary biliary cirrhosis and biochemical response to ursodeoxycholic acid. Gastroenterology. 2006;130(3):715–20.
68. Corpechot C, Chazouillères O, Poupon R. Early primary biliary cirrhosis: biochemical response to treatment and prediction of long-term outcome. J Hepatol. 2011;55(6):1361–7.
69. Kumagi T, Guindi M, Fischer SE, Arenovich T, Abdalian R, Coltescu C, et al. Baseline ductopenia and treatment response predict long-term histological progression in primary biliary cirrhosis. Am J Gastroenterol. 2010;105(10):2186–94.
70. Lammers WJ, Hirschfield GM, Corpechot C, Nevens F, Lindor KD, Janssen HLA, et al. Development and validation of a scoring system to predict outcomes of patients with primary biliary cirrhosis receiving ursodeoxycholic acid therapy. Gastroenterology. 2015;149(7):1804–1812.e4.
71. Carbone M, Sharp SJ, Flack S, Paximadas D, Spiess K, Adgey C, et al. The UK-PBC risk scores: derivation and validation of a scoring system for long-term prediction of end-stage liver disease in primary biliary cholangitis. Hepatology. 2016;63(3):930–50.
72. Tanaka A, Harada K, Ebinuma H, Komori A, Yokokawa J, Yoshizawa K, et al. Primary biliary cirrhosis—autoimmune hepatitis overlap syndrome: a rationale for corticosteroids use based on a nationwide retrospective study in Japan. Hepatol Res. 2011;41(9):877–86.
73. Chazouillères O, Wendum D, Serfaty L, Rosmorduc O, Poupon R. Long-term outcome and response to therapy of primary biliary cirrhosis-autoimmune hepatitis overlap syndrome. J Hepatol. 2006;44(2):400–6.
74. Nevens F, Andreone P, Mazzella G, Strasser SI, Bowlus C, Invernizzi P, et al. A placebo-controlled trial of obeticholic acid in primary biliary cholangitis. N Engl J Med. 2016;375(7):631–43.
75. Trauner M, Nevens F, Shiffman ML, Drenth JPH, Bowlus CL, Vargas V, et al. Long-term efficacy and safety of obeticholic acid for patients with primary biliary cholangitis: 3-year results of an international open-label extension study. Lancet Gastroenterol Hepatol. 2019;4(6):445–53.
76. Corpechot C, Chazouillères O, Rousseau A, Le Gruyer A, Habersetzer F, Mathurin P, et al. A placebo-controlled trial of bezafibrate in primary biliary cholangitis. N Engl J Med. 2018;378(23):2171–81.
77. Ishak K, Baptista A, Bianchi L, Callea F, De Groote J, Gudat F, et al. Histological grading and staging of chronic hepatitis. J Hepatol. 1995;22(6):696–9.
78. Gossard AA, Lindor KD. Development of autoimmune hepatitis in primary biliary cirrhosis. Liver Int. 2007;27(8):1086–90.
79. Saito H, Rai T, Takahashi A, Kanno Y, Monoe K, Irisawa A, et al. Clinicolaboratory characteristics of Japanese patients with primary biliary cirrhosis-autoimmune hepatitis overlap. Fukushima J Med Sci. 2006;52(2):71–7.
80. Alric L, Thebault S, Selves J, Peron J-M, Mejdoubi S, Fortenfant F, et al. Characterization of overlap syndrome between primary biliary cirrhosis and autoimmune hepatitis according to antimitochondrial antibodies status. Gastroenterol Clin Biol. 2007;31(1):11–6.
81. Amarapurkar DN, Patel ND. Spectrum of autoimmune liver diseases in western India. J Gastroenterol Hepatol. 2007;22(12):2112–7.

82. Gheorghe L, Iacob S, Gheorghe C, Iacob R, Simionov I, Vadan R, et al. Frequency and predictive factors for overlap syndrome between autoimmune hepatitis and primary cholestatic liver disease. Eur J Gastroenterol Hepatol. 2004;16(6):585–92.
83. Zhang H, Yang J, Zhu R, Zheng Y, Zhou Y, Dai W, et al. Combination therapy of ursodeoxycholic acid and budesonide for PBC-AIH overlap syndrome: a meta-analysis. Drug Des Devel Ther. 2015;9:567–74.
84. Silveira MG, Talwalkar JA, Angulo P, Lindor KD. Overlap of autoimmune hepatitis and primary biliary cirrhosis: long-term outcomes. Am J Gastroenterol. 2007;102(6):1244–50.
85. Boberg KM, Aadland E, Jahnsen J, Raknerud N, Stiris M, Bell H. Incidence and prevalence of primary biliary cirrhosis, primary sclerosing cholangitis, and autoimmune hepatitis in a Norwegian population. Scand J Gastroenterol. 1998;33(1):99–103.
86. Olsson R, Glaumann H, Almer S, Broomé U, Lebrun B, Bergquist A, et al. High prevalence of small duct primary sclerosing cholangitis among patients with overlapping autoimmune hepatitis and primary sclerosing cholangitis. Eur J Intern Med. 2009;20(2):190–6.
87. Perdigoto R, Carpenter HA, Czaja AJ. Frequency and significance of chronic ulcerative colitis in severe corticosteroid-treated autoimmune hepatitis. J Hepatol. 1992;14(2–3):325–31.
88. Czaja AJ, Carpenter HA, Santrach PJ, Moore SB. Autoimmune cholangitis within the spectrum of autoimmune liver disease. Hepatology. 2000;31(6):1231–8.
89. Bhanji RA, Mason AL, Girgis S, Montano-Loza AJ. Liver transplantation for overlap syndromes of autoimmune liver diseases. Liver Int. 2013;33(2):210–9.
90. Shoenfeld Y, Blank M, Abu-Shakra M, Amital H, Barzilai O, Berkun Y, et al. The mosaic of autoimmunity: prediction, autoantibodies, and therapy in autoimmune diseases—2008. Isr Med Assoc J. 2008;10(1):13–9.
91. Efe C, Wahlin S, Ozaslan E, Berlot AH, Purnak T, Muratori L, et al. Autoimmune hepatitis/ primary biliary cirrhosis overlap syndrome and associated extrahepatic autoimmune diseases. Eur J Gastroenterol Hepatol. 2012;24(5):531–4.
92. Wong G-W, Yeong T, Lawrence D, Yeoman AD, Verma S, Heneghan MA. Concurrent extrahepatic autoimmunity in autoimmune hepatitis: implications for diagnosis, clinical course and long-term outcomes. Liver Int. 2017;37(3):449–57.
93. Gershwin ME, Selmi C, Worman HJ, Gold EB, Watnik M, Utts J, et al. Risk factors and comorbidities in primary biliary cirrhosis: a controlled interview-based study of 1032 patients. Hepatology. 2005;42(5):1194–202.
94. Floreani A, Franceschet I, Cazzagon N, Spinazzè A, Buja A, Furlan P, et al. Extrahepatic autoimmune conditions associated with primary biliary cirrhosis. Clin Rev Allergy Immunol. 2015;48(2–3):192–7.
95. Floreani A, Mangini C, Reig A, Franceschet I, Cazzagon N, Perini L, et al. Thyroid dysfunction in primary biliary cholangitis: a comparative study at two European centers. Am J Gastroenterol. 2017;112(1):114–9.
96. Neuhauser M, Bjornsson E, Treeprasertsuk S, Enders F, Silveira M, Talwalkar J, et al. Autoimmune hepatitis-PBC overlap syndrome: a simplified scoring system may assist in the diagnosis. Am J Gastroenterol. 2010;105(2):345–53.
97. Mills P, MacSween RN, Watkinson G. Arthritis and primary biliary cirrhosis. Br Med J. 1977;2(6096):1224.
98. Parikh-Patel A, Gold E, Mackay IR, Gershwin ME. The geoepidemiology of primary biliary cirrhosis: contrasts and comparisons with the spectrum of autoimmune diseases. Clin Immunol. 1999;91(2):206–18.
99. Teufel A, Weinmann A, Kahaly GJ, Centner C, Piendl A, Wörns M, et al. Concurrent autoimmune diseases in patients with autoimmune hepatitis. J Clin Gastroenterol. 2010;44(3):208–13.
100. Aabakken L, Karlsen TH, Albert J, Arvanitakis M, Chazouilleres O, Dumonceau J-M, et al. Role of endoscopy in primary sclerosing cholangitis: European Society of Gastrointestinal Endoscopy (ESGE) and European Association for the Study of the Liver (EASL) clinical guideline. Endoscopy. 2017;49(6):588–608.
101. Shoenfeld Y, Isenberg DA. The mosaic of autoimmunity. Immunol Today. 1989;10(4):123–6.

102. Amital H, Gershwin ME, Shoenfeld Y. Reshaping the mosaic of autoimmunity. Semin Arthritis Rheum. 2006;35(6):341–3.
103. Rubel LR, Seeff LB, Patel V. Primary biliary cirrhosis-primary sclerosing cholangitis overlap syndrome. Arch Pathol Lab Med. 1984;108(5):360–1.
104. Burak K, Angulo P, Pasha TM, Egan K, Petz J, Lindor KD. Incidence and risk factors for cholangiocarcinoma in primary sclerosing cholangitis. Am J Gastroenterol. 2004;99(3):523–6.
105. Kingham JGC, Abbasi A. Co-existence of primary biliary cirrhosis and primary sclerosing cholangitis: a rare overlap syndrome put in perspective. Eur J Gastroenterol Hepatol. 2005;17(10):1077–80.
106. Jeevagan A. Overlap of primary biliary cirrhosis and primary sclerosing cholangitis—a rare coincidence or a new syndrome. Int J Gen Med. 2010;3:143–6.
107. Oliveira EMG, Oliveira PM, Becker V, Dellavance A, Andrade LEC, Lanzoni V, et al. Overlapping of primary biliary cirrhosis and small duct primary sclerosing cholangitis: first case report. J Clin Med Res. 2012;4(6):429–33.
108. Floreani A, Franceschet I, Cazzagon N. Primary biliary cirrhosis: overlaps with other autoimmune disorders. Semin Liver Dis. 2014 Aug;34(3):352–60.

Part IV

Secondary Cholangiopathies

Inflammatory Cholangitis

12

Erik Rosa-Rizzotto, Diego Caroli, and Laura Scribano

12.1 Introduction

Cholangitis is a systemic process characterized by an inflammation of one or more bile ducts; acute cholangitis is a severe, potentially life-threatening medical emergency characterized by a bacterial infection superimposed on an obstruction of the biliary tree, most commonly caused by a gallstones [1]. Before the recent advancements in critical care and management with less invasive approaches to decompress the bile system, the mortality rate for acute cholangitis was reported to be higher than 50% [2, 3]. From the figures reported in the 1970s [2, 3] since the 1980s, the mortality rates are actually less than 10% [4, 5]. The management of cholangitis has radically changed from surgical approach in the nineteenth century to an endoscopic approach, generally endoscopic retrograde cholangiopancreatography (ERCP), which has become the treatment of choice [6, 7].

It is well known that choledocholithiasis, a condition characterized by the presence of one or more gallstones in the common bile duct, is the most frequent cause of cholangitis in Western countries. In fact, bile duct stones constitute the single most common obstructive cause predisposing to cholangitis, accounting for ~80% of cases [8, 9]. Sir Berkeley Moynihan (1865–1936), full professor of Clinical Surgery at the University of Leeds, said: "Every gallstone is a tomb-stone erected to the evil memory of the germs that lie dead within it." Jean-Martin Charcot, a French neurologist and professor of Pathology, first described cholangitis in 1877 and coined the term "hepatic fever" to describe the disease. The cardinal clinical

E. Rosa-Rizzotto (✉) · D. Caroli · L. Scribano
Department of Medicine, Gastroenterology Unit, St. Anthony Hospital, Azienda Ospedale-Università, Padova, Italy
e-mail: erik.rosarizzotto@aopd.veneto.it; Diego.caroli@aopd.Veneto.it; Laura.scribano@aopd.Veneto.it

© Springer Nature Switzerland AG 2021
A. Floreani (ed.), *Diseases of the Liver and Biliary Tree*,
https://doi.org/10.1007/978-3-030-65908-0_12

features of cholangitis, namely, right upper quadrant abdominal pain, fever with chills, and jaundice, are, therefore, known as the Charcot's triad [10].

Early diagnosis is critical for determining the type and timetable of treatment and the prognosis. The Tokyo Consensus guidelines furnish clinical guidance for clinicians regarding the diagnosis, severity grading, and treatment of acute cholangitis [11, 12]. A working knowledge of its common etiologies and diagnostic criteria can assist the clinician in assessing the cause and the severity of the disease, making a prompt diagnosis and determining the appropriate treatment. Diagnosis of cholangitis is based on clinical features, laboratory test results, and radiologic investigations.

12.2   The Pathophysiology of Biliary Tree Inflammations

Partial or complete obstruction of the bile duct and subsequent infection is generally the primary factor triggering the development of acute cholangitis [13]. Physiologically, the continuous flow of bile and the innate immune defenses of the biliary epithelial cells keep the biliary tree sterile. An infection within this closed system results in bacterial colonization and increased intraluminal pressure in the biliary tree exceeding 25 cm H_2O leading to a breakdown of innate defenses [14–16]. Bacteremia can also lead to hematogenous seeding [15]. A competent sphincter of Oddi normally prevents intestinal contents from refluxing into the bile duct, and an anterograde flow of bile periodically flushes the biliary system, keeping it free of organisms. In addition, components of bile, including bile salts and immunoglobulin A (IgA), have antibacterial properties. Bile salts are bacteriostatic and directly promote sterility of the biliary tree and limit the growth of bacteria within the duodenum [16, 17]. Tight junctions between hepatocytes separate the bile canaliculi from hepatic sinusoids, thereby protecting the biliary tree from bacteremia. Finally, Kupffer cells within the hepatic sinusoids keep the biliary system sterile via phagocytosis [18].

Complete biliary obstruction creates a state of immune dysfunction [19]. Several studies indicate that the absence of bile salts and IgA in the intestine leads to an alteration in the bacterial flora colonizing the small intestine. Under normal circumstances, bacterial colonization of the duodenum and jejunum is limited [20, 21], but other studies have shown that this is not the case in bile duct-ligated rats; in this experimental model, a shift in the small bowel flora with a predominance of *E. coli* has been shown [22]. In addition to an alteration in the bacterial flora of the duodenum, intestinal bacteria are more likely to translocate in bile duct-ligated rodents [23]. Increased translocation may in part be caused by the absence of bile salts, which have a detergent effect on bacterial endotoxins; their absence may be responsible for increased translocation of endotoxin from the gut [24]. Furthermore, biliary obstruction results in increased intraductal pressures that disrupt the tight junctions between the hepatic cellular architecture leading, in turn, to a reflux of bacteria into the bloodstream [25].

12.3 The Causes of Obstruction and the Etiology of Inflammation

Choledocholithiasis is the most common underlying cause of cholangitis in Western countries [8, 9, 26]. Bile duct stones typically cause intermittent obstruction that allows bacteria to enter the bile duct and can act as a site for bacterial adhesion and growth. Most bile duct stones migrate from the gallbladder. Up to 15% of patients with symptomatic cholelithiasis also have choledocholithiasis [27, 28]. Primary de novo bile duct stones are usually pigmented bilirubin stones thought to result from bile stasis and low-level infection. De novo bile duct stones are more commonly noted in Asian populations and in elderly individuals with dilated bile ducts due to postsurgical alterations or periampullary duodenal diverticula [28, 29].

Other causes of biliary obstruction, such as benign and malignant stenosis, extrinsic compression from pancreatitis, biliary stent obstruction, and parasitic infection, may also place the patient at greater risk for developing cholangitis. Mirizzi syndrome, a condition in which the common bile duct is obstructed extrinsically by impacted calculi or stones in the gallbladder neck or cystic duct, and Lemmel syndrome, an obstructive jaundice caused by periampullary duodenal diverticulum compressing the intrapancreatic common bile duct causing cholestasis and resultant infection, are other possible causes [11].

Although rare, there are increasing reports on sclerosing cholangiopathies in the literature. Secondary sclerosing cholangitis is a chronic cholestatic biliary disease characterized by biliary inflammation, obliterative fibrosis of the bile ducts, stricture formation, and progressive destruction of the biliary tree. It can be caused by infectious, immune-mediated, toxic, obstructive, or ischemic injury. A variety of specific etiologies have been identified in the past. Unless diagnosed in a timely manner, clinical outcomes are generally less favorable for the secondary with respect to primary sclerosing cholangitis [30]. Table 12.1 outlines the most common causes of biliary obstruction leading to cholangitis.

Cholangitis is usually caused by enteric bacteria. Indeed, bile cultures are positive in more than 80% of patients with cholangitis. Nevertheless, the rates of bacteremia are variable, ranging between 20% and 80% in patients with cholangitis. Polymicrobial isolates are found in 30–90% of patients; they are more frequent in individuals who present postoperative biliary tree abnormalities or who have undergone prior biliary tree manipulation [2, 9, 31–35]. The most common organisms are *E. coli* (25–50%), *Klebsiella* (15–20%), and *Enterobacter* species (5–10%) [9]. *Enterococcus*, which is the most common Gram-positive bacterium causing cholangitis, is found in 10–20% of patients. Anaerobes, which may be present in 5–10% of patients, are usually found in mixed infections. The most commonly isolated anaerobic pathogen is *Bacteroides,* followed by *Clostridia* organisms [11]. Elderly patients and individuals with surgically altered anatomy, including biliodigestive anastomosis, are more likely to have anaerobic mixed infections [9, 34, 35].

Hepatobiliary parasites, including *Ascaris, Opisthorchis, Clonorchis,* and *Fasciola,* which are important causes of biliary obstruction, especially in Asian individuals, lead to cholangitis via superimposed bacterial infection [32]. Viral

Table 12.1 Causes of acute cholangitis

Gallstones	Bile duct strictures	Infection	Intervention on biliary tree
– Secondary choledocholithiasis – Primary bile duct stones – Complicated stones (e.g., Mirizzi syndrome)	*Benign* – Postoperative: orthotopic liver transplant (anastomotic/nonanastomotic), complicated cholecystectomy, – Pancreatitis: acute (edema), chronic (scarring, fibrosis) – Congenital anomalies: choledochal cysts, biliary atresia – Lemmel syndrome *Malignant* – Pancreatic cancer – Cholangiocarcinoma – Ampullary/duodenal neoplasm—Gallbladder carcinoma – Metastatic lymph nodes – Ampullary cancer – Duodenal cancer	*Parasitic infection* Ascariasis, liver flukes (*Opisthorchis, Clonorchis, Fasciola*) *Others* – Viral infection (AIDS cholangiopathy) – Recurrent pyogenic cholangitis (oriental cholangiopathies) – Fungal infection (candida cholangitis)	– ERCP with incomplete drainage – Percutaneous transhepatic cholangiography (PTC) – Hemobilia – Bile duct stent obstruction

infection of the biliary tract has been reported in patients with hepatitis C and human immunodeficiency virus (HIV) [33]. AIDS cholangiopathy in patients with HIV caused by *Cryptosporidium*, microsporidia, *Cyclospora*, or *Cytomegalovirus* infection is less common at present, thanks to the development of effective retroviral therapy [34]. Although Candida from the biliary tract is rarely isolated, it has been reported in immunosuppressed patients at risk for candidemia [35].

12.4 Clinical Presentation and Diagnosis

Inflammatory diseases of the bile ducts are complex pathological conditions that may be complicated by other overlapping, not entirely defined conditions [36]. Acute cholangitis (as well as suppurative or ascending cholangitis) was firstly identified as a disorder associated with recurrent fever, abdominal pain, and jaundice. The grouping of symptoms was first termed "hepatic fever" by Dr. Jean-Martin Charcot in 1887, and it is now traditionally referred to as Charcot's triad. In 1959, Reynolds added new features to the trilogy, that is, lethargy/mental confusion and shock, indicative of ongoing biliary sepsis, which were termed as "Reynolds' pentad" [13]. One study, however, investigating the diagnostic relevance of the Charcot's triad, found that only 21% of patients with acute cholangitis presented all three criteria, indicating a suboptimal diagnostic utility. In general, Charcot's triad exhibits a high specificity (95.9%), but a low sensitivity (26.4%) [37]. Reynolds' pentad (the Charcot's triad+septic shock and altered mental status) has, instead, been reported in only 4–8% of patients with severe cholangitis [38].

The Tokyo Guidelines (TG) (see Table 12.2), originally published in 2007 and revised in 2013 and 2018, set out to provide a data-driven diagnostic framework for the clinical diagnosis of acute cholangitis. Based on three domains referring to clinical, laboratory, and imaging findings, diagnoses formulated in accordance with its framework tend to be accurate in 90% of cases [39–43].

Severity grading criteria for acute cholangitis were incorporated into the TG13 version of the guidelines. Grade III is defined, according to TG13, as acute cholangitis associated with onset of dysfunction in one or more organs/systems. Grade II (moderate) is associated with any two of the following: abnormal WBC count, high fever, being over 38°C, hyperbilirubinemia, and/or hypoalbuminemia. Grade I (mild) refers to those situations in which the criteria of the other two grades are not met at the initial diagnosis. It has been shown that mortality increases significantly with rising severity stages, ranging from 1% for grade I to 5% or more for grade III [42, 43].

The commonly used biomarkers for acute cholangitis, including elevation in white blood cell count and elevated serum levels of bilirubin, alkaline phosphatase, aspartate aminotransferase, and alanine aminotransferase, should be tested routinely in all suspect cases [43]. Serum alkaline phosphatase is the most indicative marker of acute cholangitis, being increased in 74–93% of cases. It also exhibits a quicker reduction following successful drainage, with respect to other markers of cholestasis, such as bilirubin, and may provide a more accurate, early indicator of adequate drainage [40].

Although abnormally elevated serum carbohydrate antigen 19–9 (CA19–9) levels have been reported in acute cholangitis secondary to choledocholithiasis

Table 12.2 Diagnostic criteria according to Tokyo Guidelines 2013

A. Systemic inflammation
– A-1. Fever higher than 38
– A-2. Laboratory evidence of inflammation (white blood cell count <4 or >10, C-reactive protein >1)
B. Cholestasis
– B-1. Jaundice (total bilirubin >2 mg/dL)
– B-2. Abnormal liver function tests (elevation >1.5 standard deviation of alkaline phosphatase, glutamate-pyruvate transaminase, aspartate aminotransferase, or alanine aminotransferase)
C. Imaging
– C-1. Biliary dilation
– C-2. Evidence of etiology of obstruction
Suspected diagnosis: One item in A 1, 1 item in either B or C
Definite diagnosis: One item in A, 1 item in B, and 1 item in C

with rapid resolution following successful treatment [41], testing CA19–9 in the context of a routine workup of acute cholangitis is not generally recommended [42].

Other markers of inflammation, including C-reactive protein and procalcitonin, are frequently elevated, and their assessment can provide additional guidance for treatment decisions and for estimating a prognosis. Using procalcitonin to diagnose and manage sepsis has recently gained much attention. In cases of acute cholangitis, procalcitonin has been shown to be a more accurate predictor of severe disease than conventional biomarkers. Furthermore, high procalcitonin levels may support the need for biliary decompression in case of acute cholangitis [43, 44].

Blood cultures are often collected as part of an initial investigation when infection is suspected. Positive blood cultures have been reported in 21–71% of acute cholangitis cases [46]. Positive cultures, however, often fail to provide additional clinically relevant information in routine cases of community-acquired intraabdominal infection. Thus, the Tokyo Guidelines, the Guidelines of the Surgical Infection Society and of the Infectious Diseases Society of America do not recommend routinely blood cultures [45, 46]. An exception is made for the toxic or immunocompromised patient or in cases of very severe infections when culture results may assist clinicians in making decisions on treatment or on modification and duration [50].

There are various modalities for imaging of the biliary tract: the most useful are endoscopic ultrasound (EUS) and magnetic resonance imaging (MRI). All harbor different benefits and caveats.

Given its low cost and wide availability, transabdominal ultrasound is still considered the first diagnostic test in suspected gallstone disease for evaluating bile duct diameter and for ruling out other abdominal infectious sources and stone-related complications. Findings of biliary ductal dilation can support the diagnosis. The sensitivity of ultrasound for detecting common bile duct stones is, however, lower than 30% [47].

Contrast-enhanced computed tomography (CT) scan can indirectly support a diagnosis of cholangitis by providing evidence of biliary stones, ductal dilation, hepatic abscess, and/or pneumobilia in suspected cases [48].

MRI has become the gold standard for defining the morphology of the bile tree and for diagnosing cholangitis. MRI's accuracy in detecting common bile duct stones is high as 90%, but it is much lower for smaller stone diameter (<6 mm) [49, 57]. Gadolinium injection is normally not necessary [50].

EUS and ERCP are invasive procedures that can provide valuable additional diagnostic information. The latter, however, is no longer used for diagnostic purposes, being actually utilized only for therapeutic interventions. Bile duct dilatation and presence of small stones can be identified by EUS [51], which have a roughly 100% sensitivity, >90% specificity, and an overall accuracy of 96.9% for detecting bile duct stones [52]. Moreover, EUS can be performed during the same session of ERCP [53]. Purulent bile from the major papilla detected during ERCP remains the gold standard for the diagnosis of acute cholangitis [50].

12.5   Antibiotic Management

New light has been shed on the role of microbial properties in the development of some forms of cholangitis. Given the high rate of positive microbial cultures from the bile of patients with cholangitis, most clinicians prefer to obtain a microbial profile before deciding the type of drainage. The most common bacterial infections in cholangitis include: *E. coli, Klebsiella pneumoniae, Pseudomonas* species, *Enterobacter, Acinetobacter* among Gram-negative bacteria, and *Enterococcus, Streptococcus,* and *Staphylococcus* among Gram-positive bacteria [54, 55]. The antibiotic should be chosen depending on multiple factors, such as the patient's prior exposure to hospital-acquired infections and the severity of symptoms [63]. For best practice, the antibiotics prescribed for cholangitis should have a broad range of antimicrobial activities and should be small enough to be excreted effectively into the bile, that is, third-generation cephalosporins, ureidopenicillins, carbapenems, and fluoroquinolones [56]. The most effective antibiotics for cholangitis patients have been found to be imipenem-cilastatin, meropenem, amikacin, cefepime, ceftriaxone, gentamicin, piperacillin-tazobactam, and levofloxacin [57, 58].

12.6   Antibiotics for Acute Cholangitis

The rates of polymicrobial-positive cultures in acute cholangitis vary from 30–78% [61, 62, 65]. The response rate to antibiotics has been found to be satisfactory in the majority of patients [59]. Antibiotic therapy has, in fact, dramatically lowered the mortality rate in these patients, falling from approximately 50% prior to the 1970s to less than 10% in the 1980s [70].

Choosing the appropriate antibiotic is vital, particularly during the early stages of acute infectious cholangitis. The majority of patients with acute bacterial cholangitis benefit from a large-spectrum antibiotics [60]. After antibiotic prescription, the decision is focused on the type of procedure for removing the biliary obstruction [69]. There are no stopping rules regarding the discontinuation of antibiotics, but after fever resolution and after insertion of biliary drainage, stopping antibiotic treatment does not seem to have adverse effects on the clinical course of the disease [61].

Short-duration antibiotic therapy (usually for 3 days) appears sufficient when an adequate drainage is achieved and after fever resolution [62]. Nevertheless, it is highly recommended to continue antibiotic therapy during the early phases of acute cholangitis [63]. Furthermore, as septic shock can develop, a broad-spectrum antibiotic must promptly be initiated (within 1–4 h) if signs of septic shock are present [64]. Oral or intravenous administration of antibiotics is equally efficient in eradicating bacteria in these patients [65].

Resistance to various antibiotics, including quinolone, carbapenems, vancomycin, and ampicillin, has been observed in isolates from patients with acute cholangitis patients [69]. Multidrug-resistant (MDR) bacteria were isolated from 29% of patients with biliary obstruction from Germany [68]. Risk factors for MDR in that study included male sex, previous antibiotic therapy, and biliary stenting [66].

12.7   Drainage Procedures

Biliary drainage is recommended for all, but the mildest cases of acute cholangitis that respond effectively to antibiotics and supportive care.

Drainage can be performed endoscopically, percutaneously, or surgically. In addition to improvements in the care of septic patients, advances in endoscopic biliary drainage have contributed to lowering the mortality of acute cholangitis [70].

Endoscopic transpapillary biliary drainage should be considered the first-line drainage procedure because it is less invasive and is linked to a lower risk of adverse events than other drainage techniques despite the risk of pancreatitis post-ERCP [67–72]. Endoscopic transpapillary biliary drainage generally leads to less postprocedure pain than percutaneous transhepatic biliary drainage (PTBD), also known as percutaneous transhepatic cholangial drainage (PTCD) [68]. PTCD places more burden on patients because it is linked to cosmetic problems, skin inflammation, or bile leakage, compromising their quality of life.

As only a single treatment session is required to remove a bile duct stone when an endoscopic transpapillary approach is used, duration of hospitalization is shorter. PTCD is a useful alternative drainage procedure in patients with an inaccessible papilla due to upper gastrointestinal tract obstruction or when a skilled pancreaticobiliary endoscopist is unavailable [69, 70]. PTCD can be used as a salvage therapy when conventional endoscopic transpapillary drainage has failed due to difficult selective biliary cannulation. Endoscopic ultrasound guided biliary drainage (EUS-BD) appears to be a useful alternative drainage technique when standard endoscopic transpapillary drainage has failed [71, 72].

Results from a randomized controlled trial (RCT) and a meta-analysis indicate that both technical and clinical success rates of EUS-BD and PTCD, as alternative drainage techniques after failed endoscopic transpapillary biliary drainage, were approximately the same (90–100%), but the rates of PTCD-related adverse events postprocedure, that is, bleeding, cholangitis, and bile leakage were higher [73–80]. Nevertheless, it should be remembered that almost all reports regarding EUS-BD are produced in high-volume centers, where highly skilled pancreaticobiliary endoscopists are operating. One national survey carried out in Spain in low-volume centers reported a technical success rate of only 67.2% among a patient population of 106 persons [74]. Actually, EUS-BD is considered a difficult procedure that requires the skills of an experienced specialized endoscopist. Otherwise, PTCD should be selected, or the patient should be transferred to a high-volume center.

12.7.1 Percutaneous Transhepatic Cholangiography

Percutaneous transhepatic cholangiography (PTC) is a safe and effective technique for biliary drainage. It is currently considered a second-line therapy after a failure of ERCP in a patient with a surgically altered anatomy or in case of unavailability of a dedicated endoscopist [75]. Procedural success has been reported up to 95% in the event of dilated hepatic ducts and up to 70% for nondilated ones. One study reported a 90% technical success rate after internal drainage and stone removal following successful cannulation [76]. Complications of the procedure, including sepsis, hemorrhage, peritonitis, and pancreatitis, have been reported in 1.2–2.5% of patients [77].

Before the routine use of transabdominal ultrasonography, needle puncture of the bile duct under fluoroscopy was the most frequent technique. Needle puncture is currently performed under ultrasonography to avoid the damage of blood vessels.

PTCD is performed through an ultrasonography-guided transhepatic puncture of the intrahepatic bile duct using an 18-G–22-G needle. After the backflow of bile has been confirmed, a guidewire is advanced into the bile duct. Finally, a 7-Fr–10-Fr catheter is placed in the bile duct under fluoroscopic control over the guidewire. It is safer to use a small-gauge (22-G) needle for the puncture in patients without biliary dilation. According to the Quality Improvement Guidelines developed by American radiologists, the success rate of drainage is considered as 86% in patients with biliary dilation and 63% in patients without.

12.7.2 Surgical Drainage

Biliary decompression and drainage is an open surgical intervention. Prolonged operations should be avoided in critically ill patients with bile duct stones, for whom simple procedures, such as T-tube placement without choledocholithotomy, are recommended [78]. At present, surgical drainage is extremely rare because of the widespread use of endoscopic drainage or PTCD for acute cholangitis therapy.

Open surgical drainage was once the mainstay treatment of biliary obstruction and cholangitis, but it is not usually used currently to treat severe acute cholangitis. A randomized trial by Lai and colleagues [79], comparing ERCP with surgical decompression, demonstrated a significantly higher rate of complications (66% vs. 34%) and mortality (32% vs. 10%) in the surgical drainage group. Endoscopic and percutaneous biliary drainage continue to constitute first- and second-line therapeutic choices. Recently, there has been an increased interest in early laparoscopic common duct exploration with cholecystectomy [80]. Studies have demonstrated that the approach is feasible, although current recommendations reserve this approach exclusively for patients with nonsevere acute cholangitis [81].

12.7.3 Endoscopic Retrograde Cholangiopancreatography

Endoscopic transpapillary biliary drainage has become the gold standard technique for both benign and malignant strictures because it is minimally invasive. There are two types of endoscopic transpapillary biliary drainage: endoscopic nasobiliary drainage (ENBD) for external drainage and endoscopic biliary stenting (EBS) for internal drainage. In the case of critically ill patient with acute cholangitis, the endoscopic technique should be carried out promptly and accurately to avoid serious complications. Endoscopists performing endoscopic transpapillary biliary drainage should be skilled in selective biliary cannulation techniques, including the double guidewire, pancreatic guidewire, and precut techniques [82].

Endoscopic transpapillary biliary drainage, which can be carried out via EBS or ENBD, is considered a first-line therapy for biliary decompression in acute cholangitis patients. Several studies have demonstrated that the two techniques are clinically equivalent, but patients who undergo nasobiliary drainage demonstrate more discomfort and greater electrolyte abnormalities [83, 84].

The advantages of the nasobiliary approach include the continuous monitoring of the bile output and flushing purulent bile. Endoscopic drainage utilizes 7-Fr–10-Fr plastic stent after selective biliary cannulation. This can be performed as an isolated procedure or together with other interventions for extraction of stones in cases of choledocholithiasis [85]. Endoscopic sphincterotomy and stent placement are commonly performed. Moreover, sphincterotomy may prevent the occlusion of pancreatic duct, thus preventing the post-ERCP pancreatitis, which occurs in 3–4% of cases [86], and reducing the duration of symptoms and hospital stay [87]. The major concern linked to endoscopic sphincterotomy is bleeding. The combination of severe sepsis, biliary obstruction, and hepatic dysfunction in acute cholangitis can lead to increased rates of hemorrhage following sphincterotomy [88], even in absence of associated coagulopathy [89]. In case of severe acute cholangitis, the Tokyo Guidelines recommend sphincterotomy combined with stone extraction and biliary drainage for patients with mild or moderate disease [90].

12.7.4 Endoscopic Ultrasound-Guided Biliary Drainage

In patients in whom endoscopic access to the ampulla is not possible due to altered surgical anatomy or failed cannulation, endoscopic ultrasound-guided biliary drainage (EUS-BD) can be an alternative to ERCP, an approach often used to limit the potential complications associated with PTC. EUS-BD can be performed in several ways, including transgastric or transjejunal intrahepatic biliary drainage, transduodenal or transgastric extrahepatic biliary drainage, or EUS-guided antegrade stenting approaches, and can be tailored to the patient's pathology. A meta-analysis on studies investigating the use of EUS-BD found a functional success rate higher than 90% in high-volume centers following failed ERCP [91]. The procedure is associated with an adverse event rate of 25%, being hemorrhage and bile leak, the most common complications; perforation and sepsis have also been reported. The current recommendation is to reserve EUS-BD for cases in which ERCP has failed and only in the hands of a trained, experienced therapeutic endoscopist [55, 90].

12.7.5 Drainage in the Case of Surgically Altered Anatomy

Patients with surgically altered anatomy, following, for example, a Roux-en-Y gastric bypass, present a unique challenge for the nonsurgical drainage of the biliary tree. Several approaches have been performed to circumvent the altered anatomy, including balloon enteroscopy-assisted ERCP, EUS-BD, and transgastric ERCP. Balloon enteroscopy-assisted ERCP is the first-line recommendation in the Tokyo Guidelines [90]. PTC, EUS-BD, and laparoscopic common bile duct exploration can provide additional techniques when a skilled endoscopist is unavailable or in case of failure of balloon enteroscopy-assisted ERCP.

References

1. Lipsett PA, Pitt HA. Acute cholangitis. Front Biosci. 2003;8:s1229–39.
2. Andrew DJ, Johnson SE. Acute suppurative cholangitis, a medical and surgical emergency. A review of 10- year experience emphasizing early recognition. Am J Gastroenterol. 1970;54(2):141–54.
3. Shimada H, Nakagawara G, Kobayashi M, Tsuchiya S, Kudo T, Morita S. Pathogenesis and clinical features of acute cholangitis accompanied by shock. Jpn J Surg. 1984;14(4):269–77.
4. Boey JH, Way LW. Acute cholangitis. Ann Surg. 1980;191:264–70.
5. Yokoe M, Hata J, Takada T, Strasberg SM, Asbun HJ, Wakabayashi G, et al. Tokyo guidelines 2018: diagnostic criteria and severity grading of acute cholecystitis (with viedos). J Hepatobiliary Pancreat Sci. 2018;25:41–54.
6. Thompson JE Jr, Pitt HA, Doty JE, Coleman J, Irving C. Broad-spectrum penicillin as an adequate therapy for acute cholangitis. Surg Gynecol Obstet. 1990;171(4):275–82.
7. Tai DI, Shen FH, Liaw YF. Abnormal pre-drainage serum creatinine as a prognostic indicator in acute cholangitis. Hepato-Gastroenterology. 1992;39(1):47–50.
8. Hanau LH, Steigbigel NH. Cholangitis: pathogenesis, diagnosis, and treatment. Curr Clin Top Infect Dis. 1995;15:153–78.
9. Hanau LH, Steigbigel NH. Acute (ascending) cholangitis. Infect Dis Clin N Am. 2000;14(3):521–46.
10. Charcot M. De la fievre hepatique symptomatique. Comparison *avec la fievre uroseptique. Lecons sur les maladies du foie des voies biliares et des reins.* [Of symptomatic hepatic fever. Comparison with uroseptic fever. Lessons on diseases of the liver, biliary tract and kidneys]. Paris: Bourneville et Sevestre; 1877. p. 176–85.
11. Tokyo Guidelines for the management of acute cholangitis and cholecystitis. Proceedings of a consensus meeting, April 2006, Tokyo, Japan. J Hepatobiliary Pancreat Surg. 2007;14(1):1–121.
12. Kiriyama S, Takada T, Strasberg SM, et al. New diagnostic criteria and severity assessment of acute cholangitis in revised Tokyo guidelines. J Hepatobiliary Pancreat Sci. 2012;19(5):548–56.
13. Reynolds BM, Dargan EL. Acute obstructive cholangitis; a distinct clinical syndrome. Ann Surg. 1959;150(2):299–303.
14. Csendes A, Sepúlveda A, Burdiles P, et al. Common bile duct pressure in patients with common bile duct stones with or without acute suppurative cholangitis. Arch Surg. 1988;123(6):697–9.
15. Raper SE, Barker ME, Jones AL, et al. Anatomic correlates of bacterial cholangiovenous reflux. Surgery. 1989;105(3):352–9.
16. Csendes A, Fernandez M, Uribe P. Bacteriology of the gallbladder bile in normal subjects. Am J Surg. 1975;129(6):629–31.
17. Carpenter HA. Bacterial and parasitic cholangitis. Mayo Clin Proc. 1998;73(5):473–8.
18. Sung JY, Costerton JW, Shaffer EA. Defense system in the biliary tract against bacterial infection. Dig Dis Sci. 1992;37(5):689–96.
19. Jiang WG, Puntis MC. Immune dysfunction in patients with obstructive jaundice, mediators and implications for treatments. HPB Surg. 1997;10(3):129–42.
20. Kalser MH, Cohen R, Arteaga I, et al. Normal viral and bacterial flora of the human small and large intestine. N Engl J Med. 1966;274(10):558–63.
21. Plaut AG, Gorbach SL, Nahas L, et al. Studies of intestinal microflora. 3. The microbial flora of human small intestinal mucosa and fluids. Gastroenterology. 1967;53(6):868–73.

22. Ding JW, Andersson R, Soltesz V, et al. Obstructive jaundice impairs reticuloendothelial function and promotes bacterial translocation in the rat. J Surg Res. 1994;57(2):238–45.
23. Clements WD, Parks R, Erwin P, et al. Role of the gut in the pathophysiology of extrahepatic biliary obstruction. Gut. 1996;39(4):587–93.
24. Shands JW, Chun PW. The dispersion of Gram-negative lipopolysaccharide by deoxycholate. J Biol Chem. 1980;225:1221–6.
25. Attasaranya S, Fogel EL, Lehman GA. Choledocholithiasis, ascending cholangitis and gallstone pancreatitis. Med Clin North Am. 2008;92:925–60.
26. Kinney TP. Management of ascending cholangitis. Gastrointest Endosc Clin N Am. 2007;17(2):289–306, vi.
27. Tazuma S. Gallstone disease: epidemiology, pathogenesis, and classification of biliary stones (common bile duct and intrahepatic). Best Pract Res Clin Gastroenterol. 2006;20(6):1075–83.
28. Kaufman HS, Magnuson TH, Lillemoe KD, et al. The role of bacteria in gallbladder and common duct stone formation. Ann Surg. 1989;209(5):584–91, [discussion: 591–2].
29. Cetta FM. Bile infection documented as initial event in the pathogenesis of brown pigment biliary stones. Hepatology. 1986;6(3):482–9.
30. Imam MH, Talwalkar JA, Lindor KD. Secondary sclerosing cholangitis: pathogenesis, diagnosis and management. Clin Liver Dis. 2013;17(2):269–77.
31. Csendes A, Mitru N, Maluenda F, et al. Counts of bacteria and pyocites of choledochal bile in controls and in patients with gallstones or common bile duct stones with or without acute cholangitis. Hepato-Gastroenterology. 1996;43(10):800–6.
32. Rana SS, Bhasin DK, Nanda M, et al. Parasitic infestations of the biliary tract. Curr Gastroenterol Rep. 2007;9(2):156–64.
33. Gupta E, Chakravarti A. Viral infections of the biliary tract. Saudi J Gastroenterol. 2008;14(3):158–60.
34. Yusuf TE, Baron TH. AIDS cholangiopathy. Curr Treat Options Gastroenterol. 2004;7(2):111–7.
35. Wig JD, Singh K, Chawla YK, et al. Cholangitis due to candidiasis of the extrahepatic biliary tract. HPB Surg. 1998;11(1):51–4.
36. Chen LY, Goldberg HI. Sclerosing cholangitis: broad spectrum of radiographic features. Gastrointest Radiol. 1984;9:39–47.
37. Kiriyama S, et al. TG13 guidelines for diagnosis and severity grading of acute cholangitis (with videos). J Hepatobiliary Pancreat Sci. 2013;20:24–34.
38. Wada K, et al. Diagnostic criteria and severity assessment of acute cholangitis: Tokyo guidelines. J Hepato-Biliary-Pancreat Surg. 2007;14:52–8.
39. Kimura Y, et al. Definitions, pathophysiology, and epidemiology of acute cholangitis and cholecystitis: Tokyo guidelines. J Hepato-Biliary-Pancreat Surg. 2007;14(1):15–26.
40. Watanapa P. Recovery patterns of liver function after complete and artial surgical biliary decompression. Am J Surg. 1996;171(2):230–4.
41. Korkmaz M, Ünal H, Selcuk H, et al. Extraordinarily elevated serum levels of CA 19-9 and rapid decrease after successful therapy: a case report and review of literature. Turk J Gastroenterol. 2010;21(4):461–3.
42. Sulzer JK, Ocuin LM. Cholangitis causes, diagnosis, and management. Surg Clin N Am. 2019;99(2):175–84.
43. Umefune G, Kogure H, et al. Procalcitonin is a useful biomarker to predict severe acute cholangitis: a single-center prospective study. J Gastroenterol. 2017;52(6):734–45.
44. Lee YS, Cho KB, et al. Procalcitonin as a decision-supporting marker of urgent biliary decompression in acute cholangitis. Dig Dis Sci. 2018;63(9):2474–9.
45. Solomkin JS, Mazuski JE, et al. Diagnosis and management of complicated intraabdominal infection in adults and children: guidelines by the Surgical Infection Society and the Infectious Diseases Society of America. Clin Infect Dis. 2010;50(2):133–64.
46. Gomi H, Solomkin JS, Schlossberg D, et al. Tokyo guidelines 2018: antimicrobial therapy for acute cholangitis and cholecystitis. J Hepatobiliary Pancreat Sci. 2018;25(1):3–16.

47. Ramchandani M, et al. Endoscopic management of acute cholangitis as a result of common bile duct stones. Dig Endosc. 2017;29(Suppl 2):78–87.
48. Kiriyama S, et al. Tokyo guidelines 2018: diagnostic criteria and severity grading of acute cholangitis (with videos). J Hepatobiliary Pancreat Sci. 2018;25(1):17–30.
49. Soto JA, et al. Detection of choledocholithiasis with MR cholangiography: comparison of three-dimensional fast spin echo and single- and multisection half-fourier rapid acquisition with relaxation enhancement sequences. Radiology. 2000;215:737–45.
50. Arrivé L, et al. MRI of cholangitis: traps and tips. Diagn Interv Imaging. 2013;94:757–70.
51. Sun Z, et al. Controversy and progress for treatment of acute cholangitis after Tokyo guidelines (TG13). Biosci Trends. 2016;10:22–6. https://doi.org/10.5582/bst.2016.01033.
52. Meeralam Y, et al. Diagnostic accuracy of EUS compared with MRCP in detecting choledocholithiasis: a meta-analysis of diagnostic test accuracy in head-to-head studies. Gastrointest Endosc. 2017;86(6):986–93.
53. Chen YI, Martel M, Barkun AN. Choledocholithiasis: should EUS replace MRCP in patients at intermediate risk? Gastrointest Endosc. 2017;86(6):994–6.
54. Gomi H, Solomkin JS, Takada T, Strasberg SM, Pitt HA, Yoshida M, et al. TG13 antimicrobial therapy for acute cholangitis and cholecystitis. J Hepatobiliary Pancreat Sci. 2013;20:60–70. https://doi.org/10.1007/s00534-012-0572-0.
55. Weber A, Huber W, Kamereck K, Winkle P, Voland P, Weidenbach H, et al. In vitro activity of moxifloxacin and piperacillin/sulbactam against pathogens of acute cholangitis. World J Gastroenterol. 2008;14:3174–8. https://doi.org/10.3748/wjg.14.3174.
56. Shenoy SM, Shenoy S, Gopal S, Tantry BV, Baliga S, Jain A. Clinicomicrobiological analysis of patients with cholangitis. Indian J Med Microbiol. 2014;32:157–60. https://doi.org/10.4103/0255-0857.129802.
57. Salvador VB, Lozada MC, Consunji RJ. Microbiology and antibiotic susceptibility of organisms in bile cultures from patients with and without cholangitis at an Asian academic medical center. Surg Infect. 2011;12:105–11.
58. Kiesslich R, Will D, Hahn M, Nafe B, Genitsariotis R, Mäurer M, et al. Ceftriaxone versus levofloxacin for antibiotic therapy in patients with acute cholangitis. Z Gastroenterol. 2003;41:5–10.
59. Lee JG. Diagnosis and management of acute cholangitis. Nat Rev Gastroenterol Hepatol. 2009;6:533–41.
60. Zimmer V, Lammert F. Acute bacterial cholangitis. Viszeralmedizin. 2015;31:166–72.
61. Kogure H, Tsujino T, Yamamoto K, Mizuno S, Yashima Y, Yagioka H, et al. Fever-based antibiotic therapy for acute cholangitis following successful endoscopic biliary drainage. J Gastroenterol. 2011;46:1411–7.
62. van Lent AU, Bartelsman JF, Tytgat GN, Speelman P, Prins JM. Duration of antibiotic therapy for cholangitis after successful endoscopic drainage of the biliary tract. Gastrointest Endosc. 2002;55:518–22.
63. Sun Z, Zhu Y, Zhu B, Xu G, Zhang N. Controversy and progress for treatment of acute cholangitis after Tokyo guidelines (TG13). Biosci Trends. 2016;10:22–6.
64. Dellinger RP, Levy MM, Rhodes A, Annane D, Gerlach H, Opal SM, et al. Surviving sepsis campaign: international guidelines for management of severe sepsis and septic shock, 2012. Intensive Care Med. 2013;39:165–228.
65. Park TY, Choi JS, Song TJ, Do JH, Choi SH, Oh HC. Early oral antibiotic switch compared with conventional intravenous antibiotic therapy for acute cholangitis with bacteremia. Dig Dis Sci. 2014;59:2790–6.
66. Schneider J, De Waha P, Hapfelmeier A, Feihl S, Römmler F, Schlag C, et al. Risk factors for increased antimicrobial resistance: a retrospective analysis of 309 acute cholangitis episodes. J Antimicrob Chemother. 2014;69:519–25.
67. Lai EC, Mok FP, Tan ES, Lo CM, Fan ST, You KT, et al. Endoscopic biliary drainage for severe acute cholangitis. N Engl J Med. 1992;24:1582–6.

68. Umeda J, Itoi T. Current status of preoperative biliary drainage. J Gastroenterol. 2015;50:940–54.
69. Takada T, Hanyu F, Kobayashi S, Uchida Y. Percutaneous transhepatic cholangial drainage: direct approach under fluoroscopic control. J Surg Oncol. 1976;8:83–97.
70. Saad WE, Wallace MJ, Wojak JC, Kundu S, Cardella JF. Quality improvement guidelines for percutaneous transhepatic cholangiography, biliary drainage, and percutaneous cholecystostomy. J Vasc Interv Radiol. 2010;21:789–95.
71. Giovannini M, Moutardier V, Pesenti C, Bories E, Lelong B, Delpero JR. Endoscopic ultrasound-guided bilioduodenal anastomosis: a new technique for biliary drainage. Endoscopy. 2001;33:898–900.
72. Itoi T, Itokawa F, Sofuni A, Kurihara T, Tsuchiya T, Ishii K, et al. Endoscopic ultrasound-guided choledochoduodenostomy in patients with failed endoscopic retrograde cholangiopancreatography. World J Gastroenterol. 2008;14:6078–82.
73. Sharaiha RZ, Khan MA, Kamal F, Tyberg A, Tombazzi CR, Ali B, et al. Efficacy and safety of EUS-guided biliary drainage in comparison with percutaneous biliary drainage when ERCP fails: a systematic review and meta-analysis. Gastrointest Endosc. 2017;85:904–14.
74. Vila JJ, Perez-Miranda M, Vazquez-Sequeiros E, Abadia MA, Perez-Millan A, Gonzalez-Huix F, et al. Initial experience with EUS-guided cholangiopancreatography for biliary and pancreatic duct drainage: a Spanish national survey. Gastrointest Endosc. 2012;76:1133–41.
75. Itoi T, Tsuyuguchi T, Takada T, et al. TG13 indications and techniques for biliary drainage in acute cholangitis (with videos). J Hepatobiliary Pancreat Sci. 2013;20(1):71–80.
76. Saad WE, Wallace MJ, Wojak JC, et al. Quality improvement guidelines for percutaneous transhepatic cholangiography, biliary drainage, and percutaneous cholecystostomy. J Vasc Interv Radiol. 2010;21(6):789–95.
77. Burke DR, Lewis CA, Cardella JF, et al. Quality improvement guidelines for percutaneous transhepatic cholangiography and biliary drainage. J Vasc Interv Radiol. 2003;14(9 Pt 2):S243–6.
78. Saltzstein EC, Peacock JB, Mercer LC. Early operation for acute biliary tract stone disease. Surgery. 1983;94:704–8.
79. Lai EC, Mok FP, Tan ES, et al. Endoscopic biliary drainage for severe acute cholangitis. N Engl J Med. 1992;326(24):1582–6.
80. Sun Z, Zhu Y, Zhu B, et al. Controversy and progress for treatment of acute cholangitis after Tokyo guidelines (TG13). Biosci Trends. 2016;10(1):22–6.
81. Atstupens K, Plaudis H, Fokins V, et al. Safe laparoscopic clearance of the common bile duct in emergently admitted patients with choledocholithiasis and cholangitis. Korean J Hepatobiliary Pancreat Surg. 2016;20(2):53–60.
82. Mukai S, Itoi T. Selective biliary cannulation techniques for endoscopic retrograde cholangiopancreatography procedures and prevention of post-endoscopic retrograde cholangiopancreatography pancreatitis. Expert Rev Gastroenterol Hepatol. 2016;10:709–22.
83. Lee DW, Chan AC, Lam YH, et al. Biliary decompression by nasobiliary catheter or biliary stent in acute suppurative cholangitis: a prospective randomized trial. Gastrointest Endosc. 2002;56(3):361–5.
84. Park SY, Park CH, Cho SB, et al. The safety and effectiveness of endoscopic biliary decompression by plastic stent placement in acute suppurative cholangitis compared with nasobiliary drainage. Gastrointest Endosc. 2008;68(6):1076–80.
85. Mukai S, Itoi T, Baron TH, et al. Indications and techniques of biliary drainage for acute cholangitis in updated Tokyo guidelines 2018. J Hepatobiliary Pancreat Sci. 2017;24(10):537–49.
86. Tarnasky PR, Cunningham JT, Hawes RH, et al. Transpapillary stenting of proximal biliary strictures: does biliary sphincterotomy reduce the risk of postprocedure pancreatitis? Gastrointest Endosc. 1997;45(1):46–51.
87. Hui CK, Lai KC, Wong WM, et al. A randomised controlled trial of endoscopic sphincterotomy in acute cholangitis without common bile duct stones. Gut. 2002;51(2):245–7.

88. Lee MH, Tsou YK, Lin CH, et al. Predictors of re-bleeding after endoscopic hemostasis for delayed post-endoscopic sphincterotomy bleeding. World J Gastroenterol. 2016;22(11):3196–201.
89. Freeman ML. Complications of endoscopic retrograde cholangiopancreatography: avoidance and management. Gastrointest Endosc Clin N Am. 2012;22(3):567–86.
90. Mukai S, Itoi T, Baron TH, et al. Indications and techniques of biliary drainage for acute cholangitis in updated Tokyo guidelines 2018. Hepatobiliary Pancreatic Sci. 2017;24(10):537–49.
91. Wang K, Zhu J, Xing L, et al. Assessment of efficacy and safety of EUS-guided biliary drainage: a systematic review. Gastrointest Endosc. 2016;83(6):1218–27.

Drug-Induced Cholangiopathies

13

Sara De Martin, Emanuela Bonaiuto, and Daniela Gabbia

13.1 Introduction

The liver plays a central role in the selective uptake, metabolism, and excretion of the majority of xenobiotics, including drugs and environmental toxins. For this reason, the liver is one of the main targets of drug toxicity, an issue representing a primary cause of failure during drug development [1]. Moreover, a wide variety of drugs and herbal remedies used in clinical practice are known to induce a broad array of liver disorders. Two of the most severe manifestations of drug-induced liver injury (DILI) are cholestatic and mixed cholestatic/hepatocellular injury, representing about 50% of cases of all hepatic drug toxicities [2, 3].

Cholestasis is a common result of DILI and is present in the 2–5% of patients hospitalized for jaundice and in up to 20% of geriatric ones [4]. Drug-induced cholestasis can occur in the form of acute liver failure or as a chronic liver disease, resembling other intrahepatic and extrahepatic cholestatic diseases [1]. Although in acute DILI an injury to bile ducts can be frequently diagnosed by liver biopsy, the loss of bile ducts occurs rarely also when cholestasis and inflammation are severe [5]. Generally, both liver biochemical parameters and jaundice improve gradually after drug discontinuation, reaching normal levels in the ensuing months. At variance, a persistence of small bile duct loss could be observed in association with inflammatory response and prolonged cholestasis [6–8]. In this case, drug-induced liver damage reflects an injury primarily to mature cholangiocytes, biliary epithelium or their progenitor cells. In some cases, a progressive and extensive loss of the

S. De Martin (✉) · D. Gabbia
Department of Pharmaceutical and Pharmacological Sciences, University of Padova, Padova, Italy
e-mail: sara.demartin@unipd.it

E. Bonaiuto
Department of Surgery, Oncology and Gastroenterology, University of Padova, Padova, Italy

© Springer Nature Switzerland AG 2021
A. Floreani (ed.), *Diseases of the Liver and Biliary Tree*,
https://doi.org/10.1007/978-3-030-65908-0_13

interlobular bile ducts may lead to the "vanishing bile duct syndrome" (VBDS), that may progress to secondary biliary cirrhosis, liver failure, and even death [8]. VBDS is a rare condition that occurs only in 0.5% of cases of small duct biliary disease [9].

Drug-induced bile duct injury could display a wide range of pathological features, ranging from asymptomatic patients that exhibit only isolated elevations in alkaline phosphatase (ALP) or γ-glutamyl transferase (γGT) and mild bile duct disorder or "ductopenia," to progressive forms of VBDS [10]. In the majority of patients, drug-induced bile duct injury affects the biliary epithelium of interlobular ducts, a condition that can mimic other cholangiopathies, such as primary biliary cholangitis or small duct primary sclerosing cholangitis [1, 11].

A number of drugs, e.g., 5-fluorouracil and fluorodeoxyuridines, cause a selective and dose-dependent damage to larger ducts. Since the liver histology of these patients displays features similar to those observed in primary sclerosing cholangitis (PSC), this drug-induced damage has been named "drug-induced sclerosing cholangitis" or "primary sclerosing cholangitis-like" [8, 11]. This disease, characterized by segmental inflammation and fibrosis, affects mainly one or more structures of the large bile ducts, e.g., the right and left hepatic ducts and the common hepatic duct, generally sparing the smaller intrahepatic ducts and the common bile duct [8, 11, 12]. In some cases, primary sclerosing cholangitis-like displays intrahepatic features affecting small ducts.

In Table 13.1, a brief classification of drug-induced chronic cholangiopathies is reported for the sake of clarity.

13.2   Drugs Inducing Chronic Cholangiopathies

Many chemicals could induce chronic damage of the biliary epithelium resulting in drug-induced cholangiopathies of various degrees. The temporal relationship between the first drug ingestion and the onset of the symptoms is one of the key factors to be considered to provide a diagnosis [1]. Indeed, this latency period may be short (ranging from hours to few days), intermediate (1–8 weeks), or very long (1–12 months) depending on the agent causing the duct injury. In this regard, all the drugs and dietary supplements used by the patient within the last 3–6 months should be taken into account for the diagnosis of drug-induced chronic cholangiopathy. Noteworthy, cholestatic injury tends to persist even after the discontinuation of the inducing agent, probably due to the slower rate of reparation and regeneration of the secretory function of cholangiocytes with respect to hepatocytes [1].

Since a patient often takes multiple medications, the specific agent causing liver injury is not always clearly definable, also considering that it's often difficult to associate a drug with one specific clinical manifestation of DILI. The DILIN prospective study, enrolling 1433 subjects with suspected drug-induced liver injury over a 10-year period (2004–2014), pointed out that the mean number of medications taken by the patients with bile duct loss within 2 months of onset of liver injury was 9.6, the median was 7.5, and the range was 1–35 [5]. Multiple pathways have been proposed as important players in drug-induced cholangiopathies, even if the

Table 13.1 Drug-induced chronic cholangiopathies

	Duct injury localization	Pathological features	Clinical features	Biochemical features
Mild bile duct injury	Intrahepatic small ducts	Mild bile duct epithelial disorder	Asymptomatic	Mild elevation in ALP or γGT
		Inflammatory response direct to cholangiocytes		
		Presence of inflammatory cells around the biliary epithelia in portal triad		
Vanishing bile duct Syndrome (VBDS)	Intrahepatic small ducts	Less than 50% of bile ducts are seen in portal area on liver biopsy	Hepatosplenomegaly, hyperlipidemia, malabsorption, xanthelasmas, xanthomas, leads to cirrhosis	ALP >3 time increased, AST/ALT 2–10 time increased, γGT increase, Hyperbilirubinemia, Hypercholesterolemia Antimitochondrial antibody absence
		Marked ductal destruction		
		Complete disappearance with portal tract inflammation, Fibrosis, Hepatocellular necrosis		
Drug-induced sclerosing cholangitis	Intrahepatic small ducts and extrahepatic large ducts	Similar pathological features of PSC with marked ductal destruction,	Jaundice develops within 3–6 months of the drug administration	ALP >3 time increased, AST/ALT 2–10 time increased, Hyperbilirubinemia, Hypercholesterolemia
		Hepatocellular necrosis		

pathogenetic mechanisms have not been completely elucidated [13]. Among them, apoptosis induced by tumor necrosis factor-α (TNF-α), inhibition of mitochondrial function, and neoantigen formation [14] can be listed. In some patients, an immune response, mainly mediated by T cells, may play a role in the development of drug-induced cholangiopathies [11], resulting in antigen recognition on biliary epithelial cells, immune cell infiltration into the bile duct area, apoptosis, and T cell-mediated cytotoxicity [11, 15].

Drug toxicity generally results in drug-induced cholestasis, whereas severe ductopenia and VBDS are less frequent [16]. However, drug-induced VBDS has been attributed to more than 40 drugs, among which chlorpromazine, amoxicillin, carba-mazepine, clindamycin, meropenem, ajmaline, phenytoin, trimethoprim–sulfa-methoxazole, arsenic derivatives, and tetracyclines are the most frequently used [13–15, 17]. A prospective study from the DILI network suggests that 7% of the observed patients (26 of 363 total DILI cases) experienced drug-induced VBDS following the use of amoxicillin/clavulanate, temozolomide, herbal products, and azithromycin [15].

Some reports regarding drug-induced VBDS display poor evidence of causal effect between drug and symptoms, and frequently the drug is only suspected to induce liver injury [9]. A categorization of drugs reporting a well-documented hepatotoxic effect has been published by Björnsson and Hoofnagle [18], even though they didn't report a specific analysis dedicated to VBDS patients.

Regarding the drug-induced sclerosing cholangitis, it has been reported that the hepatic artery infusion chemotherapy of fluoropyrimidines (e.g., 5-fluorouracil, fluorodeoxyuridine) can mimic the pathological features of PSC [12]. Patients with liver-predominant metastatic colon cancer treated with these agents have an incidence of drug-induced sclerosing cholangitis up to 1 out of 5 [19–22]. Even the arterial embolization for the treatment of hepatocarcinoma could lead to an extensive destruction of the biliary tract with sclerosis and stenosis [12]. Furthermore, a case report described a case of a 44-year-old woman with a liver cavernous hemangioma who underwent transcatheter arterial chemoembolization (TACE) with bleomycin-iodinated oil and developed sclerosing cholangitis 6 years after treatment [23].

A retrospective study conducted on 102 patients diagnosed with DILI during 2010–2012 identified ten patients (all females) with the probable diagnosis of sclerosing cholangitis due to the administration of amoxicillin-clavulanate, sevoflurane, amiodarone, infliximab, green tea extract, venlafaxine, and atorvastatin [24].

Drug-induced sclerosing cholangitis is a quite frequent complication of scolicidal solution for the treatment of hydatid disease, a parasitic infestation due to a tapeworm of the genus Echinococcus characterized by liver and biliary cysts [11]. Hypertonic saline 20%, silver nitrate 0.5%, povidone iodine 1%, and 5% formalin are injected directly in the hydatid cysts to treat tapeworm infestation. A prolonged therapy, a particular sensitivity to these scolicidal agents or a communication between the cyst and the biliary tree, could result in caustic drug-induced sclerosing cholangitis [25].

Another drug that has been postulated to cause drug-induced sclerosing cholangitis is ketamine. Indeed, ketamine addicted subjects could suffer from epigastric pain and increased ALP or γGT related to the dilatation of the common bile duct [26–29].

A report published in 2013 reported the case of a 34-year-old woman who was given celecoxib for treating acute epigastric abdominal pain. After a 3-week treatment, biochemical markers of liver function were abnormal, with a total bilirubin of 3.4 units/L, and liver biopsy pointed out sclerosing cholangitis. Since these parameters normalized 1 month after cessation of the drug, cholangitis was imputed to celecoxib administration [30].

A list of the drugs reported to induce cholestasis with duct injury, VBDS, and primary sclerosing cholangitis-like is reported in Table 13.2.

Table 13.2 Drugs reported to cause chronic cholestasis and ductopenia

Drug	Reference
Cholestasis with mild bile duct injury	
Androgenic anabolic steroids	[31]
Carmustine	[32]
Dextropropoxyphene	[33]
Gold therapy	[34]
Methylenedianiline	[35]
Paraquat	[36]
Pioglitazone	[37, 38]
Tenoxicam	[39]
Vanishing bile duct syndrome (Ductopenia)	
Aceprometazine	[1]
Ajmaline	[10, 40]
Amineptine	[41]
Amiodarone	[42, 43]
Amitriptyline	[41]
Amoxicillin/clavulanic acid	[44–49]
Ampicillin	[50, 51]
Azathioprine	[52, 53]
Barbiturates	[54]
Benoxaprofen	[55, 56]
Carbamazepine	[57–60]
Carbutamide	[10]
Chlorothiazide	[61]
Chlorpromazine	[62–64]
Chlorpropamide	[65]
Cimetidine	[66]
Ciprofloxacin	[64, 67]
Clindamycin	[68]
Cyamemazine	[12]
Cyproheptadine	[69, 70]
D-penicillamine	[71]
Diclofenac	[72]
Erythromycin	[73]
Estradiol	[74, 75]
Fenofibrate	[76]
Flucloxacillin	[16, 77, 78]
Glycyrrhizin	[79, 80]
Haloperidol	[10, 81]
Ibuprofen	[82–85]
Imipramine	[81, 86]
Macrolides antibiotics	[87]
Meropenem	[88]
Phenytoin	[89]
Prochlorperazine	[90, 91]

(continued)

Table 13.2 (continued)

Drug	Reference
Quinolones (others)	[17, 92–94]
Terbinafine	[95–97]
Tetracyclines	[98, 99]
Thiabendazole	[100]
Tiopronin	[79]
Trifluoperazine	[101]
Tolbutamide	[102]
Trimethoprim-sulfamethoxazole	[103, 104]
Troleandomycin	[10]
Zonisamide	[105]
Drug-induced sclerosing cholangitis	
Docetaxel	[106]
Formaldehyde	[25]
Floxuridine	[19–22, 107, 108]
Hypertonic saline	[25]
Ketamine	[26–29]
Methimazole	[109]
Pembrolizumab	[110]
Povidone iodine solution	[25]
Silver nitrate	[25]
Various herbal supplements	[24]

13.3 Drug-Induced Bile Duct Injury and Vanishing Bile Duct Syndrome (VBDS)

13.3.1 Pathophysiology

The progressive and extensive destruction and disappearance of intrahepatic bile ducts induced by drug administration may lead to the "vanishing bile duct syndrome" (VBDS) [13]. The pathogenesis of this rare syndrome is poorly understood and could also be associated with many conditions other than drug toxicity, including ischemia, infection, autoimmune disease, transplant rejection, and cancer [111]. In this context, it is not always simple to promptly identify the causative relation between VBDS and one specific agent, although this syndrome is mainly associated with some drugs, such as amoxicillin-clavulanic acid [45, 46, 48, 77], flucloxacillin [77, 112], chlorpromazine [62], carbamazepine [57, 58], and meropenem [88].

The pathophysiological mechanisms involved in bile duct loss and VBDS remain not completely understood, but some general features have been identified. Bile duct loss was related to the perpetuation of liver damage (94%) and leads to a high liver-related morbidity and mortality (26%). Drug-induced VBDS could be considered as a T cell-mediated hypersensitivity reaction of the liver to the administration of certain drugs [11]. Bonkovsky and collaborators observed that patients with bile duct loss generally developed an immune-mediated moderate-to-severe acute cholestatic liver damage [5]. In some cases, VBDS is associated with severe cutaneous reactions (e.g., toxic epidermal necrolysis, Stevens–Johnson or DRESS syndrome), that are triggered by the expression of immunogenic proteins and drug metabolites- or drug-protein adducts on the cell surface of keratinocytes. The effect observed on keratinocytes led to the hypothesis that VBDS could be induced by a similar idiosyncratic hypersensitivity reaction that triggers cholangiocytes. Further supporting this hypothesis, it has been observed that the major causes of idiosyncratic cholestatic hepatitis frequently induce the VBDS, whereas those inducing acute hepatocellular injury and liver failure rarely lead to its development [5]. Moreover, patients repeatedly exposed to a drug could experience a shortening of the latency period, and also eosinophilia and lymphocyte sensitization have been observed [8].

Even though low-molecular weight compounds (<1 kDa), such as small drugs or metal ions, were thought to be unable to induce an immune response on their own, experimental and clinical evidences demonstrate that they are able to trigger the immune system to activate T cells. Two main theories have been formulated to explain T cell stimulation due to drug exposure: the *hapten model* and the *p-i concept* [11, 113]. According to the first model, chemically reactive low-molecular weight compounds, named *haptens*, bind covalently to endogenous proteins or peptides to form hapten-carrier complexes that are processed and presented to reactive T cells inducing the immune response. The p-i concept postulates that even if a drug is chemically inert and couldn't bind covalently to proteins, it could bind to human leukocyte antigen (HLA) class I molecules, priming the T cell receptor (TCR) interaction and activating T cell-mediated immune cascade [113]. HLA molecules are highly variable proteins ubiquitously expressed in all cells, whose primary function is the regulation of T cell-mediated immunity. HLA class I molecules present intracellular antigens to CD8+ T-cytotoxic cells. Antigen presenting cells (APCs) take up, process and present extracellular proteins on HLA class II molecules to stimulate the proliferation of CD4+ T-helper cells [11]. Antigen presentation operated by APC, leading to T cell activation, is further sustained by co-stimulatory molecules, such as proteins expressed by damaged cells and infectious organisms, and pro-inflammatory cytokines. Although cholangiocytes have long been considered a passive structure with the mere task of leading the bile to the intestine, many studies demonstrated their immunomodulatory role in hepatobiliary diseases. These cells constitutively express HLA class I molecules, while it has been noticed that the expression of HLA class II molecules is induced by cholestatic disease and after liver transplant rejection.

Combining together the hapten model and the p-i concept, it could be postulated that the type of drug-induced immune reaction depends on the type of immunogenicity: covalent binding of haptens is due to their chemical properties, whereas non-covalent HLA interactions depend on their structure. Moreover, the same drug can induce liver damage by both mechanisms [114–116]. In addition to the chemical and structural features of the drug, other two factors could affect drug hypersensitivity, i.e., individual's genotype and epigenetic aspects, such as environmental conditions [117]. In some patients, these three factors, named "the triangle of susceptibility to drug hypersensitivity," combine together to determine a metabolic-immunologic idiosyncrasy towards certain drugs, leading to altered toxic metabolite production or aberrant T cell-mediated reaction. The involvement of genetic HLA variability in bile duct toxicity of various drugs is well documented by many studies. For example, patients carrying the HLA-DRB1*1501-DRB5*0101-DQB*O602 haplotype are more prone to exhibit a cholestatic or mixed-type liver damage than hepatocellular hepatitis [12, 47, 49, 118].

In addition to idiosyncratic mechanisms, other pathways are probably involved in the development of drug-induced bile duct injury and VBDS. Inflammatory cells of portal tract secrete cytokines that contribute to the destruction of small bile ducts by increasing HLA expression, worsening the peribiliary vascularization, negatively affecting bile duct proliferation, and injuring the basement membrane extracellular matrix [12]. Another mechanism that has been proposed to play a role in the development of bile duct damage is the biliary excretion of toxic metabolites that cause bile duct epithelium damage [1].

Furthermore, cholestasis can be induced by increased concentrations of toxic drug and/or metabolites due to genetic alterations of metabolizing enzymes or transporters, or a hepatic decrease of the antioxidant defense, such as reduced glutathione concentration [119]. Numerous drugs, known to induced cholestasis, are indeed substrates for ATP-dependent canalicular transporters responsible for drug excretion into the bile, among which there are the bile salt export pump (BSEP), the Breast Cancer Resistance Protein (BCRP), the multidrug resistance-1 protein (MDR1), the multidrug resistance-associated protein-2 (c), and the multidrug resistance protein 3 (MDR3) ([1] and refs. therein). Even pro-inflammatory cytokines (e.g., TNF-α and IL-6) have been demonstrated to alter the hepatic expression of cytochrome P450 enzymes and biliary transporters [120, 121], further sustaining drug-induced bile duct injury [62, 63] and resulting in a critical "second hit" [122]. This phenomenon was theorized by Pirmohamed and collaborators with the *danger hypothesis*, in addition to the hapten hypothesis, to explain development of idiosyncratic drug toxic reactions. This theory stated that a drug-protein complex requires the presence of co-stimulatory signals, e.g., pro-inflammatory cytokines, to propagate the immune response [122].

13.3.2 Diagnosis

Various drugs or toxins have been involved in the development of a peculiar form of liver damage mainly affecting bile ducts, often associated with prolonged cholestasis and sometimes complicated by biliary cirrhosis [123]. The clinical features of toxin or drug-induced small bile duct injury generally include an acute phase of hepatocholangiolitis of highly variable severity, followed in a minority of cases by cholestasis, also characterized by variable severity and duration.

Symptoms at presentation are usually those of an acute, often mild hepatitis, or are similar to those of acute suppurative cholangitis (fever, shivering and upper abdominal pain, preceding the occurrence of jaundice). Furthermore, fatigue and upper abdominal symptoms may be prominent, together with the presence of dark urine and pale stools [12]. Symptoms may either be relatively mild and resolve after a short period, or be associated with profound anorexia, fatigue, and pruritus and last for a prolonged period of time.

Liver biochemistry usually shows a mild increase in aminotransferase values, alkaline phosphatase, and γ-glutamyl transpeptidase. Hypereosinophilia may be present and sometimes renal failure can occur, due to interstitial nephritis [44].

The results of a single study, analyzing sequential liver biopsies obtained from a small group of patients with drug-induced bile duct injury, indicate that features of acute cholangitis are almost invariably present in the early stages, while ductular and periductular degenerative changes characterize the late stages. According to the same study, ductopenia is present in most patients, probably as a consequence of initial cholangitis, but it is not predictive of clinical and biochemical progression [10].

The clinical presentation of drug-induced VBDS can be variable, since some cases present acute jaundice, persistent pruritus, and fatigue shortly after drug exposure, while others have a late onset [17].

The typical features for diagnosing drug-induced VBDS are the persistent elevation of ALP and bilirubin for more than 6 months, with normal or close to normal serum aminotransferase levels, and the lack of evidence of biliary disorders, such as PBC, PSC, or malignancy.

The standard diagnostic histopathological observation for VBDS is the loss of 50% or more of the intrahepatic bile ducts on a slice containing at least ten portal tracts. A moderate form can be diagnosed when the loss, although significant, regards less than 50% of the ducts. The diagnosis can be supported by immunostaining with the marker proteins cytokeratin 7 and 19. Imaging can help in discriminating between VBDS and neoplastic conditions or primary biliary disorders.

13.3.3 Therapy

Therapy of toxin- or drug-induced bile duct injury is essentially limited to the treatment of symptoms and the consequences of prolonged cholestasis. Corticosteroids have been invariably ineffective. The use of bile acid ursodeoxycholic acid (UDCA) has been extensively studied in cholestatic diseases, such as PBC and PSC, and is FDA-approved for PBC treatment [124].

VBDS treatment is based on the identification of the essential cause, and the first intervention is the discontinuation of perturbing agent as soon as possible, although many patients with VBDS respond to other pharmacological treatments with or without the removal of the injury-causing agent on the basis of the specific clinical scenario. Treatment of cholestasis and pruritus is fundamental in the clinical practice. In particular, the use of UDCA and cholestyramine may be used for ameliorating the patient's symptoms [125]. Other drugs useful for the control of pruritus due to severe cholestasis include antihistamines, rifampicin, phenobarbital, and opioid analogs [125].

For some patients, the clinical prognosis is poor, with progression to biliary cirrhosis and end-stage liver disease, including the need for liver transplantation [4].

13.4   Drug-Induced Sclerosing Cholangitis

13.4.1 Pathophysiology

A number of studies indicate that there are drugs inducing sclerosing cholangitis of intra- or/and extrahepatic bile ducts characterized by segmental inflammation, fibrosis, and strictures ([126] and refs. therein). Interestingly, an analysis of the patients affected by drug-induced sclerosing cholangitis revealed that they are preferentially females [24]. In general, since this adverse drug reaction is very uncommon and literature reported mostly case reports, very little is known about the mechanism(s) by which the different drugs could induce the development of sclerosing cholangitis.

The hepatic artery infusion of fluoropyrimidines has demonstrated low systemic toxicity, nevertheless the blood flow scan often revealed abnormalities associated to bile duct damage that could indicate an ischemic nature of the injury [11]. In an experimental rabbit model, it has been observed that 5-fluorouracil disrupted the endothelial sheet, patchy exposing the subendothelium and forming a matrix for thrombus initiation [127]. Moreover, other studies have revealed that 5-fluorouracil causes a rapid depletion of pO2 in erythrocytes, thus increasing 2,3-bisphosphoglycerate production that further sustains deoxygenation and increases deoxyhemoglobin level. These effects lead to an ionic misbalance of erythrocyte membranes and diminish their capability of delivering oxygen, causing ischemic damage to the tissues [128].

Ketamine, a non-competitive N-methyl-D-aspartate receptor (NMDAR) antagonist, is reported to cause secondary sclerosing cholangitis but the mechanisms by which this drug leads to cholestasis and biliary abnormalities have not been understood so far. Since this drug induces the ureter smooth muscle relaxation through NMDAR inhibition, explaining the hydronephrosis observed in ketamine abusers, it has been hypothesized that this effect could also be effective in the biliary tract, thus causing biliary dilatation and damage [27].

13.4.2 Diagnosis

Drug-induced sclerosing cholangitis normally occurs to one or more strictures of the large bile ducts, in particular the common hepatic duct and the right and left hepatic ducts, sparing the common bile duct and the smaller intrahepatic ducts [8, 12]. At the acute stage, transient cholangitis is usually observed, before the appearance of worsening cholestasis secondary to biliary sclerosis. The main symptoms are upper abdominal pain, jaundice, anorexia, and weight loss. Magnetic resonance can be of help in evidencing continuous irregularities associated to intra- and/or extrahepatic bile duct dilatation [24]. The histopathological changes are not specific and correspond to typical features of chronic cholestasis resembling peculiar histological changes of primary sclerosing cholangitis, such as fibrous obliterating cholangitis, characterized by different degrees of involution and atrophy of the ducts, sometimes with ductopenia [8, 12].

In a study analyzing different DILI cases, it has been observed that the cholestatic phenotype of the sclerosing cholangitis group was more severe (more patients had jaundice and underwent hospitalization) than that of the others and, in addition, the time to resolution of liver tests was significantly prolonged in these patients [24].

13.4.3 Therapy and Outcome

The outcome of drug-induced sclerosing cholangitis is variable, since most cases are nearly reversible, but some lead to severe hepatic failure [19, 21, 108]. Although the development of drug-induced PSC is usually associated to anticancer chemotherapy, it has been shown that other drugs, such as antibiotics, anesthetics, and others can lead to a bile duct injury with PSC features [24]. The pharmacological management of sclerosing cholangitis induced by chemotherapy comprises the addition of intra-arterial steroids and the selective use of UDCA, although it has been noticed that dose reduction of the chemotherapeutic agent or its discontinuation when liver function markers increase can avoid the development of strictures. Biliary stenting can be considered as an option in presence of jaundice secondary to severe strictures [21].

13.5   Conclusion

Drug-induced bile duct injury is a side effect of a number of different therapeutic options, that can be either easy to manage and characterized by a good outcome, or mostly unpredictable and even potentially fatal. Such adverse reactions remain an important issue in drug development since, although high throughput screening and animal studies can be used to evaluate potentially toxic molecules, these assays are often poorly able to predict whether a candidate drug can cause drug-induced cholangiopathy or, in general, drug-induced hypersensitivity. A more precise characterization of the molecular pathophysiological mechanism(s) of drug-induced cholangiopathy, together with retrospective gene profiling of susceptible patients may help a more reliable prediction of DILI, with the aim of identifying patients who are at risk of developing this adverse drug reaction characterized by difficulties in treatment and uncertain outcome.

References

1. Padda MS, Sanchez M, Akhtar AJ, Boyer JL. Drug-induced cholestasis. Hepatology. 2011;53(4):1377–87.
2. Bohan A, Boyer JL. Mechanisms of hepatic transport of drugs: implications for cholestatic drug reactions. Semin Liver Dis. 2002;22(2):123–36.
3. Björnsson E, Olsson R. Outcome and prognostic markers in severe drug-induced liver disease. Hepatology. 2005;42(2):481–9.

4. Reau NS, Jensen DM. Vanishing bile duct syndrome. Clin Liver Dis. 2008;12(1):203–17, x.
5. Bonkovsky HL, Kleiner DE, Gu J, Odin JA, Russo MW, Navarro VM, et al. Clinical presentations and outcomes of bile duct loss caused by drugs and herbal and dietary supplements. Hepatology. 2017;65(4):1267–77.
6. Lazaridis KN, LaRusso NF. The cholangiopathies. Mayo Clin Proc. 2015;90(6):791–800.
7. O'Hara SP, Tabibian JH, Splinter PL, LaRusso NF. The dynamic biliary epithelia: molecules, pathways, and disease. J Hepatol. 2013;58(3):575–82.
8. Desmet VJ. Vanishing bile duct syndrome in drug-induced liver disease. J Hepatol. 1997;26(Suppl 1):31–5.
9. Björnsson ES, Jonasson JG. Idiosyncratic drug-induced liver injury associated with bile duct loss and vanishing bile duct syndrome: rare but has severe consequences. Hepatology. 2017;65(4):1091–3.
10. Degott C, Feldmann G, Larrey D, Durand-Schneider A-M, Grange D, Machayekhi J-P, et al. Drug-induced prolonged cholestasis in adults: a histological semiquantitative study demonstrating progressive ductopenia. Hepatology. 1992;15(2):244–51.
11. Visentin M, Lenggenhager D, Gai Z, Kullak-Ublick GA. Drug-induced bile duct injury. Biochim Biophys Acta Mol basis Dis. 2018;1864(4 Pt B):1498–506.
12. Geubel AP, Sempoux CL. Drug and toxin-induced bile duct disorders. J Gastroenterol Hepatol. 2000;15(11):1232–8.
13. Greca RD, Cunha-Silva M, Costa LBE, Costa JGF, Mazo DFC, Sevá-Pereira T, et al. Vanishing bile duct syndrome related to DILI and Hodgkin lymphoma overlap: a rare and severe case. Ann Hepatol. 2020;19(1):107–12.
14. Hussaini SH, Farrington EA. Idiosyncratic drug-induced liver injury: an overview. Expert Opin Drug Saf. 2007;6(6):673–84.
15. Sundaram V, Björnsson ES. Drug-induced cholestasis. Hepatol Commun. 2017;1(8):726–35.
16. Hashim A, Barnabas A, Miquel R, Agarwal K. Successful liver transplantation for drug-induced vanishing bile duct syndrome. BMJ Case Rep. 2020;13(1):e233052.
17. Levine C, Trivedi A, Thung SN, Perumalswami PV. Severe ductopenia and cholestasis from levofloxacin drug-induced liver injury: a case report and review. Semin Liver Dis. 2014;34(2):246–51.
18. Björnsson ES, Hoofnagle JH. Categorization of drugs implicated in causing liver injury: critical assessment based on published case reports. Hepatology. 2016;63(2):590–603.
19. Ko YJ, Karanicolas PJ. Hepatic arterial infusion pump chemotherapy for colorectal liver metastases: an old technology in a new era. Curr Oncol. 2014;21(1):e116–21.
20. Daly JM, Kemeny N, Oderman P, Botet J. Long-term hepatic arterial infusion chemotherapy. Anatomic considerations, operative technique, and treatment morbidity. Arch Surg. 1984;119(8):936–41.
21. Ito K, Ito H, Kemeny NE, Gonen M, Allen PJ, Paty PB, et al. Biliary sclerosis after hepatic arterial infusion pump chemotherapy for patients with colorectal cancer liver metastasis: incidence, clinical features, and risk factors. Ann Surg Oncol. 2012;19(5):1609–17.
22. Kemeny N, Seiter K, Niedzwiecki D, Chapman D, Sigurdson E, Cohen A, et al. A randomized trial of intrahepatic infusion of fluorodeoxyuridine with dexamethasone versus fluorodeoxyuridine alone in the treatment of metastatic colorectal cancer. Cancer. 1992;69(2):327–34.
23. Jin S, Shi X-J, Sun X-D, Wang S-Y, Wang G-Y. Sclerosing cholangitis secondary to bleomycin-iodinated embolization for liver hemangioma. World J Gastroenterol. 2014;20(46):17680–5.
24. Gudnason HO, Björnsson HK, Gardarsdottir M, Thorisson HM, Olafsson S, Bergmann OM, et al. Secondary sclerosing cholangitis in patients with drug-induced liver injury. Dig Liver Dis. 2015;47(6):502–7.
25. Sahin M, Eryilmaz R, Bulbuloglu E. The effect of scolicidal agents on liver and biliary tree (experimental study). J Invest Surg. 2004;17(6):323–6.
26. Seto W-K, Ng M, Chan P, Ng IO-L, Cheung SC-W, Hung IF-N, et al. Ketamine-induced cholangiopathy: a case report. Am J Gastroenterol. 2011;106(5):1004–5.
27. Lo RSC, Krishnamoorthy R, Freeman JG, Austin AS. Cholestasis and biliary dilatation associated with chronic ketamine abuse: a case series. Singap Med J. 2011;52(3):e52 5.

28. Wong SW, Lee KF, Wong J, Ng WWC, Cheung YS, Lai PBS. Dilated common bile ducts mimicking choledochal cysts in ketamine abusers. Hong Kong Med J. 2009;15(1):53–6.
29. Turkish A, Luo JJ, Lefkowitch JH. Ketamine abuse, biliary tract disease, and secondary sclerosing cholangitis. Hepatology. 2013;58(2):825–7.
30. Nayudu SK, Badipatla S, Niazi M, Balar B. Cholestatic hepatitis with small duct injury associated with celecoxib. Case Rep Med. 2013;2013:e315479. https://www.hindawi.com/journals/crim/2013/315479/. Accessed 3 Apr 2020.
31. Androgenic steroids. In: LiverTox: clinical and research information on drug-induced liver injury. Bethesda, MD: National Institute of Diabetes and Digestive and Kidney Diseases; 2012. http://www.ncbi.nlm.nih.gov/books/NBK548931/. Accessed 27 Apr 2020.
32. Carmustine. In: LiverTox: clinical and research information on drug-induced liver injury. Bethesda, MD: National Institute of Diabetes and Digestive and Kidney Diseases; 2012. http://www.ncbi.nlm.nih.gov/books/NBK548307/. Accessed 27 Apr 2020.
33. Rosenberg WM, Ryley NG, Trowell JM, McGee JO, Chapman RW. Dextropropoxyphene induced hepatotoxicity: a report of nine cases. J Hepatol. 1993;19(3):470–4.
34. Gold preparations. In: LiverTox: clinical and research information on drug-induced liver injury. Bethesda, MD: National Institute of Diabetes and Digestive and Kidney Diseases; 2012. http://www.ncbi.nlm.nih.gov/books/NBK548786/. Accessed 27 Apr 2020.
35. Zimmerman HJ, Lewis JH. Drug-induced cholestasis. Med Toxicol. 1987;2(2):112–60.
36. Bataller R, Bragulat E, Nogué S, Görbig MN, Bruguera M, Rodés J. Prolonged cholestasis after acute paraquat poisoning through skin absorption. Am J Gastroenterol. 2000;95(5):1340–3.
37. Masubuchi Y. Metabolic and non-metabolic factors determining troglitazone hepatotoxicity: a review. Drug Metab Pharmacokinet. 2006;21(5):347–56.
38. Patel H, Sonawane Y, Jagtap R, Dhangar K, Thapliyal N, Surana S, et al. Structural insight of glitazone for hepato-toxicity: resolving mystery by PASS. Bioorg Med Chem Lett. 2015;25(9):1938–46.
39. Trak-Smayra V, Cazals-Hatem D, Asselah T, Duchatelle V, Degott C. Prolonged cholestasis and ductopenia associated with tenoxicam. J Hepatol. 2003;39(1):125–8.
40. Mullish BH, Fofaria RK, Smith BC, Lloyd K, Lloyd J, Goldin RD, et al. Severe cholestatic jaundice after a single administration of ajmaline; a case report and review of the literature. BMC Gastroenterol. 2014;14:60.
41. Amitriptyline. In: LiverTox: clinical and research information on drug-induced liver injury. Bethesda, MD: National Institute of Diabetes and Digestive and Kidney Diseases; 2012. http://www.ncbi.nlm.nih.gov/books/NBK548410/. Accessed 27 Apr 2020.
42. Ortega-Alonso A, Andrade RJ. Chronic liver injury induced by drugs and toxins. J Dig Dis. 2018;19(9):514–21.
43. Amiodarone. In: LiverTox: clinical and research information on drug-induced liver injury. Bethesda, MD: National Institute of Diabetes and Digestive and Kidney Diseases; 2012. http://www.ncbi.nlm.nih.gov/books/NBK548109/. Accessed 27 Apr 2020.
44. Hautekeete ML, Brenard R, Horsmans Y, Henrion J, Verbist L, Derue G, et al. Liver injury related to amoxycillin-clavulanic acid: interlobular bile-duct lesions and extrahepatic manifestations. J Hepatol. 1995;22(1):71–7.
45. Smith LA, Ignacio JRA, Winesett MP, Kaiser GC, Lacson AG, Gilbert-Barness E, et al. Vanishing bile duct syndrome: amoxicillin-clavulanic acid associated intra-hepatic cholestasis responsive to ursodeoxycholic acid. J Pediatr Gastroenterol Nutr. 2005;41(4):469–73.
46. Richardet JP, Mallat A, Zafrani ES, Blazquez M, Bognel JC, Campillo B. Prolonged cholestasis with ductopenia after administration of amoxicillin/clavulanic acid. Dig Dis Sci. 1999;44(10):1997–2000.
47. O'Donohue J, Oien K, Donaldson P, Underhill J, Clare M, MacSween R, et al. Co-amoxiclav jaundice: clinical and histological features and HLA class II association. Gut. 2000;47(5):717–20.
48. deLemos AS, Ghabril M, Rockey DC, Gu J, Barnhart HX, Fontana RJ, et al. Amoxicillin–clavulanate-induced liver injury. Dig Dis Sci. 2016;61(8):2406–16.

49. Hautekeete ML, Horsmans Y, Van Waeyenberge C, Demanet C, Henrion J, Verbist L, et al. HLA association of amoxicillin-clavulanate--induced hepatitis. Gastroenterology. 1999;117(5):1181-6.

50. Cavanzo FJ, Garcia CF, Botero RC. Chronic cholestasis, paucity of bile ducts, red cell aplasia, and the Stevens-Johnson syndrome. An ampicillin-associated case. Gastroenterology. 1990;99(3):854–6.

51. Ampicillin. In: LiverTox: clinical and research information on drug-induced liver injury. Bethesda, MD: National Institute of Diabetes and Digestive and Kidney Diseases; 2012. http://www.ncbi.nlm.nih.gov/books/NBK547894/. Accessed 27 Apr 2020.

52. Dev HY, et al. Reversible cholestasis with bile duct injury following azathioprine therapy. A case report. Liver. 1991;11:89. https://www.ncbi.nlm.nih.gov/pubmed/2051906. Accessed 27 Apr 2020.

53. Azathioprine. In: LiverTox: clinical and research information on drug-induced liver injury. Bethesda, MD: National Institute of Diabetes and Digestive and Kidney Diseases; 2012. http://www.ncbi.nlm.nih.gov/books/NBK548332/. Accessed 27 Apr 2020.

54. Pagliaro L, Campesi G, Aguglia F. Barbiturate jaundice. Report of a case due to a barbital-containing drug, with positive rechallenge to phenobarbital. Gastroenterology. 1969;56(5):938–43.

55. Babbs C, Warnes TW. Primary biliary cirrhosis after benoxaprofen. Br Med J (Clin Res Ed). 1986;293(6541):241.

56. Nonsteroidal antiinflammatory drugs (NSAIDs). In: LiverTox: clinical and research information on drug-induced liver injury. Bethesda, MD: National Institute of Diabetes and Digestive and Kidney Diseases; 2012. http://www.ncbi.nlm.nih.gov/books/NBK548614/. Accessed 27 Apr 2020.

57. Ramos AMO, Gayotto LCC, Clemente CM, Mello ES, Luz KG, Freitas ML. Reversible vanishing bile duct syndrome induced by carbamazepine. Eur J Gastroenterol Hepatol. 2002;14(9):1019–22.

58. Forbes GM, Jeffrey GP, Shilkin KB, Reed WD. Carbamazepine hepatotoxicity: another cause of the vanishing bile duct syndrome. Gastroenterology. 1992;102(4 Pt 1):1385–8.

59. de Galoscy C, Horsmans Y, Rahier J, Geubel AP. Vanishing bile duct syndrome occurring after carbamazepine administration: a second case report. J Clin Gastroenterol. 1994;19(3):269–71.

60. Levy M, Goodman MW, Van Dyne BJ, Sumner HW. Granulomatous hepatitis secondary to carbamazepine. Ann Intern Med. 1981;95(1):64–5.

61. Husebye KO. Jaundice with persisting pericholangiolitic inflammation in a patient treated with chlorothiazide. Dig Dis Sci. 1964;9(6):439–46.

62. Moradpour D, Altorfer J, Flury R, Greminger P, Meyenberger C, Jost R, et al. Chlorpromazine-induced vanishing bile duct syndrome leading to biliary cirrhosis. Hepatology. 1994;20(6):1437–41.

63. Chlorpromazine. In: LiverTox: clinical and research information on drug-induced liver injury. Bethesda, MD: National Institute of Diabetes and Digestive and Kidney Diseases; 2012. http://www.ncbi.nlm.nih.gov/books/NBK548793/. Accessed 27 Apr 2020.

64. Ishak KG, Irey NS. Hepatic injury associated with the phenothiazines. Clinicopathologic and follow-up study of 36 patients. Arch Pathol. 1972;93(4):283–304.

65. Geubel AP, Nakad A, Rahier J, Dive C. Prolonged cholestasis and disappearance of interlobular bile ducts following chlorpropamide and erythromycin ethylsuccinate. Case of drug interaction? Liver. 1988;8(6):350–3.

66. Cimetidine. In: LiverTox: clinical and research information on drug-induced liver injury. Bethesda, MD: National Institute of Diabetes and Digestive and Kidney Diseases; 2012. http://www.ncbi.nlm.nih.gov/books/NBK548130/. Accessed 27 Apr 2020.

67. Ciprofloxacin. In: LiverTox: clinical and research information on drug-induced liver injury. Bethesda, MD: National Institute of Diabetes and Digestive and Kidney Diseases; 2012. http://www.ncbi.nlm.nih.gov/books/NBK548066/. Accessed 27 Apr 2020.

68. Clindamycin. In: LiverTox: clinical and research information on drug-induced liver injury. Bethesda, MD: National Institute of Diabetes and Digestive and Kidney Diseases; 2012. http://www.ncbi.nlm.nih.gov/books/NBK548292/. Accessed 27 Apr 2020.

69. Larrey D, Geneve J, Pessayre D, Machayekhi JP, Degott C, Benhamou JP. Prolonged cholestasis after cyproheptadine-induced acute hepatitis. J Clin Gastroenterol. 1987;9(1):102–4.

70. Cyproheptadine. In: LiverTox: clinical and research information on drug-induced liver injury. Bethesda, MD: National Institute of Diabetes and Digestive and Kidney Diseases; 2012. http://www.ncbi.nlm.nih.gov/books/NBK548422/. Accessed 27 Apr 2020.

71. Penicillamine. In: LiverTox: clinical and research information on drug-induced liver injury. Bethesda, MD: National Institute of Diabetes and Digestive and Kidney Diseases; 2012. http://www.ncbi.nlm.nih.gov/books/NBK548246/. Accessed 27 Apr 2020.

72. Kawasaki Y, Matsubara K, Hashimoto K, Tanigawa K, Kage M, Iwata A, et al. Nonsteroidal anti-inflammatory drug-induced vanishing bile duct syndrome treated with plasmapheresis. J Pediatr Gastroenterol Nutr. 2013;57(5):e30–1.

73. Erythromycin. In: LiverTox: clinical and research information on drug-induced liver injury. Bethesda, MD: National Institute of Diabetes and Digestive and Kidney Diseases; 2012. http://www.ncbi.nlm.nih.gov/books/NBK547881/. Accessed 27 Apr 2020.

74. Lieberman DA, Keeffe EB, Stenzel P. Severe and prolonged oral contraceptive jaundice. J Clin Gastroenterol. 1984;6(2):145–8.

75. Estrogens and oral contraceptives. In: LiverTox: clinical and research information on drug-induced liver injury. Bethesda, MD: National Institute of Diabetes and Digestive and Kidney Diseases; 2012. http://www.ncbi.nlm.nih.gov/books/NBK548539/. Accessed 27 Apr 2020.

76. Fenofibrate. In: LiverTox: clinical and research information on drug-induced liver injury. Bethesda, MD: National Institute of Diabetes and Digestive and Kidney Diseases; 2012. http://www.ncbi.nlm.nih.gov/books/NBK548607/. Accessed 27 Apr 2020.

77. Davies MH, Harrison RF, Elias E, Hübscher SG. Antibiotic-associated acute vanishing bile duct syndrome: a pattern associated with severe, prolonged, intrahepatic cholestasis. J Hepatol. 1994;20(1):112–6.

78. Eckstein RP, Dowsett JF, Lunzer MR. Flucloxacillin induced liver disease: histopathological findings at biopsy and autopsy. Pathology. 1993;25(3):223–8.

79. Chitturi S, Farrell GC. Drug-induced cholestasis. Semin Gastrointest Dis. 2001;12(2):113–24.

80. Ishii M, Miyazaki Y, Yamamoto T, Miura M, Ueno Y, Takahashi T, et al. A case of drug-induced ductopenia resulting in fatal biliary cirrhosis. Liver. 1993;13(4):227–31.

81. He K, Cai L, Shi Q, Liu H, Woolf TF. Inhibition of MDR3 activity in human hepatocytes by drugs associated with liver injury. Chem Res Toxicol. 2015;28(10):1987–90.

82. Alam I, Ferrell LD, Bass NM. Vanishing bile duct syndrome temporally associated with ibuprofen use. Am J Gastroenterol. 1996;91(8):1626–30.

83. Basturk A, Artan R, Yılmaz A, Gelen MT, Duman O. Acute vanishing bile duct syndrome after the use of ibuprofen. Arab J Gastroenterol. 2016;17(3):137–9.

84. Kim H, Yang HK, Kim SH, Park JH. Ibuprofen associated acute vanishing bile duct syndrome and toxic epidermal necrolysis in an infant. Yonsei Med J. 2014;55(3):834–7.

85. Xie W, Wang Q, Gao Y, Pan CQ. Vanishing bile duct syndrome with hyperlipidemia after ibuprofen therapy in an adult patient: a case report. BMC Gastroenterol. 2018;18(1):142.

86. Imipramine. In: LiverTox: clinical and research information on drug-induced liver injury. Bethesda, MD: National Institute of Diabetes and Digestive and Kidney Diseases; 2012. http://www.ncbi.nlm.nih.gov/books/NBK547884/. Accessed 27 Apr 2020.

87. Macrolide Antibiotics. In: LiverTox: clinical and research information on drug-induced liver injury. Bethesda, MD: National Institute of Diabetes and Digestive and Kidney Diseases; 2012. http://www.ncbi.nlm.nih.gov/books/NBK548398/. Accessed 27 Apr 2020.

88. Schumaker AL, Okulicz JF. Meropenem-induced vanishing bile duct syndrome. Pharmacotherapy. 2010;30(9):953.

89. Phenytoin. In: LiverTox: clinical and research information on drug-induced liver injury. Bethesda, MD: National Institute of Diabetes and Digestive and Kidney Diseases; 2012. http://www.ncbi.nlm.nih.gov/books/NBK548889/. Accessed 27 Apr 2020.

90. Lok AS, Ng IO. Prochlorperazine-induced chronic cholestasis. J Hepatol. 1988;6(3):369–73.
91. Prochlorperazine. In: LiverTox: clinical and research information on drug-induced liver injury. Bethesda, MD: National Institute of Diabetes and Digestive and Kidney Diseases; 2012. http://www.ncbi.nlm.nih.gov/books/NBK548122/. Accessed 27 Apr 2020.
92. Orman ES, Conjeevaram HS, Vuppalanchi R, Freston JW, Rochon J, Kleiner DE, et al. Clinical and histopathologic features of fluoroquinolone-induced liver injury. Clin Gastroenterol Hepatol. 2011;9(6):517–523.e3.
93. Moxifloxacin. In: LiverTox: clinical and research information on drug-induced liver injury. Bethesda, MD: National Institute of Diabetes and Digestive and Kidney Diseases; 2012. http://www.ncbi.nlm.nih.gov/books/NBK548166/. Accessed 27 Apr 2020.
94. Robinson W, Habr F, Manlolo J, Bhattacharya B. Moxifloxacin associated vanishing bile duct syndrome. J Clin Gastroenterol. 2010;44(1):72–3.
95. Mallat A, Zafrani ES, Metreau JM, Dhumeaux D. Terbinafine-induced prolonged cholestasis with reduction of interlobular bile ducts. Dig Dis Sci. 1997;42(7):1486–8.
96. van 'tWout JW, Herrmann WA, de Vries RA, Stricker BH. Terbinafine-associated hepatic injury. J Hepatol. 1994;21(1):115–7.
97. Terbinafine. In: LiverTox: clinical and research information on drug-induced liver injury. Bethesda, MD: National Institute of Diabetes and Digestive and Kidney Diseases; 2012. http://www.ncbi.nlm.nih.gov/books/NBK548617/. Accessed 27 Apr 2020.
98. Farrell GC. Drug-induced hepatic injury. J Gastroenterol Hepatol. 1997;12(9–10):S242–50.
99. Doxycycline. In: LiverTox: clinical and research information on drug-induced liver injury. Bethesda, MD: National Institute of Diabetes and Digestive and Kidney Diseases; 2012. http://www.ncbi.nlm.nih.gov/books/NBK548353/. Accessed 27 Apr 2020.
100. Roy MA, Nugent FW, Aretz HT. Micronodular cirrhosis after thiabendazole. Dig Dis Sci. 1989;34(6):938–41.
101. Trifluoperazine. In: LiverTox: clinical and research information on drug-induced liver injury. Bethesda, MD: National Institute of Diabetes and Digestive and Kidney Diseases; 2012. http://www.ncbi.nlm.nih.gov/books/NBK548927/. Accessed 27 Apr 2020.
102. Erlinger S. Drug-induced cholestasis. J Hepatol. 1997;26(Suppl 1):1–4.
103. Faria LC, Resende CC, Couto CA, Couto OFM, Fonseca LPC, Ferrari TCA. Severe and prolonged cholestasis caused by trimethoprim-sulfamethoxazole: a case report. Clinics (Sao Paulo). 2009;64(1):71–4.
104. Kowdley KV, Keeffe EB, Fawaz KA. Prolonged cholestasis due to trimethoprim sulfamethoxazole. Gastroenterology. 1992;102(6):2148–50.
105. Vuppalanchi R, Chalasani N, Saxena R. Restoration of bile ducts in drug-induced vanishing bile duct syndrome due to zonisamide. Am J Surg Pathol. 2006;30(12):1619–23.
106. Horsley-Silva JL, Dow EN, Menias CO, Smith ML, Carballido EM, Lindor KD, et al. Docetaxel induced sclerosing cholangitis. Dig Dis Sci. 2015;60(12):3814–6.
107. Floxuridine. In: LiverTox: clinical and research information on drug-induced liver injury. Bethesda, MD: National Institute of Diabetes and Digestive and Kidney Diseases; 2012. http://www.ncbi.nlm.nih.gov/books/NBK548421/. Accessed 27 Apr 2020.
108. Ludwig J, Kim CH, Wiesner RH, Krom RA. Floxuridine-induced sclerosing cholangitis: an ischemic cholangiopathy? Hepatology. 1989;9(2):215–8.
109. Schwab GP, Wetscher GJ, Vogl W, Redmond E. Methimazole-induced cholestatic liver injury, mimicking sclerosing cholangitis. Langenbecks Arch Chir. 1996;381(4):225–7.
110. Matsumoto S, Watanabe K, Kobayashi N, Irie K, Yamanaka S, Kaneko T. Pembrolizumab-induced secondary sclerosing cholangitis in a non-small cell lung cancer patient. Respirol Case Rep. 2020;8(5):e00560.
111. Karnsakul W, Arkachaisri T, Atisook K, Wisuthsarewong W, Sattawatthamrong Y, Aanpreung P. Vanishing bile duct syndrome in a child with toxic epidermal necrolysis: an interplay of unbalanced immune regulatory mechanisms. Ann Hepatol. 2006;5(2):116–9.
112. Olsson R, Wiholm BE, Sand C, Zettergren L, Hultcrantz R, Myrhed M. Liver damage from flucloxacillin, cloxacillin and dicloxacillin. J Hepatol. 1992;15(1–2):154–61.

113. Pichler WJ. The p-i concept: pharmacological interaction of drugs with immune receptors. World Allergy Organ J. 2008;1(6):96–102.
114. Barbatis C, Woods J, Morton JA, Fleming KA, McMichael A, McGee JO. Immunohistochemical analysis of HLA (A, B, C) antigens in liver disease using a monoclonal antibody. Gut. 1981;22(12):985–91.
115. Feng J, Li M, Gu W, Tang H, Yu S. The aberrant expression of HLA-DR in intrahepatic bile ducts in patients with biliary atresia: an immunohistochemistry and immune electron microscopy study. J Pediatr Surg. 2004;39(11):1658–62.
116. Demetris AJ, Lasky S, Van Thiel DH, Starzl TE, Whiteside T. Induction of DR/IA antigens in human liver allografts. An immunocytochemical and clinicopathologic analysis of twenty failed grafts. Transplantation. 1985;40(5):504–9.
117. Ogese MO, Ahmed S, Alferivic A, Betts CJ, Dickinson A, Faulkner L, et al. New approaches to investigate drug-induced hypersensitivity. Chem Res Toxicol. 2017;30(1):239–59.
118. Nicoletti P, Aithal GP, Bjornsson ES, Andrade RJ, Sawle A, Arrese M, et al. Association of liver injury from specific drugs, or groups of drugs, with polymorphisms in HLA and other genes in a genome-wide association study. Gastroenterology. 2017;152(5):1078–89.
119. Liu Z-X, Kaplowitz N. Immune-mediated drug-induced liver disease. Clin Liver Dis. 2002;6(3):755–74.
120. Trauner M, Arrese M, Lee H, Boyer JL, Karpen SJ. Endotoxin downregulates rat hepatic ntcp gene expression via decreased activity of critical transcription factors. J Clin Invest. 1998;101(10):2092–100.
121. Fardel O, Le Vée M. Regulation of human hepatic drug transporter expression by pro-inflammatory cytokines. Expert Opin Drug Metab Toxicol. 2009;5(12):1469–81.
122. Pirmohamed M, Naisbitt DJ, Gordon F, Park BK. The danger hypothesis--potential role in idiosyncratic drug reactions. Toxicology. 2002;181–182:55–63.
123. Ali AH, Tabibian JH, Lindor KD. Update on pharmacotherapies for cholestatic liver disease. Hepatol Commun. 2017;1(1):7–17.
124. European Association for the Study of the Liver. EASL clinical practice guidelines: management of cholestatic liver diseases. J Hepatol. 2009;51(2):237–67.
125. Bakhit M, McCarty TR, Park S, Njei B, Cho M, Karagozian R, et al. Vanishing bile duct syndrome in Hodgkin's lymphoma: a single center experience and clinical pearls. J Clin Gastroenterol. 2016;50(8):688.
126. Brooling J, Leal R. Secondary sclerosing cholangitis: a review of recent literature. Curr Gastroenterol Rep. 2017;19(9):1–7.
127. Cwikiel M, Zhang B, Eskilsson J, Wieslander JB, Albertsson M. The influence of 5-fluorouracil on the endothelium in small arteries. An electron microscopic study in rabbits. Scanning Microsc. 1995;9(2):561–76.
128. Spasojević I, Jelić S, Zakrzewska J, Bačić G. Decreased oxygen transfer capacity of erythrocytes as a cause of 5-fluorouracil related ischemia. Molecules. 2008;14(1):53–67.

Part V
Neoplasms of the Biliary Tree

Cholangiocarcinoma

14

Alberto Lasagni, Mario Strazzabosco, Maria Guido,
Luca Fabris, and Massimiliano Cadamuro

14.1 Introduction

Cholangiocarcinoma (CCA) includes a group of different epithelial cancers with features of biliary tract differentiation arising from any tract of the biliary tree. They present particular similarities but also substantial inter-tumour and intra-tumour differences that affect pathogenesis and outcome, and histologically, they are, with rare exceptions, adenocarcinomas. CCA is a rare cancer accounting about 3% of all gastrointestinal malignancies, while it is the second primary liver cancer for mortality, overcoming hepatocellular carcinoma (HCC) [1]. Based on its anatomical location,

A. Lasagni
General Medicine Division, Azienda Ospedale-Università di Padova, Padova, Italy
e-mail: alberto.lasagni@aopd.veneto.it

M. Strazzabosco
Digestive Disease Section, Yale University, New Haven, CT, USA
e-mail: mario.strazzabosco@yale.edu

M. Guido
Department of Pathology, Treviso Regional Hospital, Azienda ULSS2 Marca Trevigiana, Treviso, Italy

Department of Medicine-DIMED, University of Padova, Padova, Italy
e-mail: mguido@unipd.it

L. Fabris (✉)
General Medicine Division, Azienda Ospedale-Università di Padova, Padova, Italy

Digestive Disease Section, Yale University, New Haven, CT, USA

Department of Molecular Medicine-DMM, University of Padova, Padova, Italy
e-mail: luca.fabris@unipd.it, luca.fabris@yale.edu

M. Cadamuro
Department of Molecular Medicine-DMM, University of Padova, Padova, Italy
e-mail: massimiliano.cadamuro@unipd.it

© Springer Nature Switzerland AG 2021
A. Floreani (ed.), *Diseases of the Liver and Biliary Tree*,
https://doi.org/10.1007/978-3-030-65908-0_14

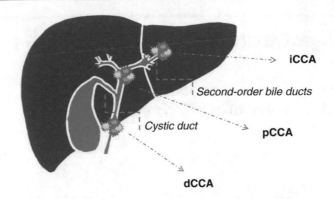

Fig. 14.1 Classifications of CCAs

CCA is classified as intrahepatic (iCCA), perihilar (pCCA), and distal (dCCA) (Fig. 14.1); iCCA is defined as involving proximally up to the second degree bile ducts, pCCA is localized from second degree bile branches of right and left bile ducts to the insertion of cystic duct into common bile duct, and dCCA includes the area till the ampulla of Vater [2, 3]. Recently, the WHO classification added a new distinct subtype: the mixed hepatocellular-cholangiocellular carcinoma, accounting for less than 1% of all liver cancers [4]. Gallbladder carcinoma is considered a different biliary tract cancer due to its different features in epidemiology, pathology, clinical presentation and management. pCCA is the most common form, accounting about the 60% of cases, followed by dCCA with 30% and lastly iCCA around 10% [5]. Currently, the three types of CCA are considered as distinct cancers since different clinical and management features. Terms as Klatskin tumour for pCCA, intra- and extrahepatic CCA represent previous codifications that are discouraged [2].

CCA is an aggressive neoplasia, mostly diagnosed at advanced stages. Most cases are sporadic but conditions leading to chronic inflammation and cholestasis have been recognized as risk factors. Diagnosis remains challenging due to absence of symptoms at the earliest stages. It is difficult to visualize owing to its anatomical localization and its desmoplastic and paucicellular character often makes inconclusive the result of cytological or pathological analysis. So, diagnostic work-up needs full integration of anamnesis, physical examination, laboratory tests including serum onco-markers, imaging studies and cytology/pathology [6]. Surgical resection with histologically negative margins is the only curative treatment, although only few patients (around 35%) present early stage disease amenable for this option. Likewise, liver transplantation is an option for a small subset of selected patients suffering from pCCA after neoadjuvant chemo-radio treatment [7].

Generally, prognosis is poor for most patients: desmoplastic nature, de novo activation of cell survival and chemoresistance pathways, high genetic variability and interaction with a rich tumour microenvironment, all contribute to the resistance of therapy. Understanding cholangiocarcinoma biology, genetic profiles and its complete interactions with the microenvironment, associated to advances in targeted, radio- and immunotherapy will lead to improvement in survival [8, 9].

14.2 Epidemiology

14.2.1 Incidence

Cholangiocarcinoma is reported to be a rare cancer representing only 3% of all gastrointestinal cancers, but the increased incidence and the absolute need of early diagnosis for good outcome are raising interest. Mean age of presentation is around 60–70 years old, rarely before 40 years old. In most cases, it is sporadic, but its incidence differs worldwide, and it is higher where specific risk factors are diffuse. In Western countries, incidence rates are low (<5/100,000) whereas in South East Asia region are higher (8/100,000) reaching a peak of around 85/100,000 in Northeast Thailand. Age-adjusted rate are highest in Hispanic and Asian populations (2.8–3.3/100,000) with a little male predominance (1.2–1.5 vs. 1.0/100,000) except in female Hispanic population (1.5/100,000) [2] (Fig. 14.2).

Several studies showed in the USA and across Europe a tenfold increase of iCCA incidence at the end of last century, reaching a plateau in the past 10 years. By contrast, incidence of pCCA/dCCA decreases at a slower rate, In particular, iCCA frequency is increasing in Western countries with a patchwork pattern and its mortality has raised by 36.3% both in the USA and European either in Asian countries. Since the mid-1990s in the UK and the USA, iCCA mortality overcame HCC becoming the first cause of death for primary liver cancer. The effective increasing of incidence rates is discussed in literature: although better diagnostic techniques are available, no significant change arose in the proportion of patients among different stage at diagnosis supporting a true increasing of incidence. Nevertheless, incidence and mortality rates of pCCA/dCCA appear decreasing in the USA and worldwide. It is difficult to evaluate real incidence of pCCA and dCCA since, historically, they were grouped with gallbladder carcinoma and then as extrahepatic disease, without specific type differentiation. Other misleading factors are frequent lack of

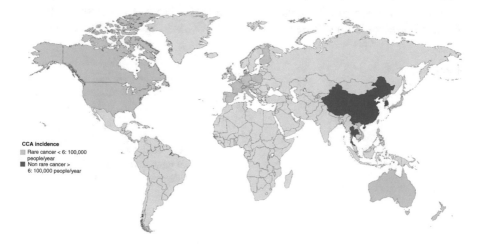

Fig. 14.2 Worldwide incidence of CCA. Low versus high incidence countries

histopathological confirmation, difficulty to determine anatomical origin in the advanced stage at diagnosis that could lead to misclassification as adenocarcinomas of upper gastrointestinal tract, and potential misclassification due to evolving edition of the World Health Organization's (WHO) International Classification of Disease for Oncology (ICD-O) coding system [10]. Besides differences in classification and improvement of diagnostic tools, several demographic phenomena could affect the real incidence of CCA subtypes. The expected obesity epidemic is supposed to increase rates, while changing burden of viral hepatitis due to new antiviral therapy will decline rates in future [9]. Finally, CCA incidence trends are a tricky issue that needs caution in interpretation and future epidemiological effort in standardizing and making accurate data record.

14.2.2 Risk Factors

Multiple factors are involved in CCA pathogenesis. The wide geographical and ethnic variability of incidence suggests the presence of genetic, environmental and cultural predispositions, even if most cases are idiopathic and no risk factor is present. CCA has been linked to different diseases, involving chronic biliary inflammation and increased cellular turnover [11] (Table 14.1). Nevertheless, papers investigating potential risk factors rarely differentiate among the different CCA subtypes, so their specific effects on iCCA, pCCA, or dCCA are unclear.

Hepatobiliary flukes, *Opisthorchis viverrini* and *Clonorchis sinensis*, are strongly associated to CCA with an odds ratio up to 27 and have been included in the list of group 1 human carcinogens by the WHO's International Agency for Research on Cancer [12]. Flukes infestation is particularly frequent in North-eastern Thailand where CCA incidence is the highest worldwide and transmission occurs through faecal-oral route via raw or poor-cooked fish, thereby the flukes populate biliary branches causing chronic irritation.

Hepatolithiasis is another endemic disease involved in CCA carcinogenesis in Asia. It is present in up to 70% of patients with CCA in Japan and Taiwan and it is

Table 14.1 Risk factors for CCA

Risk factors
Hepatobiliary flukes
Hepatolithiasis
Cirrhosis
Viral chronic hepatitis (B and C)
Primary sclerosing cholangitis
Fibrocystic liver disease (congenital hepatic fibrosis, Caroli disease, choledochal cysts …)
Metabolic syndrome and obesity
Diabetes mellitus
Toxins (e.g. alcohol, thorotrast, dioxin)
Genetic polymorphisms (e.g. ABCC2, MTHFR, KLRK1)

estimated a lifelong risk of CCA up to 10% in patients with intrahepatic biliary stones. Similarly, primary sclerosing cholangitis (PSC), bile stasis and recurrent subclinical episodes of cholangitis are thought to contribute and sustain oncogenesis.

Cirrhosis and viral chronic hepatitis C and B have been recognized as independent risk factors for CCA, especially iCCA. Regarding viral hepatitis, their effect is more consistent for virus C in the Western countries and for virus B in South East Asia, linked to their endemic areas. Their tumourigenic potential is mainly associated to hepatocellular carcinoma (HCC) but not only: according to a meta-analysis the odds ratio to develop iCCA is 22.9 (95% CI 18.2–28.8) for cirrhosis, 5.1 (95% CI 2.9–8.9) for HBV, and 4.8 (95% CI 2.4–9.7) for HCV [13]. Similar to HCC, chronic inflammation promotes carcinogenesis through secretion of inflammatory cytokines, acceleration in cellular turnover and distortion in the hepatic architecture due to fibrosis.

Primary sclerosing cholangitis (PSC) is a leading risk factor, primarily for pCCA, due to chronic inflammation with bile stasis, sclerosing and proliferative epithelial processes [14]. PSC patients anticipate the development of CCA of about 30 years with respect to the general population; the diagnosis is often in the fourth decade, and their lifetime risk is around 20%. Furthermore, most of CCA diagnosis falls in the first 2 years from diagnosis. So, patients with PSC need a strict surveillance through a multimodal diagnostic approach based on the repetition of serum markers (CA19.9) and imaging investigations, magnetic resonance (MR) and ultrasound (US). Prospective studies about risk stratification among patients with PSC and regarding the timing of follow-up are actually lacking. It may be a possibility to re-evaluate a patient every 6–12 months alternating MR and US imaging studies [15].

Fibrocystic liver disease, including different congenital rare diseases characterized by biliary dysgenesis, counts CCA development as the most feared complication. Congenital hepatic fibrosis and biliary duct dilation (Caroli syndrome), including Caroli disease and choledochal cysts, are associated to a lifetime incidence of CCA ranging between 6% and 30% with a mean age of diagnosis of 32 years old [16, 17]. Cholestasis, flowing of pancreatic enzymes and biliary inflammation, secondary to pancreato-biliary ducts abnormalities can lead to carcinogenesis.

In recent meta-analysis, metabolic syndrome, diabetes and obesity have been also associated to increased risk of developing iCCA [13, 18]. Among toxins, alcohol consumption is an independent risk factor with an overall OR of 2.8 for iCCA [13], whereas data on smoking are controversial.

All these risk factors are responsible for the induction of chronic inflammation involving the biliary tree, a process that may be favoured by local intrahepatic accumulation of bile acids, even without clear cholestasis [19]. Ultimately, several case-control studies involving small number of patients have pointed out some genetic polymorphisms as risk factor for CCA, in particular of genes encoding for proteins involved in detoxification (ABCC2, CYP1A2, NAT2), DNA repair (MTHFR, TYMS, GSTO1, XRCC1), and immunological surveillance (KLRK1, MICA, PTGS2) [11].

14.3 Pathogenesis

Microscopically, CCA can present several variants but typically, it is an adenocarcinoma with neoplastic glands or tubules enveloped by desmoplastic reaction. Tumour cells are cuboidal to columnar and mucin-producing but may differ in degree of atypia. CCAs arise from malignant transformation of cholangiocytes, progenitor cells, or by trans-differentiation of neoplastic hepatocytes [20]. Carcinogenesis involves specific modifications at subcellular level in order to give a survival advantage to the malignant cell. These processes regulate cell cycle, survival, differentiation, proliferation, control on genome integrity, and apoptosis. In CCA, many genetic changes have been pinpointed as possible target of treatments by inhibiting specific intracellular signal pathways. Recent studies suggested that some of these genetic mutations may be similar with those found in HCC, supporting the hypothesis of common cell ancestors [21]. Furthermore, both wide variability of genetic aberrations and malignant microenvironment determine a vortex of continuous genetic evolution resulting in drug resistance. Nevertheless, data dealing with this topic are still incomplete and need confirmation. Among genetic aberrations in CCA, the genes that appeared to be the most involved in tumour pathogenesis are listed in Table 14.2 [2, 9].

Many pathways are hyperactivated in iCCA but, for now, none has been found dominant, and sufficient to drive carcinogenesis. It is well accepted that a prolonged inflammation is actively involved in malignant transition; indeed, JAK/STAT pathway, a downstream axis involved in several inflammatory-induced responses, is activated in the 50% of CCA, and IL-6, a known trophic cytokine for

Table 14.2 Genetic aberrations in CCA

Genetic aberrations in CCA			
Class of aberration	Target	Type of aberration	Associated features
Mutations	KRAS	Activating mutation	Present in 5–54% of CCA. More aggressive phenotype.
	TP53	Loss of function	Present in 30% of CCA
Copy number variations	8q, 17q, 20q	Chromosomal gain	
	3p, 4q, 9p, 17q	Chromosomal deletion	
Protein fusions	FGFR2 (kinase domain)		Especially in iCCA
	PRKACA-PRKACB		Especially in pCC/dCCA
Epigenome changes	IDH1-2	Hypermethylation	
	P16		
	SOCS3		
	RASSF1A		
	p14ARF		
	miR200c		Poor prognosis

cholangiocytes, is overexpressed, possibly for the epigenetic silencing of SOCS-3. Moreover, in neoplastic cholangiocytes, several members of EGFR family, responsible for the activation of the MAPK-ERK signalling pathway involved in cell proliferation, have been found mutated. Furthermore, 12–58% of CCA showed an increased expression of c-MET, the tyrosine kinase receptor for hepatocyte growth factor, and finally, several developmental pathways, such as Notch, AKT or Hedgehog signalling pathways are actively involved in the pathogenesis of CCA, acting as adjuvant in hepatocyte malignant transformation or giving them survival advantages [21, 22].

Recently, a genetic study classified CCA in two molecular subgroups: inflammation (40%) and proliferation (60%) with different molecular profiles and clinical outcomes [23]. The first type showed a dominance of inflammation with activation of cytokine-induced pathways and overexpression of IL-6, IL-10 and IL-17 and the permanent activation of STAT3. In the second group, is preeminent the activation of proliferative pathways, such as RAS/MAPK, MET with high level amplifications at 11q13 and deletions at 14q, that correlates with a poor outcome. Further confirmations of this classification are needed before introduction in clinical practice.

As above-mentioned, a prominent actor in CCA is desmoplastic stroma surrounding malignant cells or tumour reactive stroma (TRS). Primarily cancer-associated fibroblasts (CAFs), tumour-associated macrophages (TAMs) and vessels (both blood and lymphatic) compose TRS. Continuous interactions between CCA and stromal cells is a driving mechanism for tumour evolution and for poor response to treatments. Extracellular vesicles containing microRNA appear an important carrier in this intercellular communication, able to trigger fibroblastic differentiation of mesenchymal stem cells that release IL-6 reinforcing CCA overgrowth [24, 25]. CAFs, putatively derived from activated hepatic stellate cells and portal fibroblasts in liver, express α-smooth muscle actin and are able to modulate key malignant processes as proliferation, migration, invasion or epithelial to mesenchymal transition (Fig. 14.3) [26]. TAMs represent the major infiltrating immune cells of the stromal microenvironment in CCA. They originate from circulating monocytes and participate to CCA carcinogenesis activating Wnt-β-catenin signalling stimulating the production of Wnt ligands. Finally, neoangiogenesis is a critical step in CCA progression but interaction between vascular and tumour cells has been poorly investigated yet [27].

14.4 Clinical Features and Pathological Classification

14.4.1 iCCA

Aspecific symptoms and signs that arise in advanced stage of disease characterize clinical course of iCCA. At beginning, iCCA usually develops without severe symptoms and the diagnosis is incidental. With progression, patients could complain malaise, weight loss, fatigue, abdominal discomfort, jaundice, hepatomegaly or palpable abdominal mass. Biliary tract obstruction is rare, whereas increasing of

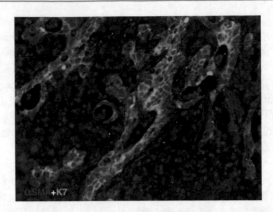

Fig. 14.3 CAF enrichment in cholangiocarcinoma. Cancer-associated fibroblasts (CAFs) closely surround neoplastic bile ducts. In archival samples from surgical resection for CCA, αSMA-positive CAFs (red) are abundantly recruited around neoplastic biliary epithelial cells (K7, green). CAFs lay in close vicinity to tumour cells and are responsible for the rich desmoplasia typical of cholangiocarcinoma. Nuclei of cells are stained with DAPI (blue). Original magnification: 20×

cholestasis enzymes may occur. Besides, night sweat is another common aspecific sign of advanced disease. In the setting of high-risk disease (e.g. cirrhosis, PSC, hepatolithiasis), clinical presentation may be a decompensation with worsening of general conditions, ascites or encephalopathy.

14.4.1.1 Histopathology

iCCA can present three different patterns of growth: mass-forming (MF-iCCA), periductal-infiltrating (PI-iCCA) or intraductal growing (IG-iCCA) (Fig. 14.4). The first type shows a sclerotic nodule with well-defined borders and a radial growth in liver parenchyma. It rates around 60% of iCCA, usually occurs in chronic non-biliary diseases and arises in peripheral small bile ducts. Most of the iCCAs are mass-forming tumour and consist in a single lesion located either in the right (35%) or left (22%) lobe, centrally (12%) or multifocally (35%). Macroscopically, it appears as solid, whitish, not capsuled mass, usually in not cirrhotic liver (70–90%). The PI-type grows in a longitudinal pattern along the bile duct, typically determining strictures, but sometimes it may invade surrounding parenchyma combining feature of PI and MF-iCCA. IG-type shows papillary growth towards duct lumina. PI and IG-iCCAs emerge from large intrahepatic bile ducts, similarly to pCCA and dCCA and are preceded by preneoplastic lesions (Table 14.3). Histologically, iCCAs are highly heterogeneous, despite the use of different nomenclatures, it is possible to summarize two main subtypes: a mixed (bile ductular) adenocarcinoma and a mucinous (bile duct) adenocarcinoma. They reflect their anatomical origin, with mixed adenocarcinoma located more peripherally than the mucinous one. Mixed iCCA presents almost exclusively MF growth pattern, is frequently

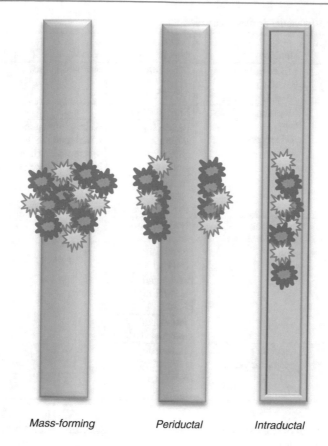

Mass-forming   Periductal   Intraductal

Fig. 14.4 Appearance of CCAs

associated with chronic liver diseases and is not preceded by preinvasive lesions. Mixed iCCA share clinical-pathological similarities with cytokeratin 19-positive hepatocellular carcinoma [4]. Mucinous iCCA could appear as all the three growing patterns, it is much stronger associated with PSC than mixed iCCA and can be preceded by preneoplastic alterations. Interestingly, mucinous iCCA shows phenotypic traits similar to pCCA and pancreatic cancers.

14.4.2 pCCA

Also known as Klatskin tumour, pCCA involves the larger biliary branches up to the common bile duct at the insertion of cystic duct level, including hepatic hilum and biliary confluence of hepatic bile ducts. Acute painless jaundice is the typical hallmark of this type of CCA in up to 90% of patients. A warning signal might be abnormal liver function tests, particularly alkaline phosphatase and serum bilirubin. Morphologically, pCCA and dCCA may appear papillary-like if they contain

Table 14.3 Histopathologic classification

Histopathologic classification	Histology	Pattern of growth	Preneoplastic lesions
iCCA (10%)	Mixed (bile ductular) adenocarcinoma	Mass-forming	Not well known
	Mucinous (bile duct type) adenocarcinoma	Mass-forming	
		Periductal infiltrating Biliary strictures	Biliary intraepithelial neoplasm, intraductal papillary neoplasm, mucinous cystic neoplasm, intraductal tubular neoplasm
		Intraductal growing Papillary growth	
pCCA (60%)	Mucinous adenocarcinoma	Nodular plus periductal infiltrating (>80%)	
		Periductal infiltrating (<10%)	
		Intraductal growing (<10%)	
dCCA (30%)	Mucinous adenocarcinoma	Periductal infiltrating	
		Intraductal growing	

important intraductal component or present a scar-like fibrosis secondary to peri-ductal invasion with stromal desmoplasia.

14.4.2.1 Histopathology

pCCAs are mucinous adenocarcinoma and appear as solid tumours, usually involving hepatic hilum, that cause circumferential stricture of the bile ducts with tendency to radial and longitudinal spreading. pCCAs adopt a nodular plus periductal-infiltrating growth pattern (Fig. 14.4) in more than 80% of cases and show early involvement of lymphatic vessels and direct invasion of liver parenchyma. Pattern similar to PI-iCCA and IG-iCCA could be also are present. IG growing pattern is typically located in the distal bile duct forming a well-defined peduncle; it is usually limited to biliary system, showing a better prognosis after resection than the other CCAs [28, 29] (Table 14.3).

14.4.3 dCCA

Distal CCA includes lesions arising on congenital choledochal cysts and at intrapancreatic bile duct portion. In some cases, advanced cancers may be misdiagnosed as pancreatic primary cancers. This subtype of CCA is often symptomatic for obstruction at early stage.

14.4.3.1 Histopathology

dCCAs are mostly mucinous adenocarcinoma, and sometimes could present PI and IG patterns (Table 14.3) (Fig. 14.4). dCCAs usually present preneoplastic lesions [8].

14.5 Diagnosis

14.5.1 iCCA

iCCA diagnosis needs a multimodal approach, and the coordinated evaluation of imaging studies, onco-markers and biopsy. Even, underlying liver disease changes the diagnostic methods.

14.5.1.1 Imaging

Upper abdominal ultrasound is a first level test to investigate suspicious liver disease; it is able to detect location and extension of biliary obstruction and liver mass. It is used also for screening during follow-up of high-risk patients: six-monthly in cirrhosis, yearly in PSC. Ultrasound is an easily available, low-cost technology with no side effect, but sensibility and specificity are low, and it is strongly operator sensitive. Lesions suspected for iCCA appears as hypoechoic masses with a possible association with peripheral bile ducts dilatation. Hyperenhancement on contrast US can improve sensibility but lacks specificity and leads to a very high rate of misdiagnosis [30]. Generally, US findings need to be confirmed by CT or MR scan [6].

The first step in diagnosis of a suspected iCCA is high quality cross-sectional imaging: a triple-phase contrast-enhanced computed tomography (CT) or multimodal magnetic resonance imaging (MRI).

On CT scan, iCCA presents typical features: hypodense hepatic lesion in the basal CT scan with irregular borders; then, peripheral rim enhancement in the arterial phase with progressive centripetal enhancement throughout all venous and late phases. This pattern is characteristic of fibrosis that is slow to acquire contrast but then withhold it. Therefore, rate and intensity of enhancement depend on the degree of fibrosis. Capsular retraction, biliary dilatation and hepatic atrophy may be present. These classical findings are present in up to 70% of iCCA. In cirrhotic liver with intrahepatic lesion, dynamic CT scan helps to differentiate iCCA from HCC. Indeed, HCC has a different contrast acquisition behaviour, characterized by rapid contrast uptake in the arterial phase and contrast washout in the venous or delayed phases [31].

MRI is the imaging technique of choice because of the best resolution of tumour extent, blood vessels and biliary ducts due to its intrinsically high tissue contrast. iCCA is visualized as a hypointense mass in T1-weighted and hyperintense in T2-weighted images. Furthermore, T2-w images allow a better definition of the fibrosis surrounding CCA that is shown as central hypodensity [32]. Dynamic images show the same CT scan contrast pattern. However, a strong enhancing rim and irregular shape in MRI contrast images suggest a mixed hepatocellular-cholangiocarcinoma. MR cholangiopancreatography (MRCP) increases the resolution of ductal systems and blood vessels and can define the exact tumour extension with the same predictive value of endoscopic retrograde cholangiopancreatography (ERCP) or percutaneous transhepatic cholangiography (PTC), being relevant to plan surgical interventions.

The role of FDG-PET and PET/CT is controversial [2, 3]. These techniques present good sensitivity but lacks on specificity. They may present many false positives in disease presenting nonspecific tissue inflammation, e.g. PSC or biliary stents. Even, false-negativity is also possible when CCA is not FDG-avid. In the staging of the disease, PET presents very good sensitivity for ruling out occult metastasis, particularly lymph node involvement. Anyway, the relevance of its role is still not well defined in the diagnostic process.

14.5.1.2 Biomarkers

Serum biomarkers could have a diagnostic value even if their sensitivity and specificity is still moderate. CA 19.9 is used also as part of screening strategy in follow-up of high-risk disease, PSC and cirrhosis. However, its increases can overlap with benign conditions as biliary obstruction and bacterial cholangitis. Some studies in PSC patients consider suspicious for iCCA, a CA19.9 cut-off of 129 IU/mL; values greater than 1000 IU/ml are instead consistent with advanced disease. Even in this setting, 10% of population presents undetectable CA19.9 levels. Biosynthesis of this marker is catalysed, in its last passages, by two proteins called Secretor and Lewis enzyme and encoded by fucosyltransferase (FUT) 2 and 3. These proteins also define individual Lewis blood group. Recent studies focused on association between variants of FUT 2-3 and different levels of CA19.9. Genotyping of FUT 2-3 may predict low, intermediate or high CA19.9 biosynthesis levels, helping to select patients suitable for screening testing CA19.9 levels. Moreover, a relevant association was found between the subgroup incapable of CA19.9 synthesis and high CEA serum levels, suggesting an influence of FUT2 genotype. Moreover, CEA is not influenced by bacterial cholangitis, thus combining FUT genotyping with CA19.9 and CEA serum levels might be a future interesting strategy for CCA screening, especially in PSC [33].

Alpha-feto protein (AFP) might be elevated in mixed HCC-CCA, other than HCC. Researches on identification of snippets of mRNA and non-coding RNA associated to iCCA in blood or other biological samples are in progress but preliminary data seem to be promising.

14.5.1.3 Biopsy

According to WHO classification of biliary tract cancer, iCCA is an adenocarcinoma, less frequently a mucinous carcinoma. More specifically, it is an adenocarcinoma with tubular and papillary structures surrounded by variable fibrous stroma. Histological diagnosis is necessary for a definitive diagnosis of iCCA. Nevertheless, in clinical practice, percutaneous biopsy is not always required for the risk of tumour seeding, that is still not well quantified, at present. Biopsy is crucial in the study of intrahepatic mass with atypical features for HCC in cirrhotic liver, or in the assessment of the best treatment in case of inoperable suspected iCCA in not cirrhotic liver. Biopsy aims to differentiate benign from malignant lesions. Differentiating iCCA from HCC and metastasis of another primary site is tricky. An immunohistochemical panel containing cytokeratin K7, K19, pCEA, hep-par 1, Moc 31 and glypican 3 showed to be useful to exclude HCC. Moreover, S100p may help to differentiate CCA from benign lesion. Sensitivity of biopsy depends on different aspects: localization, size, and expertise of the pathologist. A negative biopsy could not exclude a diagnosis because of the possibility of sampling mistakes.

14.5.2 pCCA

Diagnostic assessment includes laboratory exams, imaging, endoscopy and pathology. Basic blood tests could outline obstructive jaundice that usually is the presenting sign of CCA and the different stage of liver insufficiency. Serum concentration of IgG4 should be obtained in order to rule out IgG4-related cholangiopathy [34, 35]. Onco-markers (CA19.9, CEA) have the same role than in iCCA; they can be elevated due to hyperbilirubinemia, thus, they need to be repeated after biliary decompression.

14.5.2.1 Imaging

On ultrasound, the presence of dilated intrahepatic ducts with abrupt stricture or cutoff at hepatic duct bifurcation could be suggestive of pCCA; lobar atrophy and vascular invasion can also be detected. Cross-sectional imaging is needed to outline pCCA location, size, morphology, caudate involvement, and volume of potential remnant liver parenchyma, hepatic artery and portal vein invasion, presence of intrahepatic, nodal or distant metastasis [6]. Contrast-enhanced CT scan or MRI presents similar accuracy for evaluation of the degree of bile duct involvement, sensitivity and specificity of major vessels or nodal invasion (Fig. 14.5). CT often is not able to recognize peritoneal metastasis and sensitivity for nodal involvement is low, while it enables a better assessment of vascular invasion. MRI coupled with MR cholangiopancreatography (MRCP) improves definition of the bile duct lesion allowing a better assessment of the extension and, even, the possibility to rule out benign causes of hilar obstruction. MRCP can give a complete reconstruction of biliary tree, also in patients with complete biliary obstruction that contraindicates guidewire placement during ERCP. Diagnostic and staging accuracy of both techniques can be affected by biliary stent placement, particularly if metallic, due to artefacts and secondary inflammatory changes. However, the number and quality of studies investigating on imaging in pCCA remain modest. FDG-PET has low sensitivity because of low FDG-avidity of pCCA, whereas PET/CT has a good specificity in detecting nodal and distant metastasis but rarely adds information to other cross-sectional imaging test [36].

14.5.2.2 Endoscopy

Endoscopic retrograde cholangiopancreatography (ERCP) is a mainstay procedure in the initial evaluation. It has both diagnostic and therapeutic potential [37].

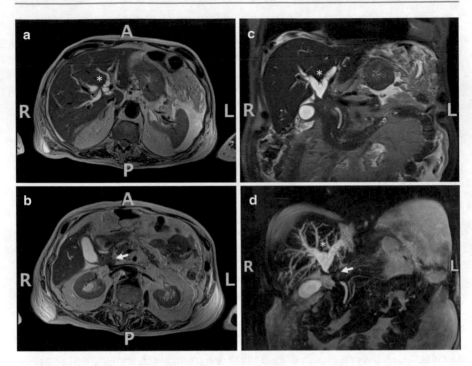

Fig. 14.5 MRCP showing pCCA/dCCA in an 80-year-old. (**a–d**) T2W axial and coronal images show bile tree dilation upstream common hepatic duct (asterisks) due to hypodense soft tissue (arrow) involving common hepatic, cystic and common bile duct

Similarly, percutaneous transhepatic cholangiography (PTC) helps to visualize strictures not accessible by ERCP. On diagnostic side, ERCP allows excellent visualization of bile ducts and biliary brushing for histologic analysis. Moreover, endoscope can carry on ultrasonography to investigate depth of mass, vascular structure invasion and eventual lymph node involvement, with the possibility of nodal fine-needle aspiration in suspicious case. Endoscopic ultrasound alone presents a higher rate of tumour detection than CT or MRI, with a preference for dCCA versus pCCA. A specific type of endoscopic ultrasound is intraductal ultrasonography (IDUS), obtained using small calibre, high frequency ultrasound probe introduced via the working channel of a standard duodenoscope. It is useful to distinguish benign from malignant strictures detecting disruption of bile duct wall; combining IDUS with ERCP increases diagnostic accuracy to more than 90%. Furthermore, in PSC patients endoscopic choledochoscopy can be useful to locate and direct biopsy on dominant strictures. Lastly, laser endomicroscopy is an emerging technology; a confocal laser probe fixed on standard ERCP catheter or choledochoscope allows the visualization of very high-resolution images of the mucosal layer [38]. Invasive cholangiography techniques are burdened by the possibility of technical failure and the risk of complications, like duodenal perforation, bile leaks, cholangitis, bleeding and pancreatitis. Tissue sampling should be avoided in patients who are possible surgical candidates for risk of tumour seeding [39].

14.5.2.3 Cytology and Pathology

Samples, obtained through endoscopic brushing, are examined by conventional cytology and fluorescence in situ hybridisation (FISH). Due to fibrotic and paucicellular nature of CCA, potentially located in inaccessible tracts of biliary tree, cytology results positive only in 40% of pCCA patients but FISH analysis could increase the sensitivity; it targets pericentromeric regions of chromosome 3, 7, 17 searching for aneusomy (gains or losses of chromosomal regions). Presence of polysomy diagnose malignancy with moderate sensitivity (50%) but good specificity (95%) [40, 41]. In PSC patients, positivity for serial polysomy identifies high-risk patients and could show lesions up to 2.7 years before they are evident at imaging [42]. Emerging techniques to improve cytological diagnostic accuracy are next-generation sequencing (NGS), study of extracellular vesicles (EVs) and circulating tumour DNA (ctDNA) or cell-free DNA. NGS can improve sensitivity of cytology and identify driver mutations, including KRAS, TP 53 and CDKN2A aberrations [43]. EVs are present in many biological fluids, including bile, where they broker intercellular communications. EVs are filled of microRNAs (miRNAs) that is associated to malignancy [24, 25]. On the other hand, EVs contain high levels of oncogenic proteins that are available for study with a separate proteomic analysis. Moreover, patients with malignant bile strictures might have a significantly greater concentration of EVs in bile than those with benign stenosis [44]. Finally, ctDNA serum concentration appeared to correlate with tumour size and stage; thus, soon, liquid biopsy may be a potential diagnostic and staging approach [45, 46].

Other types of biopsy, percutaneous or laparoscopic, are discouraged for high risk of tumour seeding [39]. Finally, definitive diagnosis is pathological also for pCCA but it is mandatory only before a systemic chemo- or radio-treatment, after exclusion of resection or transplantation protocols.

14.5.3 dCCA

On ultrasound, suspected dCCA appears as dilated intra- and extrahepatic ducts. Diagnostic work-up overlaps with pCCA.

14.5.3.1 Differential Diagnosis
Main differential diagnosis are listed in Table 14.4.

14.6 Staging

14.6.1 iCCA

Histologic tumour grading ranges from well differentiated to undifferentiated according to the presence of gland components; this classification is shared by all CCAs (Table 14.5). Tumour grade is an important independent prognostic factor of survival and recurrence.

Table 14.4 Main differential diagnosis

	iCCA	pCCA	dCCA
Benignancies	• Bile ducts proliferation	• Benign strictures (PSC, IgG4-related) • Choledocholithiasis	
Malignancies	• Primary liver cancer (HCC, epithelioid hemangioendothelioma) • Metastasis	• Extension of gallbladder cancer or iCCA	• Extension of gallbladder cancer or iCCA • Pancreatic adenocarcinoma

Table 14.5 Grading classification [48]

Grading classification	
G1	Well differentiated
G2	Moderately differentiated
G3	Poorly differentiated
G4	Undifferentiated

Recently, iCCA gained its own staging system [47–49]. In fact, up to the seventh edition of the American Joint Committee on Cancer/International Union Against Cancer (AJCC/IUCC) staging manual in 2010, it was classified as primary liver cancer, according to HCC staging criteria. In order to decide treatment, pathologists are waiting for a different staging system accounting of the several differences between iCCA and HCC. In particular, tumour dimension is not a prognostic factor for CCA and growth patterns are different from HCC. The Tumour-Node-Metastasis (TNM) classification has been validated by using multivariate analysis of outcome and survival data from single- and multi-centre studies. Current classification, the eighth edition, is effective from the beginning of 2018. T classification of invasive iCCA is based on the presence of single vs. multiple tumours, vascular invasion and peritoneal perforation. Satellitosis, intrahepatic metastasis and multifocal lesions are considered multiple tumours. Vascular invasion is present when either major vessels, portal vein or sovrahepatic veins, or microscopic intraparenchymal blood vessel are interested. Besides, direct invasion of adjacent organ, as colon, stomach, duodenum, common bile duct, diaphragm, abdominal wall, is still considered a T3 disease not a metastasis. The N classification includes involvement of regional lymph nodes as N1 disease. Collecting at least 6 lymph nodes is suggested for complete N staging. For right liver (Segments 5–8), regional nodes are hilar, peri-duodenal and peripancreatic lymph nodes, whereas for left liver (Segments 2–4) hilar and gastro-hepatic. Instead, celiac, periaortic and caval lymph nodes involvement counts as distal metastasis, M1 disease. iCCA spread disease can involve intrahepatic metastasis classified, as said, in T subgroup and to peritoneum, distal lymph nodes, lungs and pleura classified as M1 disease (Tables 14.6 and 14.7).

Clinical staging is mainly based on extensive imaging procedure aiming to fully define local but also distal extension of the disease. In cirrhotic patients, it is necessary to calculate Child–Pugh class and MELD score. When a surgical treatment of complete resection is possible and residual liver is sufficient, a surgical exploration

Table 14.6 TNM classification [48]

TNM classification	iCCA	pCCA	dCCA
Tx	Primary tumour cannot be assessed		
Tis	Intraductal tumour	Carcinoma in situ/high grade dysplasia	
T1	A: Single tumour ≤5 cm without vascular invasion	Tumour confined to the bile duct, extended up to the muscle layer or fibrous tissue	Tumour invades the bile duct wall with a depth <5 mm
	B: Single tumour >5 cm without vascular invasion		
T2	Single tumour with vascular invasion or multiple tumours	2A: Tumour invades beyond the wall of the bile duct to surrounding adipose tissue	Tumour invades the bile duct wall with a depth of 5–12 mm
		2B: Tumour invades adjacent hepatic parenchyma	
T3	Tumour perforating visceral peritoneum	Tumour invades unilateral branches of the portal vein or hepatic artery	Tumour invades the bile duct wall with a depth >12 mm
T4	Tumour involving local extrahepatic structures by direct invasion	Tumour invades the main portal vein or its branches bilaterally, or the common hepatic artery; or unilateral second-order biliary radicals with contralateral portal vein or hepatic artery involvement	Tumour involves the celiac axis, superior mesenteric artery, and/or common hepatic artery
Nx	Regional lymph nodes cannot be assessed		
N0	Regional lymph nodes metastasis absent		
N1	Regional lymph nodes metastasis present	One to three positive regional lymph nodes	
N2		Four or more positive lymph nodes from the sites described for N1	
M0	Distal metastasis absent		
M1	Distal metastasis present		

Table 14.7 Anatomic-prognostic staging intrahepatic cholangiocarcinoma [48]

Anatomic-prognostic staging iCCA			
Stage 0	Tis	N0	M0
Stage 1a	T1a	N0	M0
Stage 1b	T1b	N0	M0
Stage 2	T2	N0	M0
Stage 3a	T3	N0	M0
Stage 3b	Any T	Any N	M0
Stage 4	Any T	Any N	M1

staging is indicated [50]. Definitive staging is carried out analysing the surgical specimen. Limitations of this staging classification are that it is derived from surgical series, thus it is most valid for surgically treated patients; furthermore, it still lacks level 1 evidence.

14.6.2 pCCA

Historically, Bismuth and Corlette first set criteria to classify pCCA according to extension along bile duct and involvement of the hilum. Afterwards, their classification was modified into four subtypes giving recommendation for type of surgical resection: in subtype I stricture involves bile duct below main hepatic confluence; in subtype II stricture involves the confluence; in subtype III the disease is extended up to main right (IIIA) or left (IIIB) hepatic duct; finally, in subtype IV pCCA involves both hepatic ducts. Limitations of this classification are that it does not consider neither vascular nor nodal involvement, becoming unsuitable to predict resectability and survival.

More frequently, pCCA is classified according to AJCC TNM staging system [47–49]. Since the seventh edition of the AJCC staging manual, it is separated from dCCA (Tables 14.6 and 14.8). T classification relies on level of disease infiltration in the surrounding structures. Involvement of adjacent liver parenchyma showed a better prognosis than vascular invasion, so it is classified as T2. Besides, T4 means a disease involving bilaterally hepatic vascular structures or the second degree of bile ducts; in some selected cases, it is still possible to consider a protocol for active treatment.

Nodal spreading increases lineally with the worsening of T grading, typically involving hilar, cystic duct, common bile duct, hepatic artery, posterior pancreato-duodenal and portal vein lymph nodes. Involvement up to three regional lymph node (N1) showed a better prognosis than more (N2).

Dissemination goes along perineural and periductal lymphatic channels, thus, liver is frequently venue of metastasis, whereas involvement of extrahepatic organs (e.g. peritoneum, bone, brain, lung) is uncommon [50].

Table 14.8 Anatomic-prognostic staging perihilar cholangiocarcinoma [48]

Anatomic-prognostic staging pCCA			
Stage 0	Tis	N0	M0
Stage 1	T1	N0	M0
Stage 2	T2a-b	N0	M0
Stage 3a	T3	N0	M0
Stage 3b	T4	N0	M0
Stage 3c	Any T	N1	M1
Stage 4a	Any T	N2	M0
Stage 4b	Any T	Any N	M1

Table 14.9 Anatomic-prognostic staging distal cholangiocarcinoma [48]

Anatomic-prognostic staging dCCA			
Stage 0	Tis	N0	M0
Stage 1	T1	N0	M0
Stage 2a	T1	N1	M0
	T2	N0	
Stage 2b	T2	N1	M0
	T3	N0-1	
Stage 3a	T1-3	N2	M0
Stage 3b	T4	N0-2	M0
Stage 4	Any T	Any N	M1

14.6.3 dCCA

Bile duct wall is made by three concentric layers: a mucosal, a subepithelial and a fibromuscular one. It lacks a serosa and it is enveloped by adventitial adipose tissue. Invasion of this tissue is classified as extension beyond the bile duct. In the last AJCC staging classification [47–49], T subgroups changed from description of anatomic extent to the depth of invasion (<5, 5–12, >12 mm), that proved to be stronger associated to overall survival.

Nodal staging is crucial for outcome and would require the excision of at least 12 regional lymph nodes. Regional lymph nodes are the same for dCCA as for carcinoma of the head of pancreas. Direct invasion can involve pancreas, duodenum, stomach, colon and omentum. Furthermore, distant metastasis is found in lung, liver and peritoneum (Tables 14.6 and 14.9).

14.7 Treatment

14.7.1 iCCA

14.7.1.1 Surgery

Surgical resection is the cornerstone of the treatment of iCCA and is the only treatment that could aim to be curative. The goal is to obtain a margin-free (R0) resection, preserving sufficient liver volume. In most series, extended hepatectomy, resection and reconstruction of extrahepatic bile duct was considered necessary to obtain R0 resection [5]. Preoperative work-up is crucial to select patient with the features to undergo surgery. Identifying morphologic subtype has a prognostic value, as defining local extent and excluding nodal or distal organs involvement. Surgery is to consider for disease at TNM stage I or II. In case of liver cirrhosis, restrictions for surgery are the same for HCC. Limited data are present on role of staging laparoscopy. Highly specialized hepatobiliary centres are able to keep perioperative mortality under 5%.

Besides, routine lymphadenectomy is another controversial point. If resection of suspicious lymph nodes is mandatory, nodal dissection is not routinely performed yet, in Western rather than East Asian countries. Some recent series showed a prevalence up to 30% of nodal involvement in patients that underwent lymphadenectomy. Since this is the most critical prognostic factor of poor outcome, lymphadenectomy is suggested together with surgery.

Outcomes still are poor and the reported median disease-free survival is 26 months while recurrence rate reaches 50–60% of patients. Relapses occur mainly on liver (e.g. 50–60%) but also at nodal or peritoneal level (e.g. 20–25%). For a small subgroup of patients with only liver recurrence, a loco-regional treatment or a re-resection could be considered. Five-year survival and overall survival after surgery vary from 15% to 40% according to most series. Several factors determine recurrence risk, the most relevant appeared to be nodal involvement and hepatic extent of the disease (Table 14.10) [51]. A multidisciplinary team should evaluate borderline stage for surgery in order to make decision about therapy. Adjuvant treatment is strongly suggested after resection, nevertheless, there is no established chemotherapy protocol, and several randomized trials are ongoing [8].

Liver transplantation (LT) for iCCA is, at the moment, not recommended neither for iCCA nor for mixed hepatocellular-CCA. Published data collect small series, different criteria of patient selection, different neoadjuvant and adjuvant treatments, and different outcomes. Anyway, overall outcomes are worse than cirrhotic or HCC patients [52, 53]. Further studies on standardized selection criteria and adjuvant/neoadjuvant treatment are needed [54].

14.7.1.2 Loco-Regional Therapy

Local extended disease, beyond surgical criteria, may be treated with loco-regional treatment aiming to relieve symptoms and perhaps to prolong survival [55]. Data are constrained by small and mixed studies but no standard of care is available yet. Radiation therapy seems to show palliative advantages and can be considered in researches for multidisciplinary, adjuvant protocols and treatment in localized

Table 14.10 Negative prognostic factors in CCA [48]

	iCCA	pCCA	dCCA
Tumour features	• Multiple tumours • Vascular invasion • Periductal-infiltrating pattern	• Histologic grading • Tumour extension • Sclerosing or nodular subtypes	• Histologic grading • Tumour extension • Vascular invasion • Lymphatic invasion • Perineural invasion
Patient features	• Chronic liver disease • High levels of CA19.9	• Chronic liver disease	• High level of CA19.9
Post-surgical features	• Lymph node involvement • Positive surgical margins	• Lymph node involvement • Positive surgical margins	• Lymph node involvement • Positive surgical margins

unresectable iCCA [56, 57]. Coping with trans-arterial chemoembolization (TACE) and radioembolization (TARE) experience for HCC, limited data showed a positive effect with acceptable toxicities also in locally advanced iCCA [58, 59]. Radiofrequency ablation is an option for small (<3 cm) single lesions when surgery is not possible [60].

14.7.1.3 Systemic Therapy

Cisplatin plus gemcitabine is the first line systemic therapy for patients in good general conditions (ECOG 0-1) with advanced metastatic disease [61]. There is no evidence of effectiveness for a second line treatment after disease progression. Research is fully working on biological therapies that could be a breakthrough in improving outcomes for unresectable disease.

14.7.2 pCCA

14.7.2.1 Surgery

Surgical resection is the treatment that ensures the best long-term survival in pCCA. Different surgical techniques have been employed according to the disease extension. This is a challenging operation, often involving liver right or left lobectomy, caudate lobectomy, bile duct removal, regional lymphadenopathy resection and Roux-en-Y hepaticojejunostomy [28, 29]. Advances in surgical techniques include implementation of extended liver lobectomy, vascular reconstruction and preoperative portal vein embolization (PVE) [62]. Long-term prognosis is poor even after resection due to loco-regional recurrence and distant metastasis (Table 14.10). Thus, patient selection through preoperative assessment is a crucial step [50]. Positive lymph nodes are not absolute surgical contraindication but worsen prognosis. Criteria to set unresectability in nonmetastatic pCCA are bilateral segmental ductal extension, unilateral atrophy with either contralateral segmental ductal or vascular, unilateral segmental ductal extension with contralateral vascular invasion. Preoperatively, patient fitness is assessed for major hepatic resection; right hepatectomy or extended resection is at risk of post-hepatectomy liver failure as a consequence of insufficient or not functional liver remnant [7], the percentage of remaining functional liver volume compared with preoperative one [63]. Its estimation is done by imaging algorithms; other available tests for functional assessment are indocyanine green clearance, galactose elimination test, lidocaine-monoethylglycinexylidide test and ^{13}C-aminopyrine breath test [64]. In healthy livers, remnant liver ≥20% is associated with good surgical outcome, whereas in steatosis or cholestasis liver remnant should be ≥30–40%. Furthermore, there are some preoperative strategies to optimize functional liver remnant. Portal vein embolization is able to cause contralateral liver hypertrophy within 3–4 weeks, but it needs a favourable vascular anatomy. Another possible technique is related to portal vein ligation and in situ liver splitting; the main advantages are the quick liver regeneration but is still burdened by high morbidity and mortality. Unfortunately, up to 50% of patients are unresectable at diagnosis and margin-free (R0) resection is achieved only in 70–80% of resected patients, showing that improvements in diagnostic and preoperative work-up still are needed. Median survival after resection is 11–38 months, 5-year survival rates after surgery range from 25% to 50% with long-term survival limited by loco-regional recurrence or distant metastasis [65]. Patients with microscopic (R1) or gross (R2) positive margins have a significantly worse prognosis with median survival ranging from 12 to 21 months. Biliary drainage before surgery is controversial [66]; obstruction impacts on functional liver remnant, on renal function and on general patient fitness, but on the other side, drainage could favour cholangitis causing a delay in treatment. PTC is usually preferred to ERCP because of a better focus on tumour spread, a faster liver enzyme normalization and less cholangitis-related complications. Another option is biliary stenting that can be utilized both in preoperative management and in palliative care [67]. In the first case, plastic or covered self-expandable metal stents are suggested because they prevent cancer progression and don't interfere with surgery or radiotherapy. In inoperable disease, uncovered metal stents, draining more than 50% liver parenchyma, showed an improvement in patient survival, but once placed, they cannot be removed. This procedure may undergo complication with infectious cholangitis, possible cholecystitis or pancreatitis and is also possible the dislocation of the devise, mostly for plastic or covered metal stents. The role of adjuvant treatment still needs further definition. Adjuvant chemotherapy or chemoradiation treatment is offered to patients with margin-positive or lymph node-positive but no standard of care has been set [9, 68].

Liver transplantation preceded by neoadjuvant radio-chemotherapy is also a possibility for highly selected patients, also in advanced T4-disease [53, 69–71]. Indications are unresectable pCCA with <3 cm radial diameter without intra-/extrahepatic metastasis. Neoadjuvant protocol involves chemotherapy (5-fluorouracil (5-FU)) with radiation (external beam radiation with or without endoluminal brachytherapy boost) followed by oral capecitabine [72]. Diagnostic laparoscopy is performed to rule out metastasis. This approach reaches the best outcome with 5-year recurrence-free survival of 68% of patients, with higher rates in PSC patients, at the same rates of transplanted patients for other indications. Liver transplantation, if possible, is the first choice in PSC in order to remove the neoplastic chronic trigger and to avoid chronic liver disease progression. Indeed, in PSC patients it is not rare to find dysplastic lesions histologically classified as CCA during liver explants.

14.7.2.2 Advanced Disease

Systemic treatment with gemcitabine and cisplatin is a possibility in patients not eligible for resection or transplantation [61]. Since CCA is frequently resistant to treatment, association therapy is suggested in clinical practice. Bilateral biliary stenting is indicated before starting systemic treatment. A metal stent is the first option if life expectancy is more than 4–6 months because it showed to improve survival and to have a minor dislocation rate rather than plastic one [73]. Another palliative possibility is endoscopic intraductal radiofrequency ablation; complication rate is acceptable, but this procedure is still under development [74].

In patients with advanced pCCA and dCCA, systemic chemotherapy did not show to improve survival [75], thus enrolment in clinical trial of new treatments could be considered.

14.7.3 dCCA

14.7.3.1 Surgery

The only curative option is surgical resection, as other types of CCA. dCCA is treated as pancreatic adenocarcinoma with a pancreaticoduodenectomy. The aim is to reach a R0 resection with a focus on assessment of margins also with intraoperative frozen sections. Neoadjuvant treatment is suggested in borderline resettable disease. In patients with involvement of a short tract of portal or mesenteric vein, resection and reconstruction is performed with similar long-term survival [76]. Lymphadenectomy is also needed during surgery. Adjuvant treatment with chemoradiation is indicated in case of R1-2 or positive lymph nodes [77]. After surgical treatment, patients show a median survival of around 2 years, while survival at 5 years ranges between 20% and 40% [78] (Table 14.10). Compared to patient with localized pancreatic adenocarcinoma, similar patient with dCCA who undergo surgery, have a better survival. Unresectable disease is treated by systemic chemotherapy with gemcitabine plus cisplatin, but prognosis is shorter than 12 months.

14.8 Future Directions

Research programmes on diagnostics are looking for new biomarkers able to impact on earlier diagnosis. Currently, investigation strands are focusing on finding of CCA genetic marks in different biologic samples (e.g. serum, bile or stool) and improving cytology using advanced techniques (e.g. spectrometry, proteome analysis).

Technological advances have improved safety and effectiveness of radiotherapy: high-resolution multiphase CT and multiparametric MRI ensure accurate disease localization and extension and allow precise radiotherapy targeting. Moreover, new radiation techniques are emerging, as 3D conformal radiotherapy, intensity-modulated radiotherapy or charged particle (proton or carbon) beams, and allow centralizing radiation only on malignant tissue, sparing healthy tissue.

Ongoing advancements on understanding molecular pathways that drive CCA progression are the key to direct research to find new approaches for systemic and adjuvant treatments able to affect its terrible prognosis. Better comprehension of tumour microenvironment, stromal cells and their secreted extracellular proteins recently updated their roles in cancer pathogenesis. They play specific role in controlling tumour growth, progression and metastatization, overcoming the concept of inanimate barrier. Marked intertumoural and intratumoural heterogeneity makes difficult to find targeted therapies. Molecular profiling studies have better described genomics and transcriptomics of different CCA subtypes. Potentially targetable genetic driver alterations have been detected in about 40% of patients. Recurrent mutations in IDH1-1, FGFR1-2-3, EPHA2 and BAP1 were noted in iCCAs, while ARID1B, ELF3, PBRM1 and PRKACA-B mutations were detected mainly in pCCA/dCCA. Therapeutic agents under ongoing or recently completed trials are summarized in Table 14.11 [8]. Several selective and non-selective inhibitors of FGFRs are currently under investigation in early phase clinical trial [9]. Inhibition of HSP90 is an alternative target to directly inhibit FGFR-kinase [79]. ROS1, ALK and MEK are other kinase fusion proteins sensitive to monoclonal inhibitors [9]. In addition, epigenetic therapies are a promising target to silence mutations like at IDH1-2 level [9, 80]. Furthermore, tumour microenvironment is a pivotal player in CCA progression and cancer-associated fibroblasts (CAFs) are involved in progression, spreading and chemoresistance [81]. CAFs are involved in crosstalk with tumour microenvironment through paracrine and autocrine signalling that rules growth and development pathways. Among innate immune cells, TAMs also play a role in CCA development. Moreover, finding of α-SMA, hallmark of CAFs, or high density of TAMs has been associated with worse prognosis in iCCA. In preclinical models, BH3 mimetic navitoclax showed promising results striking CAFs [82], whereas depletion of TAMs or inhibition of Wnt signalling might reduce

Table 14.11 Therapeutic agents under clinical trials (Adapted from [8])

Class	Drug	Target
Chemotherapeutic agents	Gemcitabine–cisplatin	
	Fluorouracil–cisplatin	
	Capecitabine	
	Gemcitabine–oxaliplatin	
	mFOLFOX	
Targeted therapies	Cetuximab, erlotinib, panitumumab	EGFR
	Bevacizumab, cediranib, sorafenib, vandetanib	VEGF
	Lapatinib	ERB2
	Selumetinib, trametinib	MEK
	Dasatinib, imatinib, pazopanib, regorafenib, sorafenib, sunitinib	Multi-tyrosine kinase
	Cabozantinib	c-MET–VEGF
	Everolimus	mTOR
	BKM120	PI3K
	Ponatinib	FGFR
	Trastuzumab	HER2
	MK2206	AKT
	AG-221	IDH2
Preclinical agents	ABT-199, navitoclax (BH3 domain)	BH3 domain
	Gefitinib	EGFR
	KB9520	ERβ agonist
	BGJ398	FGFR2–PPHLN1 fusion gene
	Cyclopamine, vismodegib	Hedgehog pathway
	Others	

proliferation and stimulate apoptosis. Tumour microenvironment creates immunosuppressive milieu allowing cancer to escape from immune system control; the exact mechanisms underlying this phenomenon remain unknown, but immunotherapy is another chapter of research with promising results. Immune checkpoints inhibitor antibodies blocking interactions at CTLA-4 or PD-1 level and their ligands showed strong and durable antitumoural activity with low toxicity in a subset of patients affected by different types of cancer [9, 83, 84].

In conclusion, in future trials patients should be stratified according to genetic drivers and disease subtypes. Extensive crosstalk and interactions among several signalling pathways confirmed once again the importance of combination therapy.

References

1. Global Burden of Disease Cancer Collaboration, Fitzmaurice C, Abate D, Abbasi N, Abbastabar H, Abd-Allah F, et al. Global, regional, and national cancer incidence, mortality, years of life lost, years lived with disability, and disability-adjusted life-years for 29 cancer groups, 1990 to 2017: a systematic analysis for the global burden of disease study. JAMA Oncol. 2019;5:1749.
2. Bridgewater J, Galle PR, Khan SA, Llovet JM, Park J-W, Patel T, et al. Guidelines for the diagnosis and management of intrahepatic cholangiocarcinoma. J Hepatol. 2014;60(6):1268–89.
3. Razumilava N, Gores GJ. Cholangiocarcinoma. Lancet. 2014;383(9935):2168–79.
4. Komuta M, Govaere O, Vandecaveye V, Akiba J, Van Steenbergen W, Verslype C, et al. Histological diversity in cholangiocellular carcinoma reflects the different cholangiocyte phenotypes. Hepatology. 2012;55(6):1876–88.
5. DeOliveira ML, Cunningham SC, Cameron JL, Kamangar F, Winter JM, Lillemoe KD, et al. Cholangiocarcinoma: thirty-one-year experience with 564 patients at a single institution. Ann Surg. 2007;245(5):755–62.
6. Oliveira IS, Kilcoyne A, Everett JM, Mino-Kenudson M, Harisinghani MG, Ganesan K. Cholangiocarcinoma: classification, diagnosis, staging, imaging features, and management. Abdom Radiol (NY). 2017;42(6):1637–49.
7. Khan AS, Dageforde LA. Cholangiocarcinoma. Surg Clin N Am. 2019;99(2):315–35.
8. Banales JM, Cardinale V, Carpino G, Marzioni M, Andersen JB, Invernizzi P, et al. Cholangiocarcinoma: current knowledge and future perspectives consensus statement from the European Network for the Study of Cholangiocarcinoma (ENS-CCA). Nat Rev Gastroenterol Hepatol. 2016;13(5):261–80.
9. Rizvi S, Khan SA, Hallemeier CL, Kelley RK, Gores GJ. Cholangiocarcinoma - evolving concepts and therapeutic strategies. Nat Rev Clin Oncol. 2018;15(2):95–111.
10. Khan SA, Emadossadaty S, Ladep NG, Thomas HC, Elliott P, Taylor-Robinson SD, et al. Rising trends in cholangiocarcinoma: is the ICD classification system misleading us? J Hepatol. 2012;56(4):848–54.
11. Tyson GL, El-Serag HB. Risk factors for cholangiocarcinoma. Hepatology. 2011;54(1):173–84.
12. Kaewpitoon N, Kaewpitoon S-J, Pengsaa P, Sripa B. Opisthorchis viverrini: the carcinogenic human liver fluke. World J Gastroenterol. 2008;14(5):666–74.
13. Palmer WC, Patel T. Are common factors involved in the pathogenesis of primary liver cancers? A meta-analysis of risk factors for intrahepatic cholangiocarcinoma. J Hepatol. 2012;57(1):69–76.
14. Chapman MH, Webster GJM, Bannoo S, Johnson GJ, Wittmann J, Pereira SP. Cholangiocarcinoma and dominant strictures in patients with primary sclerosing cholangitis: a 25-year single-centre experience. Eur J Gastroenterol Hepatol. 2012;24(9):1051–8.
15. Razumilava N, Gores GJ, Lindor KD. Cancer surveillance in patients with primary sclerosing cholangitis. Hepatology. 2011;54(5):1842–52.

16. He X-D, Wang L, Liu W, Liu Q, Qu Q, Li B-L, et al. The risk of carcinogenesis in congenital choledochal cyst patients: an analysis of 214 cases. Ann Hepatol. 2014;13(6):819–26.
17. Labib PL, Goodchild G, Pereira SP. Molecular pathogenesis of cholangiocarcinoma. BMC Cancer. 2019;19:185. https://www.ncbi.nlm.nih.gov/pmc/articles/PMC6394015/. Accessed 28 Jan 2020.
18. Welzel TM, Graubard BI, Zeuzem S, El-Serag HB, Davila JA, McGlynn KA. Metabolic syndrome increases the risk of primary liver cancer in the United States: a study in the SEER-Medicare database. Hepatology. 2011;54(2):463–71.
19. Lozano E, Sanchez-Vicente L, Monte MJ, Herraez E, Briz O, Banales JM, et al. Cocarcinogenic effects of intrahepatic bile acid accumulation in cholangiocarcinoma development. Mol Cancer Res. 2014;12(1):91–100.
20. Dill MT, Tornillo L, Fritzius T, Terracciano L, Semela D, Bettler B, et al. Constitutive Notch2 signaling induces hepatic tumors in mice. Hepatology. 2013;57(4):1607–19.
21. Andersen JB, Thorgeirsson SS. Genetic profiling of intrahepatic cholangiocarcinoma. Curr Opin Gastroenterol. 2012;28(3):266–72.
22. Borger DR, Tanabe KK, Fan KC, Lopez HU, Fantin VR, Straley KS, et al. Frequent mutation of isocitrate dehydrogenase (IDH)1 and IDH2 in cholangiocarcinoma identified through broad-based tumor genotyping. Oncologist. 2012;17(1):72–9.
23. Sia D, Hoshida Y, Villanueva A, Roayaie S, Ferrer J, Tabak B, et al. Integrative molecular analysis of intrahepatic cholangiocarcinoma reveals 2 classes that have different outcomes. Gastroenterology. 2013;144(4):829–40.
24. Arbelaiz A, Azkargorta M, Krawczyk M, Santos-Laso A, Lapitz A, Perugorria MJ, et al. Serum extracellular vesicles contain protein biomarkers for primary sclerosing cholangitis and cholangiocarcinoma. Hepatology. 2017;66(4):1125–43.
25. Takahashi K, Yan I, Wen H-J, Patel T. microRNAs in liver disease: from diagnostics to therapeutics. Clin Biochem. 2013;46(10–11):946–52.
26. Cadamuro M, Nardo G, Indraccolo S, Dall'olmo L, Sambado L, Moserle L, et al. Platelet-derived growth factor-D and Rho GTPases regulate recruitment of cancer-associated fibroblasts in cholangiocarcinoma. Hepatology. 2013;58(3):1042–53.
27. Thelen A, Scholz A, Weichert W, Wiedenmann B, Neuhaus P, Gessner R, et al. Tumor-associated angiogenesis and lymphangiogenesis correlate with progression of intrahepatic cholangiocarcinoma. Am J Gastroenterol. 2010;105(5):1123–32.
28. Poruk KE, Pawlik TM, Weiss MJ. Perioperative management of hilar cholangiocarcinoma. J Gastrointest Surg. 2015;19(10):1889–99.
29. Mansour JC, Aloia TA, Crane CH, Heimbach JK, Nagino M, Vauthey J-N. Hilar cholangiocarcinoma: expert consensus statement. HPB (Oxford). 2015;17(8):691–9.
30. Galassi M, Iavarone M, Rossi S, Bota S, Vavassori S, Rosa L, et al. Patterns of appearance and risk of misdiagnosis of intrahepatic cholangiocarcinoma in cirrhosis at contrast enhanced ultrasound. Liver Int. 2013;33(5):771–9.
31. Iavarone M, Piscaglia F, Vavassori S, Galassi M, Sangiovanni A, Venerandi L, et al. Contrast enhanced CT-scan to diagnose intrahepatic cholangiocarcinoma in patients with cirrhosis. J Hepatol. 2013;58(6):1188–93.
32. Rimola J, Forner A, Reig M, Vilana R, de Lope CR, Ayuso C, et al. Cholangiocarcinoma in cirrhosis: absence of contrast washout in delayed phases by magnetic resonance imaging avoids misdiagnosis of hepatocellular carcinoma. Hepatology. 2009;50(3):791–8.
33. Wannhoff A, Gotthardt DN. Recent developments in the research on biomarkers of cholangiocarcinoma in primary sclerosing cholangitis. Clin Res Hepatol Gastroenterol. 2019;43(3):236–43.
34. Kato A, Naitoh I, Miyabe K, Hayashi K, Kondo H, Yoshida M, et al. Differential diagnosis of cholangiocarcinoma and IgG4-related sclerosing cholangitis by fluorescence in situ hybridization using transpapillary forceps biopsy specimens. J Hepatobili Pancreat Sci. 2018;25(3):188–94.
35. Kamisawa T, Nakazawa T, Tazuma S, Zen Y, Tanaka A, Ohara H, et al. Clinical practice guidelines for IgG4-related sclerosing cholangitis. J Hepatobili Pancreat Sci. 2019;26(1):9–42.

36. Ruys AT, van Beem BE, Engelbrecht MRW, Bipat S, Stoker J, Van Gulik TM. Radiological staging in patients with hilar cholangiocarcinoma: a systematic review and meta-analysis. Br J Radiol. 2012;85(1017):1255–62.
37. Tamada K, Ushio J, Sugano K. Endoscopic diagnosis of extrahepatic bile duct carcinoma: advances and current limitations. World J Clin Oncol. 2011;2(5):203–16.
38. Meining A, Chen YK, Pleskow D, Stevens P, Shah RJ, Chuttani R, et al. Direct visualization of indeterminate pancreaticobiliary strictures with probe-based confocal laser endomicroscopy: a multicenter experience. Gastrointest Endosc. 2011;74(5):961–8.
39. Heimbach JK, Sanchez W, Rosen CB, Gores GJ. Trans-peritoneal fine needle aspiration biopsy of hilar cholangiocarcinoma is associated with disease dissemination. HPB (Oxford). 2011;13(5):356–60.
40. Gonda TA, Viterbo D, Gausman V, Kipp C, Sethi A, Poneros JM, et al. Mutation profile and fluorescence in situ hybridization analyses increase detection of malignancies in biliary strictures. Clin Gastroenterol Hepatol. 2017;15(6):913–919.e1.
41. Gonda TA, Glick MP, Sethi A, Poneros JM, Palmas W, Iqbal S, et al. Polysomy and p16 deletion by fluorescence in situ hybridization in the diagnosis of indeterminate biliary strictures. Gastrointest Endosc. 2012;75(1):74–9.
42. Barr Fritcher EG, Kipp BR, Voss JS, Clayton AC, Lindor KD, Halling KC, et al. Primary sclerosing cholangitis patients with serial polysomy fluorescence in situ hybridization results are at increased risk of cholangiocarcinoma. Am J Gastroenterol. 2011;106(11):2023–8.
43. Dudley JC, Zheng Z, McDonald T, Le LP, Dias-Santagata D, Borger D, et al. Next-generation sequencing and fluorescence in situ hybridization have comparable performance characteristics in the analysis of pancreaticobiliary brushings for malignancy. J Mol Diagn. 2016;18(1):124–30.
44. Severino V, Dumonceau J-M, Delhaye M, Moll S, Annessi-Ramseyer I, Robin X, et al. Extracellular vesicles in bile as markers of malignant biliary stenoses. Gastroenterology. 2017;153(2):495–504.e8.
45. Wan JCM, Massie C, Garcia-Corbacho J, Mouliere F, Brenton JD, Caldas C, et al. Liquid biopsies come of age: towards implementation of circulating tumour DNA. Nat Rev Cancer. 2017;17(4):223–38.
46. Yang JD, Yab TC, Taylor WR, Foote PH, Ali HA, Lavu S, et al. Detection of cholangiocarcinoma by assay of methylated DNA markers in plasma. Gastroenterology. 2017;152(5):S1041–2.
47. Edge SB, American Joint Committee on Cancer, editors. AJCC cancer staging manual. 7th ed. New York, NY: Springer; 2010. 648 p.
48. Amin MB, Edge S, Greene F, Byrd DR, Brookland RK, Washington MK, et al., editors. AJCC cancer staging manual. 8th ed. Cham: Springer International Publishing; 2017. https://www.springer.com/gp/book/9783319406176. Accessed 27 Feb 2020.
49. Chun YS, Pawlik TM, Vauthey J-N. 8th Edition of the AJCC Cancer staging manual: pancreas and hepatobiliary cancers. Ann Surg Oncol. 2018;25(4):845–7.
50. Bird N, Elmasry M, Jones R, Elniel M, Kelly M, Palmer D, et al. Role of staging laparoscopy in the stratification of patients with perihilar cholangiocarcinoma. Br J Surg. 2017;104(4):418–25.
51. Ribero D, Pinna AD, Guglielmi A, Ponti A, Nuzzo G, Giulini SM, et al. Surgical approach for long-term survival of patients with intrahepatic cholangiocarcinoma: a multi-institutional analysis of 434 patients. Arch Surg. 2012;147(12):1107–13.
52. Sapisochin G, Fidelman N, Roberts JP, Yao FY. Mixed hepatocellular cholangiocarcinoma and intrahepatic cholangiocarcinoma in patients undergoing transplantation for hepatocellular carcinoma. Liver Transpl. 2011;17(8):934–42.
53. Goldaracena N, Gorgen A, Sapisochin G. Current status of liver transplantation for cholangiocarcinoma. Liver Transpl. 2018;24(2):294–303.
54. Lunsford KE, Javle M, Heyne K, Shroff RT, Abdel-Wahab R, Gupta N, et al. Liver transplantation for locally advanced intrahepatic cholangiocarcinoma treated with neoadjuvant therapy: a prospective case-series. Lancet Gastroenterol Hepatol. 2018;3(5):337–48.

55. Kolarich AR, Shah JL, George TJ, Hughes SJ, Shaw CM, Geller BS, et al. Non-surgical management of patients with intrahepatic cholangiocarcinoma in the United States, 2004-2015: an NCDB analysis. J Gastrointest Oncol. 2018;9(3):536–45.
56. Shao F, Qi W, Meng FT, Qiu L, Huang Q. Role of palliative radiotherapy in unresectable intrahepatic cholangiocarcinoma: population-based analysis with propensity score matching. Cancer Manag Res. 2018;10:1497–506.
57. Hong TS, Wo JY, Yeap BY, Ben-Josef E, McDonnell EI, Blaszkowsky LS, et al. Multi-institutional phase II study of high-dose hypofractionated proton beam therapy in patients with localized, unresectable hepatocellular carcinoma and intrahepatic cholangiocarcinoma. J Clin Oncol. 2016;34(5):460–8.
58. Kiefer MV, Albert M, McNally M, Robertson M, Sun W, Fraker D, et al. Chemoembolization of intrahepatic cholangiocarcinoma with cisplatinum, doxorubicin, mitomycin C, ethiodol, and polyvinyl alcohol: a 2-center study. Cancer. 2011;117(7):1498–505.
59. Kuhlmann JB, Euringer W, Spangenberg HC, Breidert M, Blum HE, Harder J, et al. Treatment of unresectable cholangiocarcinoma: conventional transarterial chemoembolization compared with drug eluting bead-transarterial chemoembolization and systemic chemotherapy. Eur J Gastroenterol Hepatol. 2012;24(4):437–43.
60. Kim JH, Won HJ, Shin YM, Kim K-A, Kim PN. Radiofrequency ablation for the treatment of primary intrahepatic cholangiocarcinoma. AJR Am J Roentgenol. 2011;196(2):W205–9.
61. Valle J, Wasan H, Palmer DH, Cunningham D, Anthoney A, Maraveyas A, et al. Cisplatin plus gemcitabine versus gemcitabine for biliary tract cancer. N Engl J Med. 2010;362(14):1273–81.
62. Hong YK, Choi SB, Lee KH, Park SW, Park YN, Choi JS, et al. The efficacy of portal vein embolization prior to right extended hemihepatectomy for hilar cholangiocellular carcinoma: a retrospective cohort study. Eur J Surg Oncol. 2011;37(3):237–44.
63. Khan AS, Garcia-Aroz S, Ansari MA, Atiq SM, Senter-Zapata M, Fowler K, et al. Assessment and optimization of liver volume before major hepatic resection: current guidelines and a narrative review. Int J Surg. 2018;52:74–81.
64. Gazzaniga GM, Cappato S, Belli FE, Bagarolo C, Filauro M. Assessment of hepatic reserve for the indication of hepatic resection: how I do it. J Hepato-Biliary-Pancreat Surg. 2005;12(1):27–30.
65. Nuzzo G, Giuliante F, Ardito F, Giovannini I, Aldrighetti L, Belli G, et al. Improvement in perioperative and long-term outcome after surgical treatment of hilar cholangiocarcinoma: results of an Italian multicenter analysis of 440 patients. Arch Surg. 2012;147(1):26–34.
66. Laurent A, Tayar C, Cherqui D. Cholangiocarcinoma: preoperative biliary drainage (Con). HPB (Oxford). 2008;10(2):126–9.
67. Kullman E, Frozanpor F, Söderlund C, Linder S, Sandström P, Lindhoff-Larsson A, et al. Covered versus uncovered self-expandable nitinol stents in the palliative treatment of malignant distal biliary obstruction: results from a randomized, multicenter study. Gastrointest Endosc. 2010;72(5):915–23.
68. Kim TH, Han S-S, Park S-J, Lee WJ, Woo SM, Moon SH, et al. Role of adjuvant chemoradiotherapy for resected extrahepatic biliary tract cancer. Int J Radiat Oncol Biol Phys. 2011;81(5):e853–9.
69. Heimbach JK, Haddock MG, Alberts SR, Nyberg SL, Ishitani MB, Rosen CB, et al. Transplantation for hilar cholangiocarcinoma. Liver Transpl. 2004;10(10 Suppl 2):S65–8.
70. Gores GJ, Darwish Murad S, Heimbach JK, Rosen CB. Liver transplantation for perihilar cholangiocarcinoma. Dig Dis. 2013;31(1):126–9.
71. Zamora-Valdes D, Heimbach JK. Liver transplant for cholangiocarcinoma. Gastroenterol Clin N Am. 2018;47(2):267–80.
72. Darwish Murad S, Kim WR, Harnois DM, Douglas DD, Burton J, Kulik LM, et al. Efficacy of neoadjuvant chemoradiation, followed by liver transplantation, for perihilar cholangiocarcinoma at 12 US centers. Gastroenterology. 2012;143(1):88–98.e3; quiz e14.
73. Sangchan A, Kongkasame W, Pugkhem A, Jenwitheesuk K, Mairiang P. Efficacy of metal and plastic stents in unresectable complex hilar cholangiocarcinoma: a randomized controlled trial. Gastrointest Endosc. 2012;76(1):93–9.

74. Wadsworth CA, Westaby D, Khan SA. Endoscopic radiofrequency ablation for cholangiocarcinoma. Curr Opin Gastroenterol. 2013;29(3):305–11.
75. Valle JW, Furuse J, Jitlal M, Beare S, Mizuno N, Wasan H, et al. Cisplatin and gemcitabine for advanced biliary tract cancer: a meta-analysis of two randomised trials. Ann Oncol. 2014;25(2):391–8.
76. Chua TC, Saxena A. Extended pancreaticoduodenectomy with vascular resection for pancreatic cancer: a systematic review. J Gastrointest Surg. 2010;14(9):1442–52.
77. Dickson PV, Behrman SW. Distal cholangiocarcinoma. Surg Clin North Am. 2014;94(2):325–42.
78. Kwon HJ, Kim SG, Chun JM, Lee WK, Hwang YJ. Prognostic factors in patients with middle and distal bile duct cancers. World J Gastroenterol. 2014;20(21):6658–65.
79. Acquaviva J, He S, Zhang C, Jimenez J-P, Nagai M, Sang J, et al. FGFR3 translocations in bladder cancer: differential sensitivity to HSP90 inhibition based on drug metabolism. Mol Cancer Res. 2014;12(7):1042–54.
80. Rohle D, Popovici-Muller J, Palaskas N, Turcan S, Grommes C, Campos C, et al. An inhibitor of mutant IDH1 delays growth and promotes differentiation of glioma cells. Science. 2013;340(6132):626–30.
81. Sirica AE. The role of cancer-associated myofibroblasts in intrahepatic cholangiocarcinoma. Nat Rev Gastroenterol Hepatol. 2011;9(1):44–54.
82. Mertens JC, Fingas CD, Christensen JD, Smoot RL, Bronk SF, Werneburg NW, et al. Therapeutic effects of deleting cancer-associated fibroblasts in cholangiocarcinoma. Cancer Res. 2013;73(2):897–907.
83. Martin-Liberal J, Ochoa de Olza M, Hierro C, Gros A, Rodon J, Tabernero J. The expanding role of immunotherapy. Cancer Treat Rev. 2017;54:74–86.
84. Feldman SA, Assadipour Y, Kriley I, Goff SL, Rosenberg SA. Adoptive cell therapy--tumor-infiltrating lymphocytes, t-cell receptors, and chimeric antigen receptors. Semin Oncol. 2015;42(4):626–39.

Part VI

Special Topics

Pregnancy and Diseases of the Biliary Tree

15

Nora Cazzagon

Abbreviations

CBD	Common bile duct
CGD	Complicated gallstones disease
ERCP	Endoscopic retrograde cholangiopancreatography
EUS	Endoscopic ultrasonography
ICP	Intrahepatic cholestasis of pregnancy
MRC	Magnetic resonance cholangiography
MRI	Magnetic resonance imaging
PBC	Primary biliary cholangitis
PSC	Primary sclerosing cholangitis
UDCA	Ursodeoxycholic acid

15.1 Gallstone Disease During Pregnancy

Gallstone disease is defined as the occurrence of symptoms or complications caused by gallstones in the gallbladder and/or in the bile ducts. There are two main types of gallstones, cholesterol gallstones, which are mainly composed by cholesterol and represent more than 90% of gallstones, and pigment stones, brown and black stones. The prevalence of cholesterol gallstones in adult population is around 20% in Europe and is even higher in Hispanic population of Central and South America and in American-Hispanics with Native American ancestry, the latter group showing the

N. Cazzagon (✉)
Department of Surgery, Oncology and Gastroenterology, University of Padova, Padova, Italy

Gastroenterology Unit, Azienda Ospedale Università Padova, Padova, Italy
e-mail: nora.cazzagon@unipd.it

© Springer Nature Switzerland AG 2021
A. Floreani (ed.), *Diseases of the Liver and Biliary Tree*,
https://doi.org/10.1007/978-3-030-65908-0_15

highest risk for cholesterol gallstones worldwide. The formation of cholesterol gall-stones is given by a failure of biliary cholesterol homeostasis primarily caused by a hepatic hypersecretion which largely depends on genetic predisposition. Other factors contributing to gallstones formations are gallbladder hypomotility, rapid phase transition and intestinal factors, such as increased absorption of cholesterol and reduced absorption of bile salts. All together, these defects promote cholesterol crystallization and gallstones formation [1]. Multiple well-established risk factors for gallstones disease have been identified, including female sex, pregnancy, multiparity, factors associated with metabolic syndrome, dietary factors, drugs and factors causing gallbladder hypomotility (Table 15.1). The prevalence of gallstones is higher in women than in men and this is, at least partially, explained by the effect of female sex hormones. Estrogen indeed increases gallstones formation by enhancing hepatic synthesis and secretion of cholesterol and by reducing bile salt synthesis through the upregulation of estrogen receptor 1 and G protein-coupled receptor 30 [2]. In addition, estrogen and progesterone can contribute to gallstones formation by inhibiting gallbladder smooth muscle contractile function, thus impairing gallbladder motility and finally determining gallbladder stasis. During pregnancy, and in particular in the late stage of pregnancy, plasma estrogens levels increase up to 100-folds compared with the respective average values during the menstrual cycle, and this is often associated with a significant increase in hepatic secretion of biliary cholesterol. As a result, bile becomes supersaturated with cholesterol and is more lithogenic. Additionally, high levels of estrogen and progesterone increase the risk of gallbladder stasis [3, 4]. These changes promote the formation of biliary sludge and gallstones in pregnant women and the incidence of gallstones disease increases greatly during the last two trimesters of pregnancy. Other factors can additionally contribute to gallstones formation in pregnant women such as weight gain, high-cholesterol and high-fat diet, insulin resistance, alteration in gut microbiota and immune function [5, 6]. Overall, the frequency of gallstones during pregnancy ranges from 1.2% to 12.2% in different studies [7–11] and biliary sludge is also

Table 15.1 Risk factors for cholesterol gallstones disease

General population	Pregnancy
Age	Increased parity
Female gender	Increased gestational age
Factors associated with metabolic syndrome • Overweight and obesity • Physical inactivity • Insulin resistance and diabetes mellitus • Nonalcoholic fatty liver disease	Prepregnancy obesity
Dietary factors • Hypercaloric diet • Hyperglycemic diet and high carbohydrate intake • Low-fiber diet	
Rapid weight loss	
Prolonged fasting	
Drugs (hormone-replacement therapy, octreotide, fibrates)	

more frequent, occurring in up to 15% of pregnant women. The frequency of gallstones is also higher in young women with multiple subsequent pregnancies, varying from 5.1% after one pregnancy to 12.3% after three or more pregnancies. A relative risk of 1.6–1.7 of developing gallstones after each pregnancy was reported in the Sirmione study [12], the Framingham study [13] and the MICOL study [14]. However, approximately one-third of pregnant women with gallstones remain asymptomatic and gallstones and biliary sludge may spontaneously resolve in the first year after delivery. Women with multiple pregnancy and short interval between subsequent pregnancies are at increased risk of gallstones formation because sludge can persist or recur. When symptoms occurs, the most commonly reported clinical presentation is the biliary cholic [15]. Acute cholecystitis, gallstones pancreatitis, and jaundice are other possible presentations of gallstones disease during pregnancy and are collectively called complicated gallstones disease (CGD), which can occur in 0.05–0.8% of pregnancies. Complicated gallstones disease represents the second most common non-gynecologic condition, following appendicitis, for acute abdomen requiring surgical intervention in pregnancy [16–19].

Biliary sludge is often diagnosed accidentally by ultrasonography conducted as part of prenatal routine care; on the other hand, asymptomatic women at high risk with parity are regularly monitored for the development of gallstones. Transabdominal **ultrasonography** is the first diagnostic test for identifying biliary sludge and gallstones because of several advantages including high sensitivity (>95% also for small gallstones), non-invasiveness, and low cost. However, ultrasonography may be insufficient to visualize the presence of gallstones in the common bile duct and thus, in these cases, second-level imaging techniques, such as magnetic resonance cholangiography (MRC), need to be performed. Although there are theoretical concerns for the fetus, including teratogenesis, tissue heating and acoustic damages, there is no evidence of actual harm about the use of magnetic resonance imaging (MRI) in pregnant women. The American College of Obstetricians and Gynecologist recommends a prudent use of MRI during pregnancy and the use of MRI is justified if this diagnostic technique is expected to answer a relevant clinical question or otherwise provide medical benefit to the patient [20]. **Endoscopic ultrasonography** (EUS) for identifying the presence of small gallstones (<5 mm) in the CBD is more sensitive than MRC and is recommended for diagnostic purpose against **endoscopic retrograde cholangiopancreatography** (ERCP), since the latter should only be performed for therapeutic purpose [21]. Recent European Society of Gastrointestinal Endoscopy (ESGE) guidelines recommend that therapeutic ERCP is safe and effective in pregnant women but need to be performed by experienced endoscopist and using as little radiation as achievable [21]. Non-radiation ERCP is a possibility to avoid fetus irradiation and appears to be safe but technically demanding.

Clinical and biochemical features of biliary cholic, acute cholecystitis, choledocholithiasis, and ascending cholangitis in pregnant women are comparable to that observed in general population, keeping in mind that a mild increase of white cell blood count and increased levels of alkaline phosphatase are two physiological findings observed in uncomplicated pregnancy.

Prevention of biliary sludge and gallstones in high-risk women is crucial in order to reduce the risk of cholecystectomy during pregnancy and postpartum period. General measures of prevention might include physical activity and dietary tips, while no indication exists for drug prescription in the setting of gallstones' prevention. **Treatment** of gallstones and biliary sludge in pregnant women is indicated only in symptomatic patients. Pain control is mandatory in biliary cholic and, in case of complicated gallstones disease, the supportive management is highly recommended if possible, reserving definitive treatment after delivery. Old reports concerning biliary surgery during pregnancy reported an increased risk of complication rate both for the mother and the fetus and, for this reason, a conservative approach was traditionally recommended, with surgical intervention used only in severe cases or after conservative treatment failure [22–24]. Nevertheless, conservative treatment is not free of risk since up to one-third of pregnant women with symptomatic biliary disease need for surgery and moreover, around half of pregnant women treated conservatively need surgical intervention within 2 years after delivery [25]. Moreover, each new episode of biliary cholic is associated with a risk of CGD (cholecystitis and pancreatitis) in 23% of patients and untreated CGD carries a significant risk of maternal and fetal adverse outcomes [26]. In the last two decades, advancements in surgical, anesthesiological, and obstetrical techniques and strategies have decreased the risk of intervention which is now considered safe and feasible with laparoscopic cholecystectomy being the treatment of choice in all trimesters [27–29]. The recent meta-analysis by Seghat and colleagues including 10,632 patients aimed to compare laparoscopic versus open cholecystectomy in pregnancy and showed that up to 91% of included patients were in the first or second trimester at the time of surgery and thus gestational age was not considered into analysis. Their results provided evidences in favor of a laparoscopic approach vs. open cholecystectomy in pregnant women during the first and second trimester [27]. A recent large cohort study using the California OSHPD 2007–2014 database, an administrative database, reported about maternal and fetal outcomes of 7597 pregnancies with gallstones within 4 months from delivery. One fourth of the included patients had CGD and this was associated with a significant increased risk of adverse birth outcomes and preterm delivery when compared with uncomplicated gallstones disease. Moreover, the risk for an adverse birth outcome was greater among those who underwent biliary system surgical or endoscopic intervention compared with patients treated conservatively. Preterm birth was also significantly associated with biliary system intervention. No significant differences in outcomes between patients treated with open vs. laparoscopic cholecystectomy were observed [30]. In conclusion, despite the intrinsic limitations, this study confirmed that CGD is relatively frequent among women which developed gallstones during pregnancy. However, there is limited and conflicting data to predict maternal and fetal outcomes or guide clinical decision making in CGD. Thus, it appears crucial, the need of prevention of gallstones development and a careful counseling of pregnant women regarding the risk of complications related to CGD and interventions.

15.2 Intrahepatic Cholestasis of Pregnancy

Intrahepatic cholestasis of pregnancy (ICP) is the most common pregnancy-specific liver disease, which classically occurs in the second or third trimester and is associated with rapid resolution following delivery. The disease is characterized by pruritus with elevated serum bile acids levels and/or elevation of liver enzymes in absence of other systemic or hepatobiliary disorders [31]. The symptoms and biochemical alterations resolve rapidly after delivery but may recur in subsequent pregnancies and with the use of hormonal contraception. Intrahepatic cholestasis of pregnancy is associated with a higher incidence of adverse outcomes of pregnancy including preterm delivery (spontaneous and iatrogenic), fetal distress, fetal asphyxia, meconium staining of the amniotic fluid, and stillbirth. Maternal serum levels of bile acids are associated with the rates of fetal complications, in particular when serum bile acids raised above 40 μmol/L.

15.2.1 Epidemiology

The reported incidence of ICP ranges between 0.2% and 2% with higher incidence in South America and northern Europe [32–36]. Moreover, incidence of ICP is increased in case of multiparity, in women older than 35 years and after in vitro fertilization.

15.2.2 Etiology

The etiology is complex and has not yet completely understood but genetic, environmental, and hormonal factors play a role in the pathogenesis of ICP. Evidences indeed support that the pathophysiology of the disease is related to the cholestatic effects of continuously rising levels of placenta-derived estrogens and progesterone in genetically predisposed women. There is an elevated sibling risk in affected women [37–39] and moreover, a significant variability of ICP frequency was also observed in different populations and this is reasonably due to a different genetic background. The genetic predisposition of ICP is based on mutations of genes codifying different hepatobiliary transporters, which are physiologically involved in the export of various bile components into the bile canaliculi. Moreover, several types of mutations of these hepatobiliary transporters are also involved in the pathogenesis of other cholestatic liver disease, such as progressive familial intrahepatic cholestasis (PFIC), benign recurrent intrahepatic cholestasis (BRIC), and low-phospholipid associated cholelithiasis (LPAC) (Fig. 15.1).

The bile salt export pump (BSEP, ABCB11) is an ATP-dependent transporter which is responsible of bile acids efflux into the bile canaliculi. The multidrug resistance protein 3 (MDR3, ABCB4) is an ATP-coupled transporter which flopped phosphatidylcholine into the bile canaliculi [40]. Phosphatidylcholine allows the formation of mixed micelles with bile acids, which protect luminal epithelium from

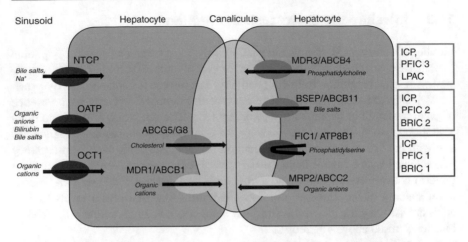

Fig. 15.1 Schematic representing transporters of bilirubin, bile salts, and phospholipids involved in bile formation and major diseases related to their mutations. *ICP* intrahepatic cholestasis of pregnancy, *PFIC* progressive familial intrahepatic cholestasis, *LPAC* low phospholipid-associated cholelithiasis, *BRIC* benign recurrent intrahepatic cholestasis, *ABC* ATP-binding cassette protein, *BSEP* bile salt export pump, *FIC* familial intrahepatic cholestasis, *MRP* multidrug resistance protein family, *MDR* multidrug resistance, *OATP* organic anion transport protein, *OCT* organic cation transporter, *NTCP* Na taurocholate co-transporting protein

detergent and toxic effects of bile salts. The multidrug resistance-associated protein 2 (MRP2, ABCC2) is another ATP-driven transporter which exports organic ion conjugates such as bilirubin, drug conjugates, and other organic ions into the bile. Cholesterol is exported by a heterodimeric complex of two membrane proteins (ABC G5/G8) and finally phosphatidylserine is exported by ATB8B1.

In intrahepatic cholestasis of pregnancy, the mutations of *ABCB4* are the most extensively studied; moreover, this gene is also mutated in PFIC3 [37, 41] and LPAC syndrome [42–45] (Fig. 15.1). Several types of mutations have been reported in different populations, including heterozygous mutations reported in mothers of children affected by PFIC3, but also in absence of PFIC; other reported mutations are single mutations, splicing mutations, and recurrent missense mutations, which were extensively reviewed [46]. Some studies have also analyzed the relationship between *ABCB4* mutations and clinical phenotype in PFIC 3, fewer have been reported for ICP [47–50]. Heterozygous mutations in *ABCB11* have been also identified in patients with ICP other than in PFIC2 and in benign recurrent intrahepatic cholestasis 2 (BRIC 2), and also some SNPs have been reported [46] (Fig. 15.1). *ATP8B1* and *ABCC2 mutations* were also suggested in ICP. Finally, a number of variants with functional effects at and around the farnesoid X receptor (*FXR*) gene, which codifies a nuclear receptor that is a key homeostatic sensor of bile acid levels in hepatocytes, has also been reported in ICP [51].

The role of sex hormones in the pathogenesis of ICP has been investigated starting from the evidence that symptoms and biochemical alterations of ICP typically occur during the second and third trimester and resolve after delivery which corresponds to physiological lowering of female hormones. In rodents, estrogens cause cholestasis through the reduction of hepatic biliary transport proteins expression and internalization of the bile acid export pump. Moreover, some studies in mice and in vitro suggested that FXR pathway is desensitized by estrogen. In ICP, the levels of sulfated progesterone metabolites at 35–41 weeks of gestation are increased and these hormones determine cholestasis and hypercholanemia acting as partial agonists of the bile acid receptor farnesoid X receptor (FXR) and competitively inhibiting hepatic bile acid uptake and efflux [52]. Moreover, these sulfate progesterone metabolites were found to be useful to predict the onset of ICP and to distinguish this entity from benign pruritus gravidarum [53]. Some environmental factors are also reported to participate to the etiology of ICP, including dietary selenium deficiency [54] and low levels of vitamin D [55].

15.2.3 Diagnosis

The diagnosis of ICP is based on the presence of pruritus, increased serum bile salt levels, and/or increase in transaminase, spontaneous and rapid resolution of symptoms and biochemical changes after delivery and absence of any underlying liver disease. **Pruritus** in ICP typically affects the palms and the soles but may occur anywhere; it often worsens at night, it could be extremely severe, eventually interfering with sleep and is not associated to specific dermatological features, except for scratching lesions. The onset of pruritus may precede or follow biochemical alterations. The pathogenesis of pruritus in ICP has not yet been clarified, but the role of lysophosphatidic acid, a pruritogen produced by autotaxin [56, 57] and bile acids, was proposed since both are elevated in the blood of women with ICP. In particular, serum autotaxin is useful in the differential diagnosis of pruritus during pregnancy by distinguishing ICP from other pruritic disorders or pre-eclampsia/HELLP syndrome with excellent sensitivity and specificity and, differently from bile acids, is not influenced by food intake [56]. **Serum bile acids** in women with ICP are commonly increased above the upper limit of normal values, which depend on fasting status and the technique used for assessment, with upper normal values around 10–14 μmol/L or 6–10 μmol/L in fasted women. Serum bile acids level above 40 μmol/L in fasting state is commonly considered a marker of severe ICP. **Transaminases** are commonly increased in ICP, with a wide range of possible elevation from 2- to 30-folds the upper limit of normal. Gamma glutamyl transferase is commonly normal in ICP, but in some cases may be elevated. Bilirubin is also increased in up to 10% of patients with ICP and when present, is characterized by a mild increase in conjugated bilirubin. Jaundice is not frequent in ICP, but it may occur. Prothrombin time (PT) prolongation is not common but it may be abnormal as a consequence of malabsorption of vitamin K, anyway it needs to be assessed at the time of delivery. As recently reported by Bicocca and colleagues, there is a lack of consensus in the diagnostic criteria of ICP between different national and regional guidelines with pruritus being the only commonly recognized criteria among all different guidelines [58]. Ultrasound examination is useful to exclude the presence of gallstones and/or bile ducts dilatations. The differential diagnosis of ICP includes benign pruritus gravidarum and the presence of other liver diseases, including viral and non-viral hepatitis.

15.2.4 Treatment

Ursodeoxycholic acid (UDCA) is recommended as first-line treatment of intrahepatic cholestasis of pregnancy. UDCA is a natural component of human bile, accounting for 1–3% of bile acids in healthy individuals and it is approved for primary biliary cholangitis (PBC), cholesterol gallstones and for preventing gallstones formation in obese patients undergoing rapid weight reduction. Several studies have confirmed the anticholestatic effect of UDCA in intrahepatic cholestasis of pregnancy that it has been shown to be effective to reduce maternal pruritus as well as decrease laboratory abnormalities [32, 59–65]. However, the effect of UDCA in improving fetal outcomes has not yet been proven. Despite the suggestion that a beneficial effect of UDCA in fetal outcome in several small studies included in one meta-analysis [65], this was not later confirmed by the recent results of the PITCHES trial where the authors did not find a significant difference in the primary composite outcome (perinatal death, preterm delivery, or neonatal unit admission for at least 4 h) between patients treated with UDCA or placebo [66]. It's worth noting that, in this trial, the inclusion criteria to diagnose ICP were the presence of pruritus and raised serum bile acids above of the upper limit of normal of the local laboratory. Thus it is possible that some included patients did not suffer of ICP, but had either pruritus without cholestasis or pruritus associated with an underlying chronic liver disease other than ICP [67].

UDCA is commonly used in the treatment of ICP and different scientific societies recommended different dosage which are summarized in Table 15.2. However, not all women treated with UDCA show a biochemical response or symptoms' improvement.

Preliminary observation suggested that *rifampicin*, used in the treatment of pruritus in cholestatic liver disease, is effective in combination with UDCA for treating women with severe ICP who do not respond to treatment with UDCA alone [68]. The mechanism of action of rifampicin in PBC is complementary to those of UDCA and includes an enhancement of bile acid detoxification and elimination.

Table 15.2 Ursodeoxycholic acid (UDCA) dose recommendations for the treatment of intrahepatic cholestasis of pregnancy in different guidelines

EASL	ACG	SMFM
UDCA 10–20 mg/kg/day with a maximum dose of 25 mg/kg/day	UDCA 10–15 mg/kg/day	Start with UDCA 300 mg twice daily, increasing to 600 mg twice daily if symptoms do not improve in 1 week

EASL European Association for the Study of the Liver, *ACG* American College of Gastroenterologist, *SMFM* The Society for Maternal-Fetal Medicine

Vitamin K supplementation in case of elevated prothrombin time is recommended by most guidelines. *Dexamethasone* is recommended to promote fetal lung maturity but is not effective to treat pruritus in ICP [59]. *Cholestyramine* is an anion exchange resin which has been suggested to improve pruritus in ICP but does not improve serum bile acid levels or liver function tests [61]; moreover, by reducing the intestinal absorption of UDCA or fat-soluble vitamins, it could increase the risk of postpartum hemorrhage. Some studies suggested that *s-adenosyl-methionine* and *antihistamines* are effective to improve pruritus in women with ICP, whereas their effect on serum biochemistry was inconsistent.

15.2.5 Maternal and Fetal Outcomes

Intrahepatic cholestasis of pregnancy is associated with an increased risk of preterm delivery ranging between 19% and 60% in different studies [69–71]. Moreover, ICP is associated with an increased risk on intrapartum fetal distress in up to 41% of pregnancy and intrauterine fetal death in 0.75–1.6% of the affected pregnancies. Two large population-based studies conducted in Sweden and the UK investigated whether fetal complications were correlated to the severity of ICP measured by bile acid levels. The authors observed that the probability of fetal complications arise when bile acid levels are ≥40 μmol/L [72, 73] while no increase in fetal risk was detected in ICP patients with bile acid levels <40 μmol/L [72]. The overall probability of fetal complications (spontaneous preterm deliveries, asphyxial events, and meconium staining of amniotic fluids, placenta and membranes) increased by 1–2% per additional μmol/L of serum bile acids [72]. ICP is usually a self-limiting benign condition for the mother, which resolves typically within 4 weeks after delivery. In some cases, liver function does not return to normal after delivery suggesting an underlying hepatobiliary disease that needs to be further investigated [74].

A Swedish population-based study, including 11,338 women with ICP and 113,893 matched women without diagnosis of ICP, assessed the risk of developing hepatobiliary disease in women with ICP and the risk of developing ICP in women with prevalent hepatobiliary disease. This study reported that women with ICP have an increased risk of later hepatobiliary disease with an increment of around 1% per year, including hepatitis C or chronic hepatitis, fibrosis or cirrhosis, and gallstone disease or cholangitis as compared to women with ICP. Moreover, ICP was more common in women with preexisting hepatitis C, chronic hepatitis, and gallstones disease. The association with ICP and other hepatobiliary disease was temporally independent, thus suggesting that part of this association is likely due to shared risk factors such as variants in the ABCB4 gene which are associated with ICP, gallstones disease, and drug-induced cholestasis [75]. The same group later reported that women with ICP are at increased risk of liver and biliary tree cancer, immune-mediated disease, i.e., diabetes mellitus, psoriasis, inflammatory polyarthropathies, and Crohn's disease and have also a small increase of cardiovascular disease compared to matched women without ICP [76].

15.3   Pregnancy in Chronic Cholestatic Liver Disease

Chronic cholestatic liver diseases include a range of different disorders in which an impaired bile formation and/or flow is caused by genetic, immunological, environmental, or other factors. The damage can occur in microscopic hepatic canaliculi, intrahepatic biliary ductules, segmental ducts or large intra- and/or extrahepatic bile ducts and, in many cases, leads to development of hepatobiliary and even systemic consequences. Primary biliary cholangitis (PBC) and primary sclerosing cholangitis (PSC) are the two most common cholestatic liver diseases which are chronic, progressive and are associated with considerable morbidity and mortality; moreover, PBC and PSC are two leading indications for liver transplantation.

Pregnancy induces changes in maternal immunity, in particular leads to a shift of Th1 cellular response to a Th2 humoral response to maintain the fetus against the immunological processes of recognition and elimination of nonself molecules [77]. It is well documented that symptoms of certain autoimmune diseases can decline during pregnancy and exacerbate after delivery. Although the mechanism underlying this phenomenon is not entirely known, several observations supported the hypothesis that sex hormones play a crucial regulatory role in this process. In particular, heightened levels of estrogen during pregnancy help to control the development, prevent rejection of the fetus and protect the mother, by expanding the regulatory T cell (Treg) compartment and by enhancing suppressive activity of Treg cells via an increased levels of FoxP3 [78].

The aim of this section is to summarize evidences regarding the impact of PBC and PSC in women fertility, the clinical course of liver disease during pregnancy, the maternal and fetal outcomes, and the suggested management of patients with PBC and PSC during pregnancy, also focusing on patients in cirrhotic stage.

Primary biliary cholangitis predilects female gender, typically occurs in postmenopausal year but growing evidence showed that typical histological features of PBC can appear much earlier and recent data observed in 25% of cases PBC is diagnosed during reproductive years. Ursodeoxycholic therapy is first-line therapy in patients with PBC and it has been shown to be effective to improve liver function tests and liver transplant free survival. In patients which do not respond to UDCA, obeticholic acid, an agonist of farnesoid X receptor, in addition to UDCA, is more effective than placebo in addition to UDCA in decreasing alkaline phosphatase and total bilirubin [79]. Moreover in patients with PBC, bezafibrate in addition to UDCA was proven to be extremely effective to induce complete biochemical response and to reduce pruritus compared to placebo and UDCA [80]. Young women with PBC diagnosed in child bearing age tend to be more symptomatic and to respond less frequently to UDCA. In the largest population-based study to date, PBC was not associated with decreased **fertility** [81]. These data were confirmed in a large case-control study by Floreani and colleagues which compared a group of 233 consecutive females along a 25 years period with 367 matched healthy women with at least one conception in their life [82]. The **clinical course of liver disease** during pregnancy was collectively reported in 67 patients with at least one pregnancy after the diagnosis of PBC or with PBC being diagnosed during pregnancy [82–84]. Trivedi et al. analyzed 50 pregnancies among 32 patients with PBC before conception and observed that 80% of patients were on biochemical remission before conception, 12% had a biochemical flare, and 30% were experiencing pruritus. During pregnancy, 71% of cases showed persistent biochemical remission while 29% of cases had biochemical flare of disease and overall, the occurrence or worsening of pruritus during pregnancy was observed in 64% of cases [83]. In the postpartum period biochemical remission was observed in around 40% of pregnancies, while 60% of cases showed a biochemical flare, whereas the frequency of pruritus came back to the reported frequency before conception (30%). Biochemical flares during pregnancy were observed both in patients with stable and active disease before conception, were independent from UDCA status and were associated to severe clinical progression in only two cases. Specifically, one woman developed portal hypertension and jaundice and another woman developed thrombocytopenia and grade 2 esophageal varices. In the remaining cases, biochemical flares were characterized by an isolated peak of alkaline phosphatase ranging between 5- and 15-fold the upper normal value and occurred in the first 5 months after delivery. The onset or worsening of pruritus during pregnancy was independently associated with the presence of an advanced histological stage at the time of diagnosis [83]. Similarly, the recent study from Williamson group reported that de novo cholestasis occurred in four (15%) women with PBC during pregnancy and cholestasis was associated with peak in bile acids during pregnancy which was significantly higher than in women without cholestasis. The possible pathogenetic mechanisms of exacerbation of pruritus and cholestasis during pregnancy may include, as described for ICP, a negative role of increased estrogen and progesterone sulfates in bile acid homeostasis and the role of autotaxin, which was shown to be elevated in PBC, in women taking oral contraceptives and also in ICP [53, 56]. Regarding major **adverse maternal outcomes**, one case of postpartum liver transplantation for liver failure and one de novo PBC was reported collectively among 81 patients with PBC in different studies [82, 83, 85–87]. **Pregnancy outcomes** in PBC patients are generally good, although miscarriages were reported in 24–38% of pregnancies [83, 86], preterm delivery in 6–33% [83, 84], and ectopic pregnancy in 2% [83]. Overall, stillbirth rate in PBC ranges between 2% and 4% in two different studies [83, 84] but **neonatal outcomes** were generally favorable [82–85] with no reported neonatal complications in babies born at term [83]. One case of chromosomal abnormalities was reported in one cirrhotic PBC patient [83].

Primary sclerosing cholangitis is an idiopathic cholestatic liver disease wherein biliary fibroinflammation typically results in multifocal intra- and/or extrahepatic bile ducts strictures alternating with dilations of bile duct segments. The disease is rare, with substantial geographic differences, with higher reported prevalence in northern Europe and North America. PSC affects patients of essentially any age, although it is more typically diagnosed in the fourth decade and is more common in male than females. PSC is associated with a concomitant inflammatory bowel disease (IBD) in 70% of patients, which are more commonly affected by ulcerative colitis. Since no medical treatment has proven to be effective to delay disease progression and liver transplant is the only effective therapy to prolong survival in patients with PSC, the natural course of PSC is generally progressive and characterized by the development of cirrhosis and its complication. The clinical course of PSC can also be characterized by the development of acute bacterial cholangitis and even recurrent cholangitis. Moreover, the disease is associated with an increased risk of development of hepatobiliary and colorectal cancer. As reported above, PSC usually occurs during a period of peak fertility and childbearing, thus the diagnosis of PSC in women of this age group often raises concerns regarding the impact of disease on fertility and pregnancy as well as the impact of pregnancy on PSC itself. Similar to PBC, studies on **fertility** and pregnancy in PSC are limited [88–93] and overall, PSC seems not to be associated with a reduction of fertility. **Clinical course** of PSC during pregnancy is generally favorable and the occurrence or worsening of pruritus is reported in a minority of women. Biochemical worsening was described in up to 20% of cases during gestational period and in 33% in postpartum period [88, 92] with IBD flares during gestation being reported in few cases [88, 92]. In one study, new onset of abdominal pain during gestation occurred in three out of ten pregnant women and it was not present before conception [88]. **Maternal outcomes** are also good in PSC and no serious adverse events were reported [84, 88, 92]. On the other hand, **pregnancy outcomes** are characterized by fetal loss in 16% of cases, not associated with advanced liver disease, preterm delivery in 8–24% of cases, and the need of cesarean section in around 30% of cases [84, 88, 92]. Reported live birth rate is as high as 88–100% in two different studies [84, 92] with no congenital abnormalities but normal development in all babies. A large population-based cohort study conducted in Sweden confirmed that maternal PSC is associated with a 3.6-fold increase in preterm birth as well as with an increased risk of cesarean section but no increase in stillbirths, neonatal deaths, small for gestational age and congenital abnormalities. Moreover, IBD status marginally affects the risk estimates [93]. However, studies conducted in pregnant patients with IBD, confirmed that an active IBD at the time of conception is associated with an increased risk of preterm delivery, miscarriages, stillbirth, and low birth weight [94, 95].

In *cirrhotic women*, pregnancy is considered a rare event due to a combination of metabolic, endocrine, nutritional, and sexual dysfunction. Disruption of the hypothalamic-pituitary axis in conjunction with alteration of estrogen metabolism leads to anovulation, amenorrhea, and infertility [96, 97]. Pregnancy could lead to a worsening of liver synthetic function and hepatic decompensation in up to 10–15% of patients due to an increase of portal hypertension and, overall, maternal mortality is as high as 1.8%. The MELD and UKELD scores are useful in pregnant women to predict the risk of hepatic decompensation. The risk of variceal hemorrhage increases in pregnant women as consequence of the increased portal hypertension and thus a variceal screening during the second trimester of pregnancy is mandatory in order to promptly establish primary prophylaxis [98, 99]. In cirrhotic patients, pregnancy outcomes are less favorable with spontaneous fetal loss reported in up to 26% of cases, preterm delivery in 39–64% of cases, and Cesarean section in 42%. Finally, fetal complications in cirrhotic women occurred in up to 48% of cases compared to 19% of non-cirrhotic women and included death, growth restriction, and prematurity [98, 99].

15.4   Management of Pregnant Women Affected by PBC and PSC

There are some points that need to be considered in the management of pregnant women with PBC and PSC and first of all is the need of a pragmatic and individualized counseling before conception, in particular in patients with portal hypertension which are at greatest risk of complications [100]. Then, during gestation a close monitoring with routine blood test and clinical assessment [74, 91, 101] is indicated. Regarding medical therapy during pregnancy, UDCA is formerly classified in the FDA class B, but experts' clinical opinion is that UDCA is generally safe during conception, pregnancy, and postpartum period including breastfeeding [83, 102] and thus EASL recommends the continued use of UDCA in pregnancy, even though supporting data are limited [74, 100]. Cholestyramine and rifampicin (third trimester onward), despite been classified in FDA pregnancy category C, are considered safe in pregnancy for the treatment of pruritus. However, clinical data are limited [61, 68] and thus recommendations regarding their use during pregnancy cannot be provided. Due to the limited data to inform a drug-related risk on the use of obeticholic acid in pregnant women, OCA should be avoided during pregnancy and breastfeeding as a precautionary measure.

As reported in the first section of the chapter, magnetic resonance cholangiography is not contraindicated during pregnancy; however, the American Association for the Study of Liver Disease (AASLD) suggests a precautional use of MRC during the second and third trimester [101], whereas the American College of Radiology doesn't provide any special consideration for any trimester of pregnancy. Similarly to the reported treatment of complicated gallstones disease, also in PSC pregnant women, ERCP is considered generally safe but a benefit-to-risk ratio needs to be assessed in each woman and should be reserved for cases in which the need for endoscopic therapy is anticipated [74, 101]. A national cohort study conducted in the USA showed that pregnancy is an independent risk factor for post-ERCP pancreatitis and the risk is higher in community hospital than in teaching centers and thus the authors recommend proper precautions for pregnant women undergoing ERPC, including transfer to a tertiary care center if appropriate [103].

In summary, in non-cirrhotic patients with PBC and PSC, fertility seems not to be reduced compared to general population, but in patients with PSC there is an increased risk of preterm delivery. In particular, patients with active IBD are at increased risk of both pregnancy and fetal adverse outcomes. Worsening of pruritus and cholestasis during gestation can occur, and in these cases, ICP needs to be excluded and an appropriate treatment established. Biochemical transient flares in postpartum period are possible and they spontaneously resolve in 1 year following delivery. UDCA treatment during pregnancy and breastfeeding is safe and should be continued. Finally, cirrhotic patients are at increased risk of serious maternal and fetal adverse outcomes, thus a proper and individualized counseling is recommended in each cirrhotic woman willing to become mother. Moreover, worsening of portal hypertension during the second and third trimester justifies the need of variceal screening in the second trimester in all cirrhotic patients.

References

1. Lammert F, Gurusamy K, Ko CW, Miquel J-F, Méndez-Sánchez N, Portincasa P, et al. Gallstones. Nat Rev Dis Prim. 2016;2(1):16024.
2. de Bari O, Wang TY, Liu M, Portincasa P, Wang DQ-H. Estrogen induces two distinct cholesterol crystallization pathways by activating ERα and GPR30 in female mice. J Lipid Res. 2015;56(9):1691–700.
3. Wang HH, Liu M, Clegg DJ, Portincasa P, Wang DQ-H. New insights into the molecular mechanisms underlying effects of estrogen on cholesterol gallstone formation. Biochim Biophys Acta. 2009;1791(11):1037–47.
4. Portincasa P, Di Ciaula A, Wang HH, Palasciano G, van Erpecum KJ, Moschetta A, et al. Coordinate regulation of gallbladder motor function in the gut-liver axis. Hepatology. 2008;47(6):2112–26.
5. Ko CW, Beresford SAA, Schulte SJ, Lee SP. Insulin resistance and incident gallbladder disease in pregnancy. Clin Gastroenterol Hepatol. 2008;6(1):76–81.
6. Wong AC, Ko CW. Carbohydrate intake as a risk factor for biliary sludge and stones during pregnancy. J Clin Gastroenterol. 2013;47(8):700–5.
7. Bolukbas FF, Bolukbas C, Horoz M, Ince AT, Uzunkoy A, Ozturk A, et al. Risk factors associated with gallstone and biliary sludge formation during pregnancy. J Gastroenterol Hepatol. 2006;21(7):1150–3.
8. Maringhini A, Marcenò MP, Lanzarone F, Caltagirone M, Fusco G, Di Cuonzo G, et al. Sludge and stones in gallbladder after pregnancy. Prevalence and risk factors. J Hepatol. 1987;5(2):218–23.
9. Valdivieso V, Covarrubias C, Siegel F, Cruz F. Pregnancy and cholelithiasis: pathogenesis and natural course of gallstones diagnosed in early puerperium. Hepatology. 1993;17(1):1–4.
10. Basso L, McCollum PT, Darling MR, Tocchi A, Tanner WA. A study of cholelithiasis during pregnancy and its relationship with age, parity, menarche, breast-feeding, dysmenorrhea, oral contraception and a maternal history of cholelithiasis. Surg Gynecol Obstet. 1992;175(1):41–6.
11. Stauffer RA, Adams A, Wygal J, Lavery JP. Gallbladder disease in pregnancy. Am J Obstet Gynecol. 1982;144(6):661–4.
12. Barbara L, Sama C, Morselli Labate AM, Taroni F, Rusticali AG, Festi D, et al. A population study on the prevalence of gallstone disease: the Sirmione study. Hepatology. 1987;7(5):913–7.
13. Friedman GD, Kannel WB, Dawber TR. The epidemiology of gallbladder disease: observations in the Framingham study. J Chronic Dis. 1966;19(3):273–92.
14. Attili AF, Capocaccia R, Carulli N, Festi D, Roda E, Barbara L, et al. Factors associated with gallstone disease in the MICOL experience. Multicenter Italian study on epidemiology of cholelithiasis. Hepatology. 1997;26(4):809–18.
15. Hay JE. Liver disease in pregnancy. Hepatology. 2008;47(3):1067–76.
16. Kuy S, Roman SA, Desai R, Sosa JA. Outcomes following cholecystectomy in pregnant and nonpregnant women. Surgery. 2009;146(2):358–66.
17. Daradkeh S, Sumrein I, Daoud F, Zaidin K, Abu-Khalaf M. Management of gallbladder stones during pregnancy: conservative treatment or laparoscopic cholecystectomy? Hepato-Gastroenterology. 1999;46(30):3074–6.
18. Swisher SG, Schmit PJ, Hunt KK, Hiyama DT, Bennion RS, Swisher EM, et al. Biliary disease during pregnancy. Am J Surg. 1994;168(6):576–9; discussion 580–1.
19. Ghumman E, Barry M, Grace PA. Management of gallstones in pregnancy. Br J Surg. 1997;84(12):1646–50.
20. American College of Obstetricians and Gynecologists' Committee on Obstetric Practice. Guidelines for diagnostic imaging during pregnancy and lactation. Obstet Gynecol. 2017;130(4):7.

21. Manes G, Paspatis G, Aabakken L, Anderloni A, Arvanitakis M, Ah-Soune P, et al. Endoscopic management of common bile duct stones: European Society of Gastrointestinal Endoscopy (ESGE) guideline. Endoscopy. 2019;51(05):472–91.
22. Saunders P, Milton PJ. Laparotomy during pregnancy: an assessment of diagnostic accuracy and fetal wastage. Br Med J. 1973;3(5872):165–7.
23. Greene J, Rogers A, Rubin L. Fetal loss after cholecystectomy during pregnancy. Can Med Assoc J. 1963;88:576–7.
24. Hiatt JR, Hiatt JC, Williams RA, Klein SR. Biliary disease in pregnancy: strategy for surgical management. Am J Surg. 1986;151(2):263–5.
25. Hedström J, Nilsson J, Andersson R, Andersson B. Changing management of gallstone-related disease in pregnancy - a retrospective cohort analysis. Scand J Gastroenterol. 2017;52(9):1016–21.
26. Glasgow RE, Visser BC, Harris HW, Patti MG, Kilpatrick SJ, Mulvihill SJ. Changing management of gallstone disease during pregnancy. Surg Endosc. 1998;12(3):241–6.
27. Sedaghat N, Cao AM, Eslick GD, Cox MR. Laparoscopic versus open cholecystectomy in pregnancy: a systematic review and meta-analysis. Surg Endosc. 2017;31(2):673–9.
28. Cox TC, Huntington CR, Blair LJ, Prasad T, Lincourt AE, Augenstein VA, et al. Laparoscopic appendectomy and cholecystectomy versus open: a study in 1999 pregnant patients. Surg Endosc. 2016;30(2):593–602.
29. Pearl J, Price R, Richardson W, Fanelli R, Society of American Gastrointestinal Endoscopic Surgeons. Guidelines for diagnosis, treatment, and use of laparoscopy for surgical problems during pregnancy. Surg Endosc. 2011;25(11):3479–92.
30. Bowie JM, Calvo RY, Bansal V, Wessels LE, Butler WJ, Sise CB, et al. Association of complicated gallstone disease in pregnancy and adverse birth outcomes. Am J Surg. 2020;220:745.
31. Williamson C, Geenes V. Intrahepatic cholestasis of pregnancy. Obstet Gynecol. 2014;124(1):120–33.
32. Laifer SA, Stiller RJ, Siddiqui DS, Dunston-Boone G, Whetham JC. Ursodeoxycholic acid for the treatment of intrahepatic cholestasis of pregnancy. J Matern Fetal Med. 2001;10(2):131–5.
33. Kenyon AP, Tribe RM, Nelson-Piercy C, Girling JC, Williamson C, Seed PT, et al. Pruritus in pregnancy: a study of anatomical distribution and prevalence in relation to the development of obstetric cholestasis. Obstet Med. 2010;3(1):25–9.
34. Lee RH, Goodwin TM, Greenspoon J, Incerpi M. The prevalence of intrahepatic cholestasis of pregnancy in a primarily Latina Los Angeles population. J Perinatol. 2006;26(9):527–32.
35. Reyes H, Aburto H, Katz R. Prevalence of intrahepatic cholestasis of pregnancy in Chile. Ann Intern Med. 1978;88:487.
36. Abedin P, Weaver JB, Egginton E. Intrahepatic cholestasis of pregnancy: prevalence and ethnic distribution. Ethn Health. 1999;4(1–2):35–7.
37. Jacquemin E, De Vree JM, Cresteil D, Sokal EM, Sturm E, Dumont M, et al. The wide spectrum of multidrug resistance 3 deficiency: from neonatal cholestasis to cirrhosis of adulthood. Gastroenterology. 2001;120(6):1448–58.
38. Eloranta M-L, Heinonen S, Mononen T, Saarikoski S. Risk of obstetric cholestasis in sisters of index patients: familial risk of obstetric cholestasis. Clin Genet. 2001;60(1):42–5.
39. Reyes H, Ribalta J, Gonzalez-Ceron M. Idiopathic cholestasis of pregnancy in a large kindred. Gut. 1976;17(9):709–13.
40. Oude Elferink RPJ, Paulusma CC. Function and pathophysiological importance of ABCB4 (MDR3 P-glycoprotein). Pflugers Arch. 2007;453(5):601–10.
41. Davit-Spraul A, Gonzales E, Baussan C, Jacquemin E. The spectrum of liver diseases related to ABCB4 gene mutations: pathophysiology and clinical aspects. Semin Liver Dis. 2010;30(2):134–46.
42. Rosmorduc O, Poupon R. Low phospholipid associated cholelithiasis: association with mutation in the MDR3/ABCB4 gene. Orphan J Rare Dis. 2007;2:29.
43. Rosmorduc O, Hermelin B, Poupon R. MDR3 gene defect in adults with symptomatic intrahepatic and gallbladder cholesterol cholelithiasis. Gastroenterology. 2001;120(6):1459–67.

44. Rosmorduc O, Hermelin B, Boelle P-Y, Parc R, Taboury J, Poupon R. ABCB4 gene mutation-associated cholelithiasis in adults. Gastroenterology. 2003;125(2):452–9.
45. Poupon R, Rosmorduc O, Boëlle PY, Chrétien Y, Corpechot C, Chazouillères O, et al. Genotype-phenotype relationships in the low-phospholipid-associated cholelithiasis syndrome: a study of 156 consecutive patients. Hepatology. 2013;58(3):1105–10.
46. Dixon PH, Williamson C. The pathophysiology of intrahepatic cholestasis of pregnancy. Clin Res Hepatol Gastroenterol. 2016;40(2):141–53.
47. Andress EJ, Nicolaou M, Romero MR, Naik S, Dixon PH, Williamson C, et al. Molecular mechanistic explanation for the spectrum of cholestatic disease caused by the S320F variant of ABCB4. Hepatology. 2014;59(5):1921–31.
48. Gautherot J, Delautier D, Maubert M-A, Aït-Slimane T, Bolbach G, Delaunay J-L, et al. Phosphorylation of ABCB4 impacts its function: insights from disease-causing mutations. Hepatology. 2014;60(2):610–21.
49. Delaunay J-L, Durand-Schneider A-M, Dossier C, Falguières T, Gautherot J, Davit-Spraul A, et al. A functional classification of ABCB4 variations causing progressive familial intrahepatic cholestasis type 3. Hepatology. 2016;63(5):1620–31.
50. Gordo-Gilart R, Andueza S, Hierro L, Martínez-Fernández P, D'Agostino D, Jara P, et al. Functional analysis of ABCB4 mutations relates clinical outcomes of progressive familial intrahepatic cholestasis type 3 to the degree of MDR3 floppase activity. Gut. 2015;64(1):147–55.
51. Van Mil SWC, Milona A, Dixon PH, Mullenbach R, Geenes VL, Chambers J, et al. Functional variants of the central bile acid sensor FXR identified in intrahepatic cholestasis of pregnancy. Gastroenterology. 2007;133(2):507–16.
52. Abu-Hayyeh S, Papacleovoulou G, Lövgren-Sandblom A, Tahir M, Oduwole O, Jamaludin NA, et al. Intrahepatic cholestasis of pregnancy levels of sulfated progesterone metabolites inhibit farnesoid X receptor resulting in a cholestatic phenotype. Hepatology. 2013;57(2):716–26.
53. Abu-Hayyeh S, Ovadia C, Lieu T, Jensen DD, Chambers J, Dixon PH, et al. Prognostic and mechanistic potential of progesterone sulfates in intrahepatic cholestasis of pregnancy and pruritus gravidarum: autoimmune, cholestatic and biliary disease. Hepatology. 2016;63(4):1287–98.
54. Reyes H, Báez ME, González MC, Hernández I, Palma J, Ribalta J, et al. Selenium, zinc and copper plasma levels in intrahepatic cholestasis of pregnancy, in normal pregnancies and in healthy individuals, in Chile. J Hepatol. 2000;32(4):542–9.
55. Wikström Shemer E, Marschall H-U. Decreased 1,25-dihydroxy vitamin D levels in women with intrahepatic cholestasis of pregnancy. Acta Obstet Gynecol Scand. 2010;89(11):1420–3.
56. Kremer AE, Bolier R, Dixon PH, Geenes V, Chambers J, Tolenaars D, et al. Autotaxin activity has a high accuracy to diagnose intrahepatic cholestasis of pregnancy. J Hepatol. 2015;62(4):897–904.
57. Reyes H, Sjövall J. Bile acids and progesterone metabolites in intrahepatic cholestasis of pregnancy. Ann Med. 2000;32(2):94–106.
58. Bicocca MJ, Sperling JD, Chauhan SP. Intrahepatic cholestasis of pregnancy: review of six national and regional guidelines. Eur J Obstet Gynecol Reprod Biol. 2018;231:180–7.
59. Glantz A, Marschall H-U, Lammert F, Mattsson L-A. Intrahepatic cholestasis of pregnancy: a randomized controlled trial comparing dexamethasone and ursodeoxycholic acid. Hepatology. 2005;42(6):1399–405.
60. Palma J, Reyes H, Ribalta J, Hernández I, Sandoval L, Almuna R, et al. Ursodeoxycholic acid in the treatment of cholestasis of pregnancy: a randomized, double-blind study controlled with placebo. J Hepatol. 1997;27(6):1022–8.
61. Kondrackiene J, Beuers U, Kupcinskas L. Efficacy and safety of ursodeoxycholic acid versus cholestyramine in intrahepatic cholestasis of pregnancy. Gastroenterology. 2005;129(3):894–901.
62. Gurung V, Middleton P, Milan SJ, Hague W, Thornton JG. Interventions for treating cholestasis in pregnancy. Cochrane Database Syst Rev. 2013;6:CD000493.

63. Chappell LC, Gurung V, Seed PT, Chambers J, Williamson C, Thornton JG, et al. Ursodeoxycholic acid versus placebo, and early term delivery versus expectant management, in women with intrahepatic cholestasis of pregnancy: semifactorial randomised clinical trial. BMJ. 2012;344:e3799.
64. Bacq Y, le Besco M, Lecuyer A-I, Gendrot C, Potin J, Andres CR, et al. Ursodeoxycholic acid therapy in intrahepatic cholestasis of pregnancy: results in real-world conditions and factors predictive of response to treatment. Dig Liver Dis. 2017;49(1):63–9.
65. Bacq Y, Sentilhes L, Reyes HB, Glantz A, Kondrackiene J, Binder T, et al. Efficacy of ursodeoxycholic acid in treating intrahepatic cholestasis of pregnancy: a meta-analysis. Gastroenterology. 2012;143(6):1492–501.
66. Chappell LC, Chambers J, Dixon PH, Dorling J, Hunter R, Bell JL, et al. Ursodeoxycholic acid versus placebo in the treatment of women with intrahepatic cholestasis of pregnancy (ICP) to improve perinatal outcomes: protocol for a randomised controlled trial (PITCHES). Lancet. 2018;19(1):657.
67. Beuers U, de Vries E. Reply to: 'UDCA therapy in intrahepatic cholestasis of pregnancy?'. J Hepatol. 2020;72(3):587–8.
68. Geenes V, Chambers J, Khurana R, Shemer EW, Sia W, Mandair D, et al. Rifampicin in the treatment of severe intrahepatic cholestasis of pregnancy. Eur J Obstet Gynecol Reprod Biol. 2015;189:59–63.
69. Bacq Y, Sapey T, Bréchot MC, Pierre F, Fignon A, Dubois F. Intrahepatic cholestasis of pregnancy: a French prospective study. Hepatology. 1997;26(2):358–64.
70. Fisk NM, Storey GN. Fetal outcome in obstetric cholestasis. Br J Obstet Gynaecol. 1988;95(11):1137–43.
71. Rioseco AJ, Ivankovic MB, Manzur A, Hamed F, Kato SR, Parer JT, et al. Intrahepatic cholestasis of pregnancy: a retrospective case-control study of perinatal outcome. Am J Obstet Gynecol. 1994;170(3):890–5.
72. Glantz A, Marschall H-U, Mattsson L-Å. Intrahepatic cholestasis of pregnancy: relationships between bile acid levels and fetal complication rates. Hepatology. 2004;40(2):467–74.
73. Geenes V, Chappell LC, Seed PT, Steer PJ, Knight M, Williamson C. Association of severe intrahepatic cholestasis of pregnancy with adverse pregnancy outcomes: a prospective population-based case-control study: Geenes et al. Hepatology. 2014;59(4):1482–91.
74. European Association for the Study of the Liver. EASL clinical practice guidelines: management of cholestatic liver diseases. J Hepatol. 2009;51(2):237–67.
75. Marschall H-U, Wikström Shemer E, Ludvigsson JF, Stephansson O. Intrahepatic cholestasis of pregnancy and associated hepatobiliary disease: a population-based cohort study. Hepatology. 2013;58(4):1385–91.
76. Wikström Shemer EA, Stephansson O, Thuresson M, Thorsell M, Ludvigsson JF, Marschall H-U. Intrahepatic cholestasis of pregnancy and cancer, immune-mediated and cardiovascular diseases: a population-based cohort study. J Hepatol. 2015;63(2):456–61.
77. Whitacre CC, Reingold SC, O'Looney PA, Blankenhorn E, Brinley F, Collier E, et al. A gender gap in autoimmunity: task force on gender, multiple sclerosis and autoimmunity*. Science. 1999;283(5406):1277–8.
78. Polanczyk MJ, Hopke C, Huan J, Vandenbark AA, Offner H. Enhanced FoxP3 expression and Treg cell function in pregnant and estrogen-treated mice. J Neuroimmunol. 2005;170(1–2):85–92.
79. Nevens F, Andreone P, Mazzella G, Strasser SI, Bowlus C, Invernizzi P, et al. A Placebo-controlled trial of obeticholic acid in primary biliary cholangitis. N Engl J Med. 2016;375(7):631–43.
80. Corpechot C, Chazouillères O, Rousseau A, Le Gruyer A, Habersetzer F, Mathurin P, et al. A placebo-controlled trial of bezafibrate in primary biliary cholangitis. N Engl J Med. 2018;378(23):2171–81.
81. Boonstra K, Kunst AE, Stadhouders PH, Tuynman HA, Poen AC, van Nieuwkerk KMJ, et al. Rising incidence and prevalence of primary biliary cirrhosis: a large population-based study. Liver Int. 2014;34(6):e31–8.

82. Floreani A, Infantolino C, Franceschet I, Tene IM, Cazzagon N, Buja A, et al. Pregnancy and primary biliary cirrhosis: a case-control study. Clin Rev Allergy Immunol. 2015;48(2–3):236–42.
83. Trivedi PJ, Kumagi T, Al-Harthy N, Coltescu C, Ward S, Cheung A, et al. Good maternal and fetal outcomes for pregnant women with primary biliary cirrhosis. Clin Gastroenterol Hepatol. 2014;12(7):1179–1185.e1.
84. Cauldwell M, Mackie F, Steer P, Henehghan M, Baalman J, Brennand J, et al. Pregnancy outcomes in women with primary biliary cholangitis and primary sclerosing cholangitis: a retrospective cohort study. BJOG. 2020;127:876–84.
85. Poupon R, Chrétien Y, Chazouillères O, Poupon RE. Pregnancy in women with ursodeoxycholic acid-treated primary biliary cirrhosis. J Hepatol. 2005;42(3):418–9.
86. Efe C, Kahramanoğlu-Aksoy E, Yilmaz B, Ozseker B, Takci S, Roach EC, et al. Pregnancy in women with primary biliary cirrhosis. Autoimmun Rev. 2014;13(9):931–5.
87. Matsubara S, Isoda N, Taniguchi N. Jaundice as the first manifestation of primary biliary cirrhosis during pregnancy: measurement of portal vein blood flow. J Obstet Gynaecol Res. 2011;37(7):963–4.
88. Janczewska I, Olsson R, Hultcrantz R, Broomé U. Pregnancy in patients with primary sclerosing cholangitis. Liver. 1996;16(5):326–30.
89. Bergquist A, Montgomery SM, Lund U, Ekbom A, Olsson R, Lindgren S, et al. Perinatal events and the risk of developing primary sclerosing cholangitis. World J Gastroenterol. 2006;12(37):6037–40.
90. Kammeijer CQ, De Man RA, De Groot CJM. Primary sclerosing cholangitis and pregnancy. Clin Pract. 2011;1(3):e55.
91. Gossard A, Lindor K. Pregnancy in primary sclerosing cholangitis. Gut. 2011;60(8):1027–8.
92. Wellge BE, Sterneck M, Teufel A, Rust C, Franke A, Schreiber S, et al. Pregnancy in primary sclerosing cholangitis. Gut. 2011;60(8):1117–21.
93. Ludvigsson JF, Bergquist A, Ajne G, Kane S, Ekbom A, Stephansson O. A population-based cohort study of pregnancy outcomes among women with primary sclerosing cholangitis. Clin Gastroenterol Hepatol. 2014;12(1):95–100.e1.
94. Stephansson O, Larsson H, Pedersen L, Kieler H, Granath F, Ludvigsson JF, et al. Crohn's disease is a risk factor for preterm birth. Clin Gastroenterol Hepatol. 2010;8(6):509–15.
95. Cornish J, Tan E, Teare J, Teoh TG, Rai R, Clark SK, et al. A meta-analysis on the influence of inflammatory bowel disease on pregnancy. Gut. 2007;56(6):830–7.
96. Cundy TF, O'Grady JG, Williams R. Recovery of menstruation and pregnancy after liver transplantation. Gut. 1990;31(3):337–8.
97. Cundy TF, Butler J, Pope RM, Saggar-Malik AK, Wheeler MJ, Williams R. Amenorrhoea in women with non-alcoholic chronic liver disease. Gut. 1991;32(2):202–6.
98. Westbrook RH, Yeoman AD, O'Grady JG, Harrison PM, Devlin J, Heneghan MA. Model for end-stage liver disease score predicts outcome in cirrhotic patients during pregnancy. Clin Gastroenterol Hepatol. 2011;9(8):694–9.
99. Shaheen AAM, Myers RP. The outcomes of pregnancy in patients with cirrhosis: a population-based study. Liver Int. 2010;30(2):275–83.
100. European Association for the Study of the Liver. EASL clinical practice guidelines: the diagnosis and management of patients with primary biliary cholangitis. J Hepatol. 2017;67(1):145–72.
101. Chapman R, Fevery J, Kalloo A, Nagorney DM, Boberg KM, Shneider B, et al. Diagnosis and management of primary sclerosing cholangitis. Hepatology. 2010;51(2):660–78.
102. de Vries E, Beuers U. Ursodeoxycholic acid in pregnancy? J Hepatol. 2019;71(6):1237–45.
103. Inamdar S, Berzin TM, Sejpal DV, Pleskow DK, Chuttani R, Sawhney MS, et al. Pregnancy is a risk factor for pancreatitis after endoscopic retrograde cholangiopancreatography in a national cohort study. Clin Gastroenterol Hepatol. 2016;14(1):107–14.

Transplant and Autoimmune Diseases

16

Martina Gambato and Francesco Paolo Russo

16.1 Primary Biliary Cholangitis

16.1.1 End-Stage Liver Disease

Some patients with PBC have a normal quality of life without liver-related complications, while others progress to cirrhosis, liver failure, and death. Nowadays 40% of patients with PBC will develop cirrhosis within 10 years, being at increased risk of liver failure and hepatocellular carcinoma [1]. One of the liver complications in patients with PBC is the development of varices; nearly 6% of patients with early-stage disease have varices [2, 3]. The 3-year survival after initial variceal bleed is about 50% [4]. Hepatocellular carcinoma occurs in 1–6% of patients with PBC per year. Fatigue and pruritus are the most common symptoms in PBC patients and often have a more negative effect on quality of life than the disease itself [5, 6]. Before the widespread use of screening liver chemistries and the availability of UDCA, PBC was not usually diagnosed until the disease had reached an advanced stage, with subsequent median survival of 6–10 years [7]. Ursodeoxycholic acid (UDCA) treatment has been associated with a reduced relative risk of liver transplantation or death [8], regardless of age, sex, or disease stage. The association remains significant in cases of incomplete biochemical response. The strong association between UDCA therapy and prolonged LT-free survival was recently shown in both a large American cohort and European international cohort [9], with adequate dose recommendations. In younger patients with PBC, there is a stronger LT-free survival benefit of UDCA than in older patients, who can present also extrahepatic factors for death, unlikely to be influenced by UDCA [9]. Accurately

M. Gambato · F. P. Russo (✉)
Multivisceral Transplant and Gastroenterology Unit, Department of Surgery, Oncology and Gastroenterology, Padova University Hospital, Padova, Italy
e-mail: francescopaolo.russo@unipd.it

© Springer Nature Switzerland AG 2021
A. Floreani (ed.), *Diseases of the Liver and Biliary Tree*,
https://doi.org/10.1007/978-3-030-65908-0_16

predicting clinical outcomes in patients with PBC is challenging. In a meta-analysis [10] of over 4800 patients with primary biliary cirrhosis, the strongest predictor of death or liver transplantation was alkaline phosphatase more than two times the upper limit of normal, 1 year after study enrolment. The Model for End-Stage Liver Disease (MELD) and Mayo Prognostic Model for PBC (Mayo R score) have been validated in PBC patients to predict the risk of death and they were used in LT setting to determine the right timing of transplant.

16.1.2 Liver Transplantation

When liver cirrhosis-induced liver failure is progressive, LT remains a definitive therapeutic option. LT is usually indicated for decompensated cirrhosis or hepatocellular carcinoma; more rarely, intractable pruritus might justify transplantation. The percentage of transplantations for PBC as compared to other etiologies decreased to less than one-fifth of its original proportion of 20%. In contrast, the absolute number of transplantations for PBC has remained virtually stable over the last 10 years. Characteristics of patients undergoing transplantation for PBC have changed over time, whereby they are now older, have higher MELD scores, and are more likely to be male than 30 years ago [11]. Although allocation criteria are country specific but in most of the regions of the world allocation for LT is currently based on the MELD criteria. This allocation system offers the possibility of standard exceptions in case the synthetic capacity of the liver underestimates the severity of the disease. In this regard, in many countries PSC patients receive priority if they suffer from recurrent cholangitis. Before the introduction of the MELD system PBC patients received systematically higher priority on the waiting list if these suffered from pruritus. Even if currently PBC disease is not a reason for a standard exception, recent data demonstrated however that in different parts of the world the mortality of PBC patients on the waiting list for LT has increased and is higher versus other indications such as PSC or HCV. This suggests that patients with PBC listed for LT should be considered for MELD exception points [12]. LT is an excellent treatment for patients with decompensated disease, with 90–95% 1-year patient survival, and 80–85% 5-year graft survival [13]. Ten-year survival rates are 75–80% and recurrence of PBC after transplant occurs in 10–40% of patients. Between 1988 and 2015, 8% of cirrhosis patients were transplanted due to PBC, based on the data from the European Liver Transplant Registry [13].

16.1.3 PBC Recurrence After LT

The first report of PBC recurrence was described in 1982 [14]. Since then, relatively sparse epidemiological data have been reported, showing medium- and long-term recurrence rates between 17% and 46%. The diagnosis of PBC recurrence is purely histological, with liver biopsies showing florid duct lesions and, in more advanced stages, granulomatosis cholangitis [15]. Early and nonspecific inflammation features such as high-grade lymphoplasmacytic portal infiltrates have been described too [16]. To date, it is not clear if they should be considered as full diagnostic criteria or just as latent signs of PBC recurrence. Immunocytochemical stains (antibody to cytocheratin-7 and antibody to C355.1) may also be useful in doubtful cases [17]. The Global PBC Study Group showed that a younger age at the time of diagnosis and LT, tacrolimus use, and severe biochemical cholestasis within the first 6 months after LT were independently associated with an increased risk of recurrence of PBC. Recurrence of PBC was associated with worse graft and overall survival after LT. However, the pathogenesis explaining the association between early abnormal liver biochemistries tests within 1 year of LT and a higher risk of recurrence of PBC still needs a definitive answer [18]. Classical pretransplant symptoms such as pruritus and jaundice are rarely observed during the post-transplant follow-up. Along the same line, fatigue and osteoporosis are nonspecific and should not be used for diagnosis. Also, xerostomia and/or xerophthalmia may resolve or persist after LT. Anti-mitochondria autoantibodies (AMA) usually persist after LT [19] and there is no correlation between the presence and the titer of AMA and the risk of development of PBC recurrence. Given that, different cofounding factors must be taken into account when looking into PBC recurrence reported rates, including but not limited to: the execution of post-LT liver biopsy as per-protocol procedure or not, the sampling error of liver biopsy, the use of less restrictive criteria for PBC recurrence diagnosis. Average time to PBC recurrence significantly varies among the studies too, being affected by several factors (mainly duration of follow-up and center experience as number of LT performed for PBC). Centers with high volume load (i.e., more than 100 patients transplanted for PBC) report an average time to recurrence between 3 and 5.5 years [20, 21]. Cumulative incidence of PBC recurrence seems to be more appropriate and to provide more useful information, varying between 21% and 37% at 10 years [15]. Post-transplant follow-up should adhere to current guidelines (European Association for the Study of the Liver) [22, 23], taking into consideration that these patients present a much higher risk of osteoporosis as well as other concomitant autoimmune diseases (i.e., thyroid dysfunction) [24]. Preliminary data suggested that prophylactic UDCA after liver transplantation might reduce the risk of recurrent PBC but this is not yet standard of care [25]. In a recently published international multicenter study of 3902 PBC patients, Harms et al. [8] found that treatment with UDCA is associated with prolonged liver transplant-free survival. Data just confirmed in a multicenter long-term study, where preventive administration of UDCA after LT for PBC showed a reduced risk of disease recurrence, and a parallel reduction in the long-term risk of graft loss, liver-related death, and all-cause death [26]. From a practical perspective, EASL guidelines suggest its use in patients with proven or likely recurrent of PBC. Obeticholic acid seems to be a promising therapy for PBC patients with inadequate response or intolerance to UDCA in the non-transplant setting. However, data are awaited to examine the effects of OCA on clinical outcome in patients with recurrent PBC.

16.2 Primary Sclerosis Cholangitis (PSC)

16.2.1 PSC as Indication for LT

The natural history of PSC is remarkable for its variability between patients. In general, PSC is a progressive disease with death or LT occurring at a mean of 12–16 years from the diagnosis [27–29]. Recent International PSC Study Group data showed that 36.7% of patients progressed to LT or death during a median follow-up of 14.5 years [4]. PSC patients showing an advanced histological stage on liver biopsy and those who have high-grade and diffuse intrahepatic biliary stricturing showed decreased overall survival and poor prognosis [28, 30]. In historical cohorts of PSC patients, liver failure and cirrhosis complications were the most common drivers for fatal outcome (64% of all deaths) [30]. Nowadays, liver transplantation is the only treatment able to modify the natural history of the disease. PSC is a well-recognized indication for liver transplantation. From ELTR data cholestatic liver disease represents 10% of all indications, in a young age range of recipients [31]. Similarly, in the USA, PSC is the fourth most common indication for LT, accounting for approximately 10% of LT [32]. In some areas, such as in the Scandinavian countries, which have a relatively low prevalence of hepatitis C and alcoholic liver disease, PSC is the leading indication accounting for 16% of the LT [33]. The indication for LT varies between patients with cirrhosis and patients with complications related to biliary tree dysfunction, such as recurrent cholangitis. So, the most important challenging point is the adequate timing of LT in PSC patients in order to obtain better survival results. Several models based on clinical, biochemical, and histological features have been developed for monitoring therapeutic interventions and has used in determining the optimal timing for LT. In the initial Mayo PSC model, patient age, serum bilirubin, hemoglobin concentration, hepatic histological stage, and presence or absence of inflammatory bowel disease (IBD) were identified as independent prognostic variables [27]. Among the other reported scores, several features have been identified as independent prognostic variables, such as age, serum alkaline phosphatase and bilirubin levels, histological stage, hepatomegaly, and splenomegaly [34, 35]. The reviewed PSC model added to serum bilirubin, other parameters of liver necrosis, like serum aspartate aminotransferase level and the presence of advanced liver disease, like history of variceal bleeding and serum albumin level [36]. In advanced stages of PSC, Child–Pugh score has been demonstrated to be useful in determining outcome after LT [37]. The policies for allocation in LT based on "sickest first" rule make optimal timing for LT in PSC patients highly challenging. PSC patients with Child–Pugh score of 10 or more associated with portal hypertension complications have more chances to receive a graft. On the other hand, patients with PSC at high risk of recurrent bacterial cholangitis and septicemia have a high incidence of morbidity. Because many of these patients have well-preserved hepatic synthetic function, the allocation policy that uses the MELD score alone may not appropriately prioritize these selected groups of patients to avoid a poor outcome. A consensus paper from Gores et al. concluded that patients who have two or more culture-proven bacteremia within a 6-month period or who have septic complications of bacterial cholangitis should be considered as a MELD exceptional case [38]. Bacteremia should be non-iatrogenic (unrelated to a procedure such as recent endoscopic retrograde cholangiogram or transhepatic cholangiogram) and should occur in a patient who does not have a biliary tube or stent; in addition, these episodes of bacterial cholangitis may occur in patients who have been treated with antibiotic therapy that has failed to suppress these septic episodes. Patients who meet the above criteria should have a calculated MELD score that is based on the serum bilirubin and creatinine concentrations and international normalized ratio. Importantly, being cholangiocarcinoma a dramatical complication of PSC, physicians should refer patients for LT earlier than they would patients with other causes of chronic liver disease. Historically CCA has been considered to be a relative contraindication for LT in many programs due to high rate of recurrence. Mayo Clinic reported the first data on LT for CCA, showing acceptable patient survival after LT in selected patients who undergo radiation and chemotherapy prior to LT. Similarly, in retrospective series, patients with early intrahepatic CCA and without an indication for liver resection showed excellent results in terms of recurrence-free survival after LT. Although the first were poor, the results of LT for PSC have shown marked improvement in the last decades. Post-transplant outcome is excellent, with patient survival more than 8% at 1 and 5 years, 77% and 62% at 10 and 20 years after LT (ELTR data). Indeed, a retrospective analysis of PSC patients using the Mayo PSC natural history model has shown that liver transplantation significantly improves patient survival compared with the estimated survival in the absence of liver LT [39]. Still, in a single-center prospective cohort [40] it was demonstrated that fatigue improves after LT. However, 44% of the 31 patients had moderate to severe fatigue at 2 years after LT. Although patient survival following LT is excellent in PSC patients, long-term graft survival is somewhat less, which seems to be related to a higher incidence of acute and chronic rejection and disease recurrence [32].

16.2.2 PSC Recurrence After LT

Recurrence of PSC following liver transplant was first reported as early as 1988 [41]. PSC has been shown to recur between 10% and 27%, with a mean interval between LT and onset of 6 months to 5 years [42], imparting significant morbidity, need for re-transplantation, and an increased mortality risk [43–45]. The etiology of recurrent PSC (rPSC) remains largely unknown but identifying possible risk factors may help to develop treatment strategies to reduce its incidence. To make diagnosis of rPSC, nonspecific bile duct injuries and strictures caused by allograft reperfusion injury, ischemia, rejection, and recurrent biliary sepsis should be excluded [46–48]. The Mayo Clinic criteria are now used as the gold standard for diagnosing rPSC [49, 50], consisting of a confirmed diagnosis of PSC prior to LT; cholangiography showing intrahepatic and/or extrahepatic biliary stricturing, irregularity after 90 days after LT or liver biopsy showing fibrous cholangitis and/or fibro-obliterative lesions with or without ductopenia, biliary fibrosis or biliary cirrhosis. Moreover, conditions such as hepatic artery thrombosis/stenosis, established ductopenic rejection, anastomotic strictures alone, non-anastomotic strictures or ischemic type biliary lesions (ITBL) within 90 days and ABO incompatibility between donor and recipient must be excluded. A recent metanalysis including 14 studies describing possible risk factors for rPSC for 2481 patients revealed 18% of rPSC after LT. They showed that colectomy before LT, CCA before LT, any episode of acute cellular rejection after LT, and laboratory MELD score were associated with the risk of rPSC. Trivedi et al. revealed a colectomy with end-ileostomy to have a more favorable outcome on graft survival and a protective effect on rPSC as opposed to ileal pouch-anal anastomosis or no colectomy [51] also investigated the association between colectomy and rPSC in a study. Moreover, Joshi et al. identified active IBD as a significant predictor for graft failure after liver transplantation [52]. Nowadays, performing a colectomy before transplantation is not routine practice and more data is needed in order to reconsider the threshold for colectomy in PSC-IBD patients with persistent intestinal inflammation and progressive liver disease that are likely to need a LT. Regarding the presence of CCA as risk factor, Gordon et al. explained this finding by the therapy for CCA because it may induce changes in the native hepatic artery, resulting in secondary sclerosing cholangitis after LT, which makes it difficult to differentiate from rPSC. However, this finding is not fully clear, because CCA is often diagnosed in the explant after LT, in patients not receiving chemotherapy. The role of acute cellular rejection on rPSC risk is not fully understood. The increase of autoimmune epitopes during rejection could explain the immune-mediated ductal damage [47] or the treatment of rejections may enhance the development of rPSC [44, 53]. Moreover, the extended donor criteria (EDC) grafts have also been reported as a significant risk factor for rPSC [54]. Recurrence of PSC post-LT appears to be a relatively benign disease, with some uncertain. Maheshwari et al. [55] using the UNOS database showed a higher re-transplantation rate and a lower survival in PSC, comparing with PBC recipients from the same study population. These data have been confirmed elsewhere [56, 57], but other studies report no effect [58]. There is no established medical therapy for rPSC. UDCA is used and associated with improvement of liver tests. Symptomatic treatment of pruritus and interventional cholangiographic treatment of biliary strictures should be considered when dominant and clinically significant strictures are present.

16.3 Autoimmune Hepatitis (AIH)

Indications for LT in AIH include decompensated cirrhosis, failure of medical treatment, fulminant AIH, liver cancer, and hepatocellular failure with a MELD score >16 points. In patients with chronic liver disease related to AIH, a lack of response to standard immunosuppression regimens is predictive for LT, especially when there is less than 50% improvement of aminotransferases within 6 months [59].

On the other hand, no clear definition for acute severe AIH exists yet. Czaja et al. [60] and Yeoman et al. [61] previously defined acute severe AIH as an acute presentation (≤26 weeks) with an INR of ≥1.5, without histological evidence of cirrhosis.

Recently, a subclassification of the acute presentation of AIH has been proposed to guide the therapeutic approach and to improve the prognostication. Possible definitions could include the following: (1) Acute AIH: icteric with no evidence of coagulopathy or encephalopathy; (2) acute severe (AS-AIH): icteric and coagulopathic (INR ≥ 1.5) but no evidence of encephalopathy; (3) AS-AIH with acute liver failure (ALF): icteric, coagulopathic (INR ≥ 1.5), and encephalopathic [62]. In 2 recent studies, 60–70% of patients with AS-AIH defined as having an acute presentation with an INR ≥ 1.5 in the absence of chronic liver disease [61] developed ALF. The histological diagnosis of AS-AIH is challenging because the findings are nonspecific and may overlap with lesions found in viral hepatitis and DILI. In contrast to classic AIH, histological features of autoimmune ALF appear to predominate in the centrilobular zone.

The findings can reflect a spectrum of severity, from diffuse lobular hepatitis to confluent centrilobular/bridging/multiacinar necrosis to sub-massive hepatocellular loss. Hofer et al. reported that centrilobular necrosis may indicate acute-onset AIH in as high as 87% of patients [63]. The US Acute Liver Failure (USALF) Study Group composed a histological classification specific for ALF. They proposed a classification based on histological variants of massive hepatic necrosis (MHN). Two specific patterns (MHN 4-centrilobular hemorrhagic necrosis and MHN 5-confluent necrosis superimposed on chronic hepatitis) were deemed to be more specific of an autoimmune etiology.

A special consideration is drug-induced liver injury (DILI) that resembles and may be difficult to differentiate from AIH. There are three main types of autoimmune DILI: (1) AIH with superimposed DILI; (2) DILI-induced AIH; (3) Immune-mediated DILI. A subgroup of idiosyncratic DILIs shows features of autoimmunity and may require liver transplantation in 4–5%. The diagnosis can be difficult because the clinical presentation, biochemistry, serology, and histology can often be indistinguishable from idiopathic AIH. Liver biopsy is strongly recommended because some features (e.g., severe features, emperipolesis, and rosette formation) are more typical for a diagnosis of idiopathic AIH [64], while eosinophil infiltration is more likely present in DILI. Centrilobular necrosis can be seen in both [65, 66]. Even though a proportion of patients with AS-AIH respond to corticosteroids, for the majority with ALF, LT remains the best option [67, 68]. Thus, patients with encephalopathy development should be considered for LT immediately [69–72]. It was demonstrated that a MELD score of ≤28 on admission, low-grade encephalopathy, absence of MHN on histology, and improvement of bilirubin and INR within 4 days of therapy were associated with higher response rates to corticosteroids [70, 73, 74]. Failure to improve Model for End-Stage Liver Disease–sodium (MELD-Na), UK Model for End-Stage Liver Disease scores or bilirubin within 7 days of corticosteroid therapy indicates a group at high risk of progressing to ALF [75, 76]. Recently, an algorithm for the management of acute AIH has been proposed [62]. Outcome after LT for patients with AIH is generally good with a 5- and 10-year approximately 75% overall survival. The results on long-term survival after LT for AIH, from the European Liver Transplant Registry (ELTR), between 1998 and 2017, were recently reported. Patients after AIH were compared with patients receiving LT for the other autoimmune liver diseases: PBC and PSC and for alcoholic liver cirrhosis. They showed that patients who underwent LT for AIH had a lower overall survival compared to patients transplanted for PBC and PSC. Patients with AIH-LT were at increased risk of death and graft loss due to infections and graft rejection compared to all other groups. AIH-LT patients were at particularly high risk for lethal fungal infections, which occurred mainly during the first 90 days post LT. Excluding patients who died within 90 days after LT, patient survival was similar between patients after AIH-LT and patients after PSC-LT.

16.3.1 AIH Recurrence After LT

Recurrence of AIH affects approximately 25% of liver allografts during the first 5 years after liver transplantation and more than 50% after 10 years of follow-up. Establishing an accurate frequency of recurrent AIH (rAIH) has been challenging. Different groups have used variable diagnostic criteria and histological features [77]. Diagnostic criteria of recurrence must include a combination of biochemical changes (elevated serum aminotransferases levels and hypergammaglobulinemia), histological features of AIH, and steroid dependency. After LT, review of the explant and correlation with pretransplant serology is mandatory. Elevated liver enzymes and immunoglobulins before LT and lymphoplasmacytic infiltration with moderate-to-severe inflammatory activity in explants may be associated with a greater likelihood of AIH recurrence after LT [77, 78]. Active disease before LT directly influences the development of rAIH, implying that recurrence may simply be a continuum of the original process. There is a need to identify patients at risk for early recurrence using protocol liver biopsies and immunoglobulin levels in order to better evaluating management strategies for prevention and treatment. In addition, increased frequency of acute and late rejection has been observed in this group of patients compared with those with non-AIH liver diseases. Immunosuppressive therapy should be pursued even if liver test results are normal. In some cohort studies, low maintenance immunosuppression and termination of corticosteroids has been associated with higher risk of rAIH [79–81]. A UK study reported that long-term corticosteroid use after LT for AIH is safe and associated with a lower incidence of rAIH compared to other series [82]. The treatment of rAIH is empiric and very much depends on the presentation, which can be variable. When patients present with asymptomatic disease and minimal changes in liver biochemistry or histology, minor adjustments with increased immunosuppression may be sufficient to suppress recurrent disease [79, 83]. When patients present with more active rAIH, however, more potent regimens tend to be employed with either an increased dose, re-starting with corticosteroids and/or addition of immunosuppressive agents. Re-transplantation may be required for patients with rAIH who present with liver failure and graft loss; this has traditionally been documented primarily in children and young adults. For example, in one North American center, 60% of children with rAIH developed cirrhosis, and evidence for rAIH was observed in all patients that required re-transplantation [84].

De novo AIH develops in LT recipients transplanted for other liver diseases. The frequency of de novo AIH has been estimated at 5–10% of pediatric recipients and 1–2% in adult recipients. It was originally described in children after LT, predominantly in those with biliary atresia [85] and subsequently found in a higher prevalence of LT recipients with PBC [86]. The incidence of de novo AIH is variable because multiple descriptions have been used in case series; however, the disease is rare and does not appear to have an impact on long-term survival. De novo AIH was described in adults transplanted for drug-induced liver disease, alcoholic cirrhosis, PSC, PBC, cryptogenic cirrhosis, and HCV-related cirrhosis in 2001 [87].

The term, "plasma cell-rich rejection" has been suggested as a substitute of "de novo AIH" because the histological features of lymphocytic cholangitis, central perivenulitis, and T cell-mediated rejection are atypical for AIH [88]. It is not clear yet if this form of graft dysfunction constitutes an autoimmune (de novo AIH) or an alloimmune—plasma cell-rich rejection—reaction. The clinical manifestations of de novo AIH are similar to those of rAIH and classical AIH. Most patients have hypergammaglobulinemia, increased serum IgG levels, and ANA, SMA, or both ANA and SMA. Portal and periportal (interface) hepatitis with lymphocytes and plasma cells are the main histological features of de novo AIH. Perivenular cell necrosis, lobular hepatitis, portal fibrosis, zonal necrosis, and centrilobular necrosis have also been reported. Recipients of female grafts or older donors have a higher prevalence of de novo AIH. Prednisone or prednisolone remains the main treatment of de novo AIH, but combined therapy with other immunosuppressive agents has also been used. In adults, prednisone or prednisolone, 30 mg daily, in conjunction with azathioprine, 1–2 mg/kg daily, is recommended. The dose of prednisone or prednisolone should be decreased during a period of 4–8 weeks to maintain a dose of 5–10 mg daily [89].

References

1. Trivedi PJ, Lammers WJ, van Buuren HR, et al. Stratification of hepatocellular carcinoma risk in primary biliary cirrhosis: a multicentre international study. Gut. 2016;65(2):321–9. https://doi.org/10.1136/gutjnl-2014-308351.
2. Ali AH, Sinakos E, Silveira MG, Jorgensen RA, Angulo P, Lindor KD. Varices in early histological stage primary biliary cirrhosis. J Clin Gastroenterol. 2011;45(7):e66–71. https://doi.org/10.1097/MCG.0b013e3181f18c4e.
3. Ikeda F, Okamoto R, Baba N, et al. Prevalence and associated factors with esophageal varices in early primary biliary cirrhosis. J Gastroenterol Hepatol. 2012;27(8):1320–8. https://doi.org/10.1111/j.1440-1746.2012.07114.x.
4. Lindor KD, Gershwin ME, Poupon R, et al. Primary biliary cirrhosis. Hepatology. 2009;50(1):291–308. https://doi.org/10.1002/hep.22906.
5. Mells GF, Pells G, Newton JL, et al. Impact of primary biliary cirrhosis on perceived quality of life: the UK-PBC national study. Hepatology. 2013;58(1):273–83. https://doi.org/10.1002/hep.26365.
6. Al-Harthy N, Kumagi T, Coltescu C, Hirschfield GM. The specificity of fatigue in primary biliary cirrhosis: evaluation of a large clinic practice. Hepatology. 2010;52(2):562–70. https://doi.org/10.1002/hep.23683.

7. Locke GR III, Therneau TM, Ludwig J, Dickson ER, Lindor KD. Time course of histological progression in primary biliary cirrhosis. Hepatology. 1996;23(1):52–6. https://doi.org/10.1002/hep.510230108.
8. Harms MH, de Veer RC, Lammers WJ, et al. Number needed to treat with ursodeoxycholic acid therapy to prevent liver transplantation or death in primary biliary cholangitis. Gut. 2019;69:1502. https://doi.org/10.1136/gutjnl-2019-319057.
9. Harms MH, van Buuren HR, Corpechot C, et al. Ursodeoxycholic acid therapy and liver transplant-free survival in patients with primary biliary cholangitis. J Hepatol. 2019;71(2):357–65. https://doi.org/10.1016/j.jhep.2019.04.001.
10. Lammers WJ, van Buuren HR, Hirschfield GM, et al. Levels of alkaline phosphatase and bilirubin are surrogate end points of outcomes of patients with primary biliary cirrhosis: an international follow-up study. Gastroenterology. 2014;147(6):1338–e15. https://doi.org/10.1053/j.gastro.2014.08.029.
11. Harms MH, Janssen QP, Adam R, et al. Trends in liver transplantation for primary biliary cholangitis in Europe over the past three decades. Aliment Pharmacol Ther. 2019;49(3):285–95. https://doi.org/10.1111/apt.15060.
12. Nevens F. PBC-transplantation and disease recurrence. Best Pract Res Clin Gastroenterol. 2018;34–35:107–11. https://doi.org/10.1016/j.bpg.2018.09.001.
13. https://www.ELTR.org.
14. Neuberger J, Portmann B, Macdougall BR, Calne RY, Williams R. Recurrence of primary biliary cirrhosis after liver transplantation. N Engl J Med. 1982;306(1):1–4.
15. Charatcharoenwitthaya P, Pimentel S, Talwalkar JA, Enders FT, Lindor KD, Krom RA, et al. Long-term survival and impact of ursodeoxycholic acid treatment for recurrent primary biliary cirrhosis after liver transplantation. Liver Transpl. 2007;13(9):1236–45.
16. Sylvestre PB, Batts KP, Burgart LJ, Poterucha JJ, Wiesner RH. Recurrence of primary biliary cirrhosis after liver transplantation: histologic estimate of incidence and natural history. Liver Transpl. 2003;9(10):1086–93.
17. Van de Water J, Gerson LB, Ferrell LD, Lake JR, Coppel RL, Batts KP, et al. Immunohistochemical evidence of disease recurrence after liver transplantation for primary biliary cirrhosis. Hepatology. 1996;24(5):1079–84.
18. Montano-Loza AJ, Hansen BE, Corpechot C, et al. Factors associated with recurrence of primary biliary cholangitis after liver transplantation and effects on graft and patient survival [published correction appears in Gastroenterology. 2020;158(1):288]. Gastroenterology. 2019;156(1):96–107.e1. https://doi.org/10.1053/j.gastro.2018.10.001.
19. Klein R, Huizenga JR, Gips CH, Berg PA. Antimitochondrial antibody profiles in patients with primary biliary cirrhosis before orthotopic liver transplantation and titres of antimitochondrial antibody-subtypes after transplantation. J Hepatol. 1994;20(2):181–9.
20. Liermann Garcia RF, Evangelista Garcia C, McMaster P, Neuberger J. Transplantation for primary biliary cirrhosis: retrospective analysis of 400 patients in a single center. Hepatology. 2001;33(1):22–7.
21. Jacob DA, Neumann UP, Bahra M, Klupp J, Puhl G, Neuhaus R, et al. Long-term follow-up after recurrence of primary biliary cirrhosis after liver transplantation in 100 patients. Clin Transpl. 2006;20(2):211–20.
22. EASL. EASL clinical practice guidelines: liver transplantation. J Hepatol. 2016;64(2):433–85.
23. EASL. EASL clinical practice guidelines: the diagnosis and management of patients with primary biliary cholangitis. J Hepatol. 2017;67(1):145–72.
24. Floreani A, Cazzagon N. PBC and related extrahepatic diseases. Best Pract Res Clin Gastroenterol. 2018;34–35:49–54.
25. Bosch A, Dumortier J, Maucort-Boulch D, et al. Preventive administration of UDCA after liver transplantation for primary biliary cirrhosis is associated with a lower risk of disease recurrence. J Hepatol. 2015;63(6):1449–58. https://doi.org/10.1016/j.jhep.2015.07.038.
26. Corpechot C, Chazouillères O, Belnou P, et al. Long-term impact of preventive UDCA therapy after transplantation for primary biliary cholangitis. J Hepatol. 2020;73(3):559–65. https://doi.org/10.1016/j.jhep.2020.03.043.

27. Wiesner RH, Grambsch PM, Dickson ER, et al. Primary sclerosing cholangitis: natural history, prognostic factors, and survival analysis. Hepatology. 1989;10:430–6.
28. Farrant JM, Hayllar KM, Wilkinson ML, et al. Natural history and prognostic variables in primary sclerosing cholangitis. Gastroenterology. 1991;100:1710–7.
29. Angulo P, Larson DR, Therneau TM, et al. Time course of histological progression in primary sclerosing cholangitis. Am J Gastroenterol. 1999;94:3310–3.
30. Broome ÅU, Olsson R, Loof L, et al. Natural history and prognostic factors in 305 Swedish patients with primary sclerosing cholangitis. Gut. 1996;38:610–5.
31. Adam R, Karam V, Delvart V, O'Grady J, Mirza D, Klempnauer J, Castaing D, Neuhaus P, Jamieson N, Salizzoni M, Pollard S, et al. Evolution of indications and results of liver transplantation in Europe. A report from the European Liver Transplant Registry (ELTR). J Hepatol. 2012;57(3):675–88. https://doi.org/10.1016/j.jhep.2012.04.015.
32. Seaberg EC, Belle SH, Beringer KC, et al. Liver transplantation in the United States from 1987-1998:updated results from the Pitt-UNOS Liver Transplant Registry. Clin Transpl. 1998:17–37.
33. Nordic Liver Transplant Registry. www.scandiatransplant.org.
34. Weismüller TJ, Trivedi PJ, Bergquist A, et al. Patient age, sex, and inflammatory bowel disease phenotype associate with course of primary sclerosing cholangitis. Gastroenterology. 2017;152:1975–84.
35. Dickson ER, Murtaugh PA, Wiesner RH, et al. Primary sclerosing cholangitis: renement and validation of survival models. Gastroenterology. 1992;103:1893–901.
36. Kim WR, Therneau TM, Wiesner RH, et al. A revised natural history model for primary sclerosing cholangitis obviates the need for liver histology. Mayo Clin Proc. 2000;75:688–94.
37. Talwalkar JA, Seaberg EC, Kim WR, et al. Predicting clinical and economic outcome after liver transplantation using the Mayo Primary Sclerosing Cholangitis Model and Child-Pugh score. Liver Transpl. 2000;6:753.
38. Gores GJ, Gish RG, Shrestha R, Wiesner RH. Model for end-stage liver disease (MELD) exception for bacterial cholangitis. Liver Transpl. 2006;12:S91–2.
39. Wiesner RH. Liver transplantation for primary biliary cirrhosis and primary sclerosing cholangitis: predicting outcomes with natural history models. Mayo Clin Proc. 1998;73:575–88.
40. Carbone M, Bufton S, Monaco A, Griffiths L, Jones DE, Neuberger JM. The effect of liver transplantation on fatigue in patients with primary biliary cirrhosis: a prospective study. J Hepatol. 2013;59(3):490–4. https://doi.org/10.1016/j.jhep.2013.04.017.
41. Lerut J, Demetris AJ, Stieber AC, et al. Intrahepatic bile duct strictures after human orthotopic liver transplantation. Recurrence of primary sclerosing cholangitis or unusual presentation of allograft rejection? Transpl Int. 1988;1:127–30.
42. Duclos-Vallee JC, Sebagh M. Recurrence of autoimmune disease, primary sclerosing cholangitis, primary biliary cirrhosis, and autoimmune hepatitis after liver transplantation. Liver Transpl. 2009;15:S25–34.
43. Egawa H, Ueda Y, Ichida T, et al. Risk factors for recurrence of primary sclerosing cholangitis after living donor liver transplantation in Japanese registry. Am J Transplant. 2011;11:518–27.
44. Alexander J, Lord JD, Yeh MM, Cuevas C, Bakthavatsalam R, Kowdley KV. Risk factors for recurrence of primary sclerosing cholangitis after liver transplantation. Liver Transpl. 2008;14:245–51.
45. Miki C, Harrison JD, Gunson BK, Buckels JA, McMaster P, Mayer AD. Inflammatory bowel disease in primary sclerosing cholangitis: an analysis of patients undergoing liver transplantation. Br J Surg. 1995;82:1114–7.
46. Khettry U, Keaveny A, Goldar-Najafi A, Lewis WD, Pomfret EA, Pomposelli JJ, et al. Liver transplantation for primary sclerosing cholangitis: a long-term clinicopathologic study. Hum Pathol. 2003;34:1127–36.
47. Jeyarajah DR, Netto GJ, Lee SP, Testa G, Abbasoglu O, Husberg BS, et al. Recurrent primary sclerosing cholangitis after orthotopic liver transplantation: is chronic rejection part of the disease process? Transplantation. 1998;66:1300–6.

48. Brandsaeter B, Schrumpf E, Clausen OP, Abildgaard A, Hafsahl G, Bjoro K. Recurrent sclerosing cholangitis or ischemic bile duct lesions—a diagnostic challenge? Liver Transpl. 2004;10:1073–4.
49. Graziadei IW, Wiesner RH, Batts KP, et al. Recurrence of primary sclerosing cholangitis following liver transplantation. Hepatology. 1999;29:1050–6.
50. Graziadei IW, Wiesner RH, Marotta PJ, et al. Long-term results of patients undergoing liver transplantation for primary sclerosing cholangitis. Hepatology. 1999;30:1121–7.
51. Trivedi PJ, Reece J, Laing RW, et al. The impact of ileal pouch-anal anastomosis on graft survival following liver transplantation for primary sclerosing cholangitis. Aliment Pharmacol Ther. 2018;48:322.
52. Joshi D, Bjarnason I, Belgaumkar A, et al. The impact of inflammatory bowel disease post-liver transplantation for primary sclerosing cholangitis. Liver Int. 2013;33:53–61.
53. Aravinthan AD, Doyle AC, Issachar A, et al. First-degree living-related donor liver transplantation in autoimmune liver diseases. Am J Transplant. 2016;16:3512–21.
54. Alabraba E, Nightingale P, Gunson B, Hubscher S, Olliff S, Mirza D, et al. A re-evaluation of the risk factors for the recurrence of primary sclerosing cholangitis in liver allografts. Liver Transpl. 2009;15:330–40.
55. Maheshwari A, Yoo HY, Thuluvath PJ. Long-term outcome of liver transplantation in patients with PSC: a comparative analysis with PBC. Am J Gastroenterol. 2004;99(3):538–42.
56. Campsen J, Zimmerman MA, Trotter JF, Wachs M, Bak T, Steinberg T, et al. Clinically recurrent primary sclerosing cholangitis following liver transplantation: a time course. Liver Transpl. 2008;14:181–5.
57. Demetris AJ, Adeyi O, Bellamy CO, Clouston A, Charlotte F, Czaja A, et al. Liver biopsy interpretation for causes of late liver allograft dysfunction. Hepatology. 2006;44:489–501.
58. Cholongitas E, Shusang V, Papatheodoridis GV, Marelli L, Manousou P, Rolando N, et al. Risk factors for recurrence of primary sclerosing cholangitis after liver transplantation. Liver Transpl. 2008;14:138–43.
59. Moncrief KJ, Savu A, Ma MM, Bain VG, Wong WW, Tandon P. The natural history of inflammatory bowel disease and primary sclerosing cholangitis after liver transplantation–a single-centre experience. Can J Gastroenterol. 2010;24:40–6.
60. Czaja AJ. Acute and acute severe (fulminant) autoimmune hepatitis. Dig Dis Sci. 2013;58:897–914.
61. Yeoman AD, Westbrook RH, Zen Y, Bernal W, Al-Chalabi T, Wendon JA, et al. Prognosis of acute severe autoimmune hepatitis (AS-AIH): the role of corticosteroids in modifying outcome. J Hepatol. 2014;61:876–82.
62. Rahim MN, Liberal R, Miquel R, Heaton ND, Heneghan MA. Acute severe autoimmune hepatitis: corticosteroids or liver transplantation? Liver Transpl. 2019;25:946–59.
63. Hofer H, Oesterreicher C, Wrba F, Ferenci P, Penner E. Centrilobular necrosis in autoimmune hepatitis: a histological feature associated with acute clinical presentation. J Clin Pathol. 2006;59:246–9.
64. Suzuki A, Brunt EM, Kleiner DE, Miquel R, Smyrk TC, Andrade RJ, et al. The use of liver biopsy evaluation in discrimination of idiopathic autoimmune hepatitis versus drug-induced liver injury. Hepatology. 2011;54:931–9.
65. Björnsson E, Talwalkar J, Treeprasertsuk S, Kamath PS, Takahashi N, Sanderson S, et al. Drug-induced autoimmune hepatitis: clinical characteristics and prognosis. Hepatology. 2010;51:2040–8.
66. Bernal W, Ma Y, Smith HM, Portmann B, Wendon J, Vergani D. The significance of autoantibodies and immunoglobulins in acute liver failure: a cohort study. J Hepatol. 2007;47:664–70.
67. Karkhanis J, Verna EC, Chang MS, Stravitz RT, Schilsky M, Lee WM, Brown RS Jr, for Acute Liver Failure Study Group. Steroid use in acute liver failure. Hepatology. 2014;59:612–21.
68. Ichai P, Duclos-Vallée JC, Guettier C, Hamida SB, Antonini T, Delvart V, et al. Usefulness of corticosteroids for the treatment of severe and fulminant forms of autoimmune hepatitis. Liver Transpl. 2007;13:996–1003.

69. European Association for the Study of the Liver. EASL clinical practice guidelines: autoimmune hepatitis. J Hepatol. 2015;63:971–1004.
70. Mendizabal M, Marciano S, Videla MG, Anders M, Zerega A, Balderramo DC, et al. Fulminant presentation of autoimmune hepatitis: clinical features and early predictors of corticosteroid treatment failure. Eur J Gastroenterol Hepatol. 2015;27:644–8.
71. Czaja AJ, Donaldson PT, Lohse AW. Antibodies to soluble liver antigen/liver pancreas and HLA risk factors for type 1 autoimmune hepatitis. Am J Gastroenterol. 2002;97:413–9.
72. Johnson PJ, McFarlane IG. Meeting report: International Autoimmune Hepatitis Group. Hepatology. 1993;18:998–1005.
73. Verma S, Gunuwan B, Mendler M, Govindrajan S, Redeker A. Factors predicting relapse and poor outcome in type I autoimmune hepatitis: role of cirrhosis development, patterns of transaminases during remission and plasma cell activity in the liver biopsy. Am J Gastroenterol. 2004;99:1510–6.
74. Miyake Y, Iwasaki Y, Terada R, Onishi T, Okamoto R, Sakai N, et al. Clinical characteristics of fulminant-type autoimmune hepatitis: an analysis of eleven cases. Aliment Pharmacol Ther. 2006;23:1347–53.
75. Yeoman AD, Westbrook RH, Zen Y, Maninchedda P, Portmann BC, Devlin J, et al. Early predictors of corticosteroid treatment failure in icteric presentations of autoimmune hepatitis. Hepatology. 2011;53:926–34.
76. De Martin E, Coilly A, Houssel-Debry P, Ollivier-Hourmand I, Heurgue-Berlot A, Artru F, et al. for FILFOIE Consortium. Treatment and prognosis of acute severe autoimmune hepatitis. J Hepatol. 2017;66(Suppl):S4.
77. Montano-Loza AJ, Mason AL, Ma M, Bastiampillai RJ, Bain VG, Tandon P. Risk factors for recurrence of autoimmune hepatitis after liver transplantation. Liver Transpl. 2009;15:1254–61.
78. Ayata G, Gordon FD, Lewis WD, et al. Liver transplantation for autoimmune hepatitis: a long-term pathologic study. Hepatology. 2000;32:185–92.
79. Prados E, Cuervas-Mons V, de la Mata M, et al. Outcome of autoimmune hepatitis after liver transplantation. Transplantation. 1998;66:1645–50.
80. Milkiewicz P, Hubscher SG, Skiba G, Hathaway M, Elias E. Recurrence of autoimmune hepatitis after liver transplantation. Transplantation. 1999;68:253–6.
81. Hubscher SG. Recurrent autoimmune hepatitis after liver transplantation: diagnostic criteria, risk factors, and outcome. Liver Transpl. 2001;7:285–91.
82. Krishnamoorthy TL, Miezynska-Kurtycz J, Hodson J, et al. Longterm corticosteroid use after liver transplantation for autoimmune hepatitis is safe and associated with a lower incidence of recurrent disease. Liver Transpl. 2016;22:34–41.
83. Khalaf H, Mourad W, El-Sheikh Y, et al. Liver transplantation for autoimmune hepatitis: a single-center experience. Transplant Proc. 2007;39:1166–70.
84. Birnbaum AH, Benkov KJ, Pittman NS, McFarlane-Ferreira Y, Rosh JR, LeLeiko NS. Recurrence of autoimmune hepatitis in children after liver transplantation. J Pediatr Gastroenterol Nutr. 1997;25:20–5.
85. Kerkar N, Hadzic N, Davies ET, et al. De-novo autoimmune hepatitis after liver transplantation. Lancet. 1998;351:409–13.
86. Montano-Loza AJ, Vargas-Vorackova F, Ma M, et al. Incidence and risk factors associated with de novo autoimmune hepatitis after liver transplantation. Liver Int. 2012;32:1426–33.
87. Heneghan MA, Portmann BC, Norris SM, Williams R, Muiesan P, Rela M, et al. Graft dysfunction mimicking autoimmune hepatitis following liver transplantation in adults. Hepatology. 2001;34:464–70.
88. Demetris AJ, Bellamy C, Hübscher SG, O'Leary J, Randhawa PS, Feng S, et al. 2016 Comprehensive update of the Banff Working Group on Liver Allograft Pathology: introduction of antibody-mediated rejection. Am J Transplant. 2016;16:2816–35.
89. Stirnimann G, Ebadi M, Czaja AJ, Montano-Loza AJ. Recurrent and de novo autoimmune hepatitis. Liver Transpl. 2019;25(1):152–66. https://doi.org/10.1002/lt.25375.

Printed in the United States
by Baker & Taylor Publisher Services